RATING SCALES IN PARKINSON'S DISEASE

RATING SCALES IN PARKINSON'S DISEASE

CLINICAL PRACTICE AND RESEARCH

Cristina Sampaio, MD, PhD
INSTITUTO DE MEDICINA MOLECULAR
FACULDADE DE MEDICINA DE LISBOA
LABORATÓRIO DE FARMACOLOGIA CLÍNICA E TERAPÊUTICA,
LISBON, PORTUGAL

Christopher G. Goetz, MD
DEPARTMENT OF NEUROLOGICAL SCIENCES
RUSH UNIVERSITY MEDICAL CENTER
CHICAGO, ILLINOIS

Anette Schrag, PhD, FRCP
UNIVERSITY DEPARTMENT OF CLINICAL NEUROSCIENCES
INSTITUTE OF NEUROLOGY
UNIVERSITY COLLEGE LONDON
LONDON, UNITED KINGDOM

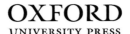

OXFORD
UNIVERSITY PRESS

OXFORD

UNIVERSITY PRESS

Oxford University Press, Inc., publishes works that further
Oxford University's objective of excellence
in research, scholarship, and education.

Oxford   New York
Auckland   Cape Town   Dar es Salaam   Hong Kong   Karachi
Kuala Lumpur   Madrid   Melbourne   Mexico City   Nairobi
New Delhi   Shanghai   Taipei   Toronto

With offices in
Argentina   Austria   Brazil   Chile   Czech Republic   France   Greece
Guatemala   Hungary   Italy   Japan   Poland   Portugal   Singapore
South Korea   Switzerland   Thailand   Turkey   Ukraine   Vietnam

Copyright © 2012 by Oxford University Press, Inc.

Published by Oxford University Press, Inc.
198 Madison Avenue, New York, New York 10016
www.oup.com

Oxford is a registered trademark of Oxford University Press

Library of Congress Cataloging-in-Publication Data
Parkinson's disease rating scales: evaluating the motor and the non-motor domains/[edited by] Cristina Sampaio,
Christopher G. Goetz, Anette Schrag.
p. ; cm.
Includes bibliographical references.
ISBN 978–0–19–978310-6 (hardcover : alk. paper)
I. Sampaio, Cristina, MD.   II. Goetz, Christopher G.   III. Schrag, Anette.
II.   [DNLM: 1. Parkinson Disease–diagnosis.   2. Parkinson Disease–complications.
3. Severity of Illness Index. WL 359]
III. LC Classification not assigned
IV. 616.8'33—dc23
V. 2011053118

1 3 5 7 9 8 6 4 2
Printed in the United States of America
on acid-free paper

To our families

CONTENTS

INTRODUCTION

FOR MANY YEARS, there has been a need to develop valid tools to evaluate the signs and symptoms of Parkinson's disease (PD). However, the understanding of all the intricacies of rating scales development was not widely available, and the first development attempts were relatively crude. Despite those limitations, a number of rating scales, mostly focusing in the motor aspects of PD became available in the 1960s to the 1980s. Examples are the Webster rating scale,[1] the Columbia University Rating Scale (CURS),[2] the New York University Parkinson's Disease Scale,[3] the Schwab and England,[4] and the Northwestern University Disability Scale (NUDS).[5] Usually the data about their validation were scattered in different publications that came into print long after the actual use of the scales. New investigators and clinicians were usually at a loss when they wanted to select a scale for their work, and direct comparison of data based on different ones was impossible.

In 1987, the Unified Parkinson Disease Rating Scale (UPDRS) was developed.[6] This was a major advance in the field, but, once again, experimental data on its validation were only published much later, during the 1990s.[7,8]

The Movement Disorders Society (MDS) recognized that the issue of measurement of PD was in need of systematization and appointed a task force in 2002 to deal with this matter. Since then, the MDS Task Force on Rating Scales for Parkinson's Disease has produced and published several critiques of the available rating scales, addressing both motor and non-motor domains of PD.[9] Additionally the task force took charge of the project to develop a new version of the UPDRS: the MDS-UPDRS.[10]

During the last decade, many instruments and validation data have been accumulated, and it is reasonable to consider these contributions in a systematic way in order to place each scale in a clinical and clinimetric context. In this volume, there is an anthological component, since the chapters on specific scales are based on the papers produced under the auspices of the MDS task force. All of them were updated for this book. To give coherence to the book, some topics had not been previously published; namely, the one on scales to evaluate cognition and pharmaco-economic evaluations in PD, and several structural chapters on methodological issues of rating scales and the historical evolution of scales in PD.

The knowledge collected in this volume about rating scales applicable to the several domains of PD is distilled in a list of "recommended" (defined systematically to allow comparison across topics) scales for each domain. It is important to note that we have restricted ourselves to just one type of measurement—clinical rating scales. Other types of measurement, for example, neurophysiological or imaging, were not considered.

As the reader will conclude, with some limitations, the scientific community has managed to produce tools that are good enough to allow the conduct of adequate scientific research. The use of rating scales imposes careful choice of scale for the purpose of the study, rigorous executional methods, adequate investigator training, and proper statistical analysis. These aspects are often ignored, but they are necessary to allow accurate interpretation of the results from using a rating scale. We hope that this book will help researchers choose the instruments in their protocols and better understand the strengths and limitations of the instruments on which they rely.

What is reviewed in this book is the state of measurement science for PD in the second decade of the twenty-first century. The majority of the rating scales are anchored in interviews or objective ratings by a trained investigator; or, less frequently, they involve questionnaires that are completed independently by the research subject. For reasons that are discussed in the book, these are relatively rudimentary methodologies. For example, ideally, research subjects would be evaluated in their everyday environment while doing their usual chores. This level of reality-checking

is theoretically possible and needs further development. (An example of technology that might create great opportunities to bring rating scales to patients' homes without crossing the barriers of privacy is "augmented reality."[11]) Meanwhile, until these technologies are truly usable in large research projects, more and more efforts are being made to transfer the evaluations to the home and work environments, even if this is done by using the same rating scales but in a Web platform.

The data in this book also show the long and hard process of developing a new rating scale. Such projects can only be carried out by a strong team with an adequate budget. Given the information gathered in the book, the development of new rating scales specifically for PD is not advisable, unless sufficient consideration is given to the shortfalls of existing scales and to the content and methodology required for proposal of a new scale. At present, a scale for the assessment of psychosis in PD is being developed, but this effort resulted from a very clear gap identified in field by the MDS critique.[12] There are a few other fields without recommended scales where an effort can be justified, but we believe the many of the tools available and summarized in the book are practicable and highly applicable already, though many need more clinimetric testing and possible further refinement.

To compose the chapters, we have collected a series of international specialists whose authority is well established in the field. The editors thank the authors for their thorough and careful preparation of the material.

In conclusion, *Parkinson's Disease: Clinical Rating Scales* provides the reader with an informative manual that directs investigators and clinicians on how to select the right tool from the different rating scales available to measure the multiple domains pertinent to PD. We encourage further advances in the development of measurement science.

—*Cristina Sampaio, Christopher G. Goetz,*
and Anette Schrag

REFERENCES

1. Webster DD. Critical analysis of the disability in Parkinson's disease. *Mod Treat.* 1968; 5:257–258.
2. Duvoisin RC. The evaluation of extrapyramidal disease. In: de Ajuriaguerra J, Gauthier G, eds. *Monoamines noyaux gris centraux et syndrome de Parkinson.* G: Georg Publication; 1971: 313–325.
3. Lieberman A, Le Brun Y, Boal D. The use of a dopaminergic receptor stimulating agent (Piribendil ET-495) in Parkinson's disease. In: Usdin E, ed. *Advances in Biochemical Psychopharmacology,* Vol. 12. New York: Raven Press; 1973:415–425.
4. Schwab RS, England AC. Projection technique for evaluating surgery in Parkinson's disease. In: Gillingham FJ, Donaldson MC, eds. *Third Symposium on Parkinson's Disease.* Edinburgh: E & S Livingstone; 1969:152–157.
5. Canter CJ, de la Torre R, Mier M. A method of evaluating disability in patients with Parkinson's disease. *J Nerv Ment Dis.* 1961;133:143–147.
6. Fahn S, Elton RL, UPDRS program members. Unified Parkinson's Disease Rating Scale. In: Fahn S, Marsden CD, Goldstein M, Calne DB, eds. *Recent Developments in Parkinson's Disease,* Vol. 2. Florham Park, NJ: Macmillan Healthcare Information; 1987:153–163, 293–304.
7. Martinez-Martin P, Gil-Nagel A, Gracia LM, et al. Unified Parkinson's Disease Rating Scale characteristics and structure. The Cooperative Multicentric Group. *Mov Disord.* 1994;9:76–83.
8. Richards M, Marder K, Cote L, et al. Interrater reliability of the Unified Parkinson's Disease Rating Scale motor examination. *Mov Disord.* 1994;9:89–91.
9. See http://www.movementdisorders.org/publications/rating_scales/ (consulted December, 2011).
10. Goetz C, Fahn S, Martinez-Martin P, et al. Movement Disorder Society–sponsored revision of the Unified Parkinson's Disease Rating Scale (MDS-UPDRS): process, format, and clinimetric testing plan. *Mov Disord.* 2007;22(1):41–47.
11. Klopfer E, Sheldon J. Augmenting your own reality: student authoring of science-based augmented reality games. *New Dir Youth Dev.* Winter 2010(128):85–94.
12. Fernandez H, Aarsland D, Fénelon G, et al. Scales to assess psychosis in Parkinson's disease: critique and recommendations. *Mov Disord.* 2008;23(4): 484–500.

CONTRIBUTORS

Guido Alves, MD, PhD
The Norwegian Centre for Movement
    Disorders
Stavanger University Hospital
Stavanger, Norway

Angelo Antonini, MD, PhD
Department for Parkinson's Disease and
    Movement Disorders
IRCCS "San Camillo" Venice
University of Padua
Padua, Italy

Amber L. Bush
Michael E. DeBakey Veterans Affairs
    Medical Center
Department of Medicine
Section of Health Services Research
Baylor College of Medicine
Houston, Texas

Carlo Colosimo, MD
Department of Neurology and Psychiatry
Sapienza University of Rome
Rome, Italy

Richard Dodel, MD, MPH
Department of Neurology
Philipps-University Marburg
Marburg, Germany

Hubert H. Fernandez, MD
Center for Neurological Restoration and
    Department of Neurology
Cleveland Clinic
Cleveland, Ohio

Maria João Forjaz, PhD
Consortium for Biomedical Research in
    Neurodegenerative Diseases (CIBERNED)
Carlos III Institute of Health
National School of Public Health
Madrid, Spain

Christopher G. Goetz, MD
Department of Neurology
Rush University Medical Center
Chicago, Illinois

Jacobus J. (Bob) van Hilten, MD, PhD
Department of Neurology
Leiden University Medical Center
Leiden, The Netherlands

Birgit Högl, MD
Department of Neurology
University Hospital
Innsbruck, Austria

Albert F. G. Leentjens, MD, PhD
Department of Psychiatry
Maastricht University Medical Centre
Maastricht, The Netherlands

Kelly E. Lyons, PhD
University of Kansas Medical Center
Parkinson's Disease and Movement
    Disorder Center
Kansas City, Kansas

J. Marinus, PhD
Department of Neurology
Leiden University Medical Center
Leiden, The Netherlands

Laura Marsh, MD
Michael E. DeBakey Veterans
    Affairs Medical Center
Departments of Psychiatry and Neurology
Baylor College of Medicine
Houston, Texas

Pablo Martinez-Martin, MD, PhD
Alzheimer Disease Research Unit and
Consortium for Biomedical Research in
    Neurodegenerative Diseases (CIBERNED)
    CIEN Foundation
Carlos III Institute of Health
Alzheimer Center Reina Sofia Foundation
Madrid, Spain

Marcelo Merello MD, PhD
Movement Disorders Section
Raul Carrea Institute for Neurological
    Research (FLENI)
Buenos Aires, Argentina

Anne Pavy-Le Traon MD, PhD
Department of Neurology and Reference
    Centre for MSA
University Hospital of Toulouse
Toulouse, France

Werner Poewe, MD
Department of Neurology
Medical University of Innsbruck
Innsbruck, Austria

Olivier Rascol, MD, PhD
Department of Clinical Pharmacology
Clinical Investigation Center
University Hospital and University
    of Toulouse III
Toulouse, France

Carmen Rodriguez-Blazquez, BS
Consortium for Biomedical
    Research in Neurodegenerative
    Diseases (CIBERNED)
Department of Applied Epidemiology
National Center of Epidemiology
Carlos III Institute of Health
Madrid, Spain

Cristina Sampaio, MD, PhD
Instituto de Medicina Molecular,
    Faculdade de Medicina de Lisboa
Laboratório de Farmacologia
    Clínica e Terapêutica
Lisboa, Portugal; and
Clinical Research Unit
CHDI Foundation
Princeton, New Jersey

Anette Schrag, PhD, FRCP
University Department of Clinical
    Neurosciences
Institute of Neurology
University College London
London, United Kingdom

Stephanie R. Shaftman, MSc, MS
Biostatistics, Bioinformatics,
  and Epidemiology
Medical University of South Carolina
Charleston, South Carolina

Sergio E. Starkstein, MD, PhD
School of Psychiatry
University of Western Australia and
  Freemantle Hospital
Freemantle, Australia

Glenn T. Stebbins, PhD
Department of Neurology
Rush University Medical Center
Chicago, Illinois

Barbara C. Tilley, PhD
Lorne Bain Distinguished University Professor
Division Director, Biostatistics
University of Texas Health Science Center
  at Houston
School of Public Health
Houston, Texas

ACKNOWLEDGMENTS

THE EDITORS AND chapter authors are deeply grateful to all that have been involved in the efforts of The Movement Disorders Society Rating Scales task force and have contributed with their dedicated work and expertise to the making of many papers that have been seminal to the structure of this book. We are in debt to all. We warmly thank Dag Aarsland, Isabelle Arnulf, Paolo Barone, Richard G. Brown,K. Ray Chaudhuri ,Kelvin L. Chou, Cynthia Comella, Carl Counsell, Ester Cubo, Bruno Dubois, Kathy Dujardin, Susanne Duerr, Marian L. Evatt, Giovanni Fabbrini, Stanley Fahn, Gilles Fénelon, Joseph H. Friedman, Joaquim Ferreira, Nir Giladi, Peter Hagell, Robert A. Hauser, Graeme Hawthorne, Vanessa Hinson, Robert G. Holloway, Alex Iranzo, Joseph Jankovic, Martine Jeukens-Visser, Bengt Jonsson, Regina Katzenschlager, Horacio Kaufmann, Katie Kompoliti, Jaime Kulisevsky, Heinz Lahrmann, Anthony E. Lang, Nancy LaPelle, Andrew Lees, Sue Leurgans, Peter A. LeWitt, Kelly E. Lyons, Paul McCrone, David Nyenhuis ,William M. McDonald, Charity G. Moore, Janis Miyasaki, Per Odin, Wolfgang Oertel, C. Warren Olanow, C. Rodriguez-Blazque, Lisa Seidl, Caroline Selai, Andrew Siderowf, Mark Stacy, Matthew B. Stern, Fabrizio Stocchi, Jeanne A. Teresi, Francois Tison, Claudia Trenkwalder, Alexander I. Tröster, Jens Peter Reese, Irene H. Richard, Evzen Ruzicka, Daniel Weintraub, Mickie Welsh, Gregor K. Wenning, Yaroslov Winter, Melvin D. Yahr, and Chengwu Yang.

PART ONE

MEASUREMENT TOOLS AND HOW TO INTERPRET THE VALIDATION DATA

1

CLINICAL RATING SCALE DEVELOPMENT

Glenn T. Stebbins

Summary

Developing a new clinical rating scale is a time-consuming process. It is often useful to look for an existing scale that can fulfill the required assessment instead of undertaking the task of developing a new one. The steps involved in developing a new rating scale include identification of the domain of interest, developing items to be used in assessing the domain, choosing a scaling method, developing and refining a preliminary scale, and developing the final scale. Defining the domain of interest and items assessing that domain usually involves consultation with experts, either professionals working in the domain of interest, or individuals with personal experience with the domain. A scaling method needs to be chosen for the instrument and can include binary, ordinal, or continuous metrics. The choice of the scaling metric to be used in the instrument depends on the characteristics of the domain and determines the level of measurement of the scale. From these steps, a preliminary scale is developed and then is subjected to development testing for refinement and final item selection. When all these steps are completed, a final scale can be created, which must then undergo clinimetric examination. Although a large amount of time and effort is required to develop a useful rating scale, the benefits extend beyond the individual investigator and support the entire clinical field.

INTRODUCTION

The purpose of any rating scale is to provide quantification of a domain of interest. The domain may include observable behavior, such as tremor of the upper extremities, or unobservable or latent constructs, such as depression. Regardless of the domain of interest, the development of a useful rating scale can be a demanding task. Prior to deciding to create a new rating scale, it is useful to first determine if there are existing scales that may meet the required assessments. If the development of a new scale is required, there are certain steps that can help assure the creation of a useful, reliable, and valid scale (Figure 1-1). Accurate and adequate definition of the domain of interest is essential. Following identification of the domain of interest, individual items assessing the domain are developed. Once the items are created, the type of measurement tool or type of scaling to be employed is decided upon. These items are then refined through iterative pilot testing. The final step is the validation of the resultant scale through assessment of reliability and validity. Many of these steps require repeated testing and

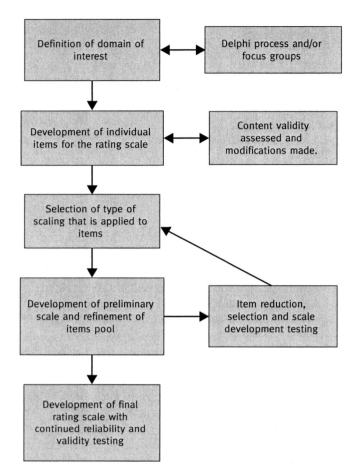

FIGURE 1-1   Process of Developing a Rating Scale.

development. Although this can be a time-consuming process, the final result of a reliable and valid instrument is well worth the effort.

Rating scales are usually collections of items that attempt to measure variables that are not objectively manifest. A classic example is the measurement of temperature. The domain of interest we assess with a thermometer is the kinetic movement of molecules within a given medium. The resultant measurement is the movement of mercury in a column of glass. The kinetic movement of molecules is the construct or domain of interest, but the movement of mercury is the measure. It is important to differentiate the domain of interest from the score on a given measurement instrument. For example, the height of the column of mercury in a thermometer is not the "true score" of temperature, but rather a proxy measure. It is also important

to understand the relationship between the domain of interest and the resultant measurement. In the case of the thermometer, even though the height of the mercury in the column is not the true score of temperature, the movement of the mercury is thought to be *caused* by the kinetic movement of the molecules.

Because rating scales are proxy measures of variables that are not objectively manifest, and because our measurement is not exact, there is error associated with any rating scale. This error is an important source of variability, and certain assumptions regarding measurement error are made. First, it is assumed that measurement error is random, such that the sum of error associated with individual items in a rating scale is zero and does not directionally influence the aggregate value of the scale. Second, it is assumed that the error associated with one item is independent from the other items of the scale. Third, it is assumed that the error is independent from the true score of the domain of interest. If these assumptions are not met, the scale is considered biased: so it is important to test rating scale for violations of these assumptions. The fields of psychometrics and clinimetrics[1] provide such assessments, and some of the techniques used in this testing are discussed in Chapter 3 of this volume.

DEVELOPING A NEW RATING SCALE

Before undertaking the task of developing a new scale, it is often useful to see if there may be existing scales that meet your needs. The best source for determining the existence of relevant scales is through a review of the literature of the domain of interest. Another resource is *Tests in Print*,[2] a listing of clinical scales. However, the scales listed in *Tests in Print* are limited to commercially available tests published in English. If a relevant scale is found, it is important to evaluate the clinimetric properties of the test to ensure that it has adequate reliability and validity (see Chapter 3 in this volume). If a relevant scale is not found, you are faced with developing a new rating scale.

The first step in developing a new rating scale is the clear delineation of the domain of interest. If one wants to develop a scale assessing the burden associated with Parkinson's disease (PD), it is important to have a clear idea of the meaning of "burden," and its specific application to patients with PD. Usually, the definition of the domain of interest can be guided by an expert knowledge of the construct. Published studies can provide a theoretical basis for defining the domain, and tapping the experiences of individuals working in or affected by the to-be-measured construct can provide important information. Two specific techniques have been found to be particularly fruitful in exploring and defining domains of interest for scale development. The first is a qualitative exploration of important constructs using focus groups. These groups are usually composed of individuals with personal experience with the condition under study. The second approach

is the use of experts in the field, termed the "Delphi approach."

Focus groups provide a method to gather information on a domain of interest from individuals who have personal experience with the condition.[3] Typically, focus groups involve five to 10 individuals with one or two moderators, and it is common to have multiple focus group sessions. Specific questions are often used to get the conversation started about the domain, but the idea of this process is to gain qualitative information on the experiences of the group members. Participation by all members of the focus group is essential, and it is important that there be no censoring of contributions. It is usual to tape-record the sessions and transcribe the results for qualitative analysis.

Focus groups are particularly informative when developing patient-reported rating scales. In this case, patients and caregivers form the groups, and the questionnaire is formatted to provoke discussion about the participants' personal experience with the domain of interest. It is often helpful to arrange for separate sessions for the patients and caregivers to promote discussion without censoring. After the two independent sessions, the two groups can be brought together for a combined session to further explore the domain.

The examination of raw data from a focus group usually follows a framework-analysis process.[4] In a framework analysis, the goal is to identify common themes that emerge from the focus group and provide a weighting of each theme's importance to the group. The first step is to become familiar with the content of the group session. By reading the transcripts and listening to the recording repeatedly, the facilitator begins to identify thematic nodes, or common themes. The themes are recorded, indexed, and compared across participants and within the group, identifying repeating or contradicting statements of the themes. These themes are then transcribed and sorted as to the relative commonality within and between sessions. These sorted themes are then used to form an inclusive definition of the overall domain of interest.

The use of experts to assist in identifying domains of interest can be as informal as talking with colleagues, or as formal an approach as the Delphi method.[5] The participants in a Delphi approach ought to include individuals who provide expertise in the various aspects of the domain of interest. To complete the Delphi exercise, the participants either complete an open-ended questionnaire about the domain or provide narratives about their views on the component elements of the domain. A listing of the characteristics of the domain is created, and the participants rank each characteristic as to its importance to the domain. The participants then discuss the rankings and are allowed to alter the order of importance as required. Following this, each participant is asked to justify their ranking and, if necessary, discuss why they do not agree with others in the panel. The ranking are again reordered as needed, and a final round of discussion and justification occurs. The results of this final discussion are then used as the expert judgements about the extent of the domain and the importance of individual aspects of the domain.

From both the focus group and the Delphi approach, a comprehensive definition of the domain of interest is developed, as well as a ranking of the individual elements of the domain. Using these definitions and rankings, individual items assessing the domain of interest can be developed. The wording for these items often will follow from the sorted themes from the focus groups or the discussions generated during the Delphi approach. So if one of the more common sorted themes from a focus group on depression in PD is a feeling of being down in the dumps, the item could simply be "I feel down in the dumps."

It is important to keep these items short, without sacrificing meaning. Additionally, it is good idea to keep the reading level for the item at the seventh grade or lower. Reading-level statistics are available on most word-processing programs, so this requirement is easily attained. At this point in the development process, it is best to have too many items that may include a certain level of redundancy. The refinement of the item pool will decrease the number of items, as well as identify redundancies. The main criterion

for these items is that they relate directly to the domain of interest.

One approach to determining whether the items generated during this process relate to the identified domain is to assess their content validity ratio (CVR).[6] Assembling a group of experts in the domain of interest (usually not the same group used in the Delphi approach), the CVR is calculated by asking the experts to review the items. The experts are asked to rate each item as either "essential" to the domain of interest, "useful in defining" the domain of interest, or "not necessary for" the domain of interest. The CVR is the ratio of the number of experts who rate the item as essential to defining the domain of interest to the total number of raters. The formula is $CVR = (Ne - N/2)/(n/2)$, where Ne equals the number of experts rating the item "essential" and N equals the total number of raters. The ratio can range of $+1.0$ to -1.0, with $+1$ representing perfect content validity and -1 representing an absence of content validity. A CVR of $+0.4$ indicates that 70% of the experts rated the item as essential to defining the domain of interest, and can be used as a threshold for rejecting items from further consideration. Care should be taken when interpreting a CVR, because the process is only as good as the quality of the expert raters.

As you are generating the large pool of items, it is a good idea to consider the scaling format to be used. This format gives substance to the items and allows for a quantification of the domain being assessed. There are many scaling formats, but the most commonly used format for rating scales involves having a stem followed by multiple-response choices. The stem is usually one item from the item pool identified through the focus group and Delphi procedures, and the multiple-response choice is the quantification of that domain item. An example of this format can be seen in Figure 1-2. When considering the scaling method, it is important to try to match the metric of the scaling to the distribution of the behavior assessed by the item. For example, if the item is assessing a continuous behavior, such as depression severity, and a scaling technique with a discrete response set of "None," "Less than once a week," "Once

FIGURE 1-2   Example of a Likert Scaled Item.

a week but not daily," and "Every day" is used, the true metric of the domain of interest is not captured. In a given situation, the discrete responses may be sufficient, but the variability of depression severity is truncated to four discreet values. This truncation of variability limits the usefulness of the quantification because all intervals of the domain are not covered.

Another consideration when matching the scaling method to the domain item is the shape of the distribution of the domain. If the domain demonstrates a linear increase in severity (Figure 1-3A), the interval between the scale values has an increased probability of being equal, representing a true interval-level measurement. However, if the severity increase is nonlinear (Figure 1-3B), the assumption of equal spacing between intervals is untenable. The degree of linearity for individual items can be assessed by item-response-theory approaches, and recommended adjustments to the scaling interval can be made.

There are other scaling methods that address the issue of domain distribution, including decreasing the width of the quantification interval, using Thurston scaling where the quantification is based directly on the theoretical distribution of the domain of interest, or using Guttman scaling where each statement assesses a higher value within the distribution of the domain of interest. However, these approaches are difficult to implement in practice and are not frequently used.

Other scaling methods are more commonly employed in developing rating scales. Each method uses varying metrics that allow for quantification of the domain of interest with differing associated sensitivity to variability. As noted in Figure 1-3, sensitivity to variability is dependent upon the interaction of the underlying distribution of the domain of interest and the scaling used in the assessment. Increased sensitivity to variability is usually a desirable trait in any measure because it reflects increased sensitivity to the construct under assessment. These more commonly used scaling metrics range from simple binary measures to continuous measures, and each metric is applicable in different situations.

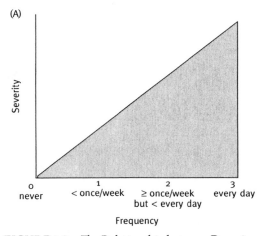

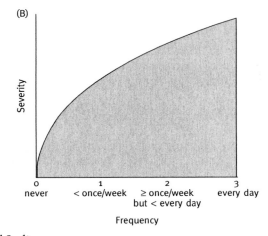

FIGURE 1-3   The Relationship between Domain and Scaling.

Binary options are the simplest, and best employed in cases where the domain is associated with little variability. Examples of such metrics include domains such as simple likes and dislikes, acceptable outcomes versus unacceptable outcomes, agreement versus disagreement, and endorsement or disapproval of summary statements. Although these outcomes assess limited ranges of variability, they are usually easy to answer and well tolerated by subjects. Furthermore, because binary responses can usually be answered quickly, the number of items in a given scale can be increased, providing a broader coverage of the domain of interest.

Likert scales are among the most commonly scaling metrics used in clinical rating scales. The item and scaling method in Figure 1-2 is an example of a Likert scale, with a stem describing the item from the domain of interest followed by ordinal response options. The response options allow for a quantification of the domain, usually ranging from a complete absence to the highest level of domain expression. The options need to reflect the distribution of domain of interest and should be ordered with relatively equal intervals between the numeric values. The number of levels of the option is also determined by the domain of interest, but ought to be relatively limited. Four levels or fewer are usually insufficient to capture the domain range, while it is difficult for most subjects to differentiate between more than 10 levels. A strength of Likert-type scaling is that each level can be tied to specific anchor that makes it easier to acquire accurate information. For example, as shown in Figure 1-2, the frequency of feeling sad or blue can be differentiated from "occurring less than once a week" to "occurring every day." This level of accuracy captures increased levels of variability in the domain of feeling sad or blue. A disadvantage of Likert-type scaling is the underlying assumption of equal intervals between the levels, an assumption that is usually difficult to prove. Unlike binary scaling, Likert scaling is usually more complex and difficult for the respondent to complete. The length of time required to complete Likert-type scales is usually greater than that required to complete binary response scales, so the maximum possible number of items on the Likert scale is lower.

A scaling method that provides quantification at the continuous level is visual analogue scaling. In this method, respondents are presented with a stem describing the domain of interest and a continuous line with descriptors of the opposite ends of the domain continuum anchoring each end of the line. The respondent marks the line at the point that represents where they fall on that continuum. The distance from the extreme, usually measured in millimeters, is the score on that item. There are numerous strengths of this type of scaling metric. Foremost among these is its ability to measure the variability of the domain of interest on a continuous level. This level of assessment increases the sensitivity of the assessment and the possibility of finding associations among variables. Additionally, the assumption of equal intervals, or an underlying linear distribution of the domain of interest, is not required, because the assessment is continuous. Finally, the time required to complete visual analogue scales is minimal, allowing an increased number of items to be included in the final construction of the scale. Unfortunately, the disadvantages of visual analogue measures are also numerous. First, determining the score for each item is time-intensive because individual measurements of the length of the line from the extreme to the mark of the respondent are required for each item. Additionally, because there is a lack of intermediate anchors along the continuum, it is difficult to assume that the same position marked by different respondents represents the same level of the domain of interest. This makes it very difficult to compare visual analogue responses across different subjects.

Regardless of the type of scaling method chosen, it is important that the same method be consistently applied in the entire scale. It is not advisable to mix binary, Likert, and visual analogue metrics in a single scale. Additionally, attention needs to be given to the time frame of assessment for the item. This gives the respondent a frame of reference for answering the item, and can limit the range of time for the assessment to a preset range. Some rating scales are based on immediate observations, while others rate lifetime traits. Usually, however, clinical rating scales are designed to assess a specific domain that can vary over time, so it is important to define the limits of the reference period. As seen in Figure 1-2, the time frame for the Likert rating of feeling sad or blue covers the past week. This interval was chosen because it is long enough to capture a meaningful range of the domain of interest, but not so long that it could be influenced by recall bias, where the respondent's response is colored by an overly long recall period.

Following the generation of the item pool and associated scaling metric, a preliminary scale can be created. Typically, this scale includes more items than are intended for the final scale. The increased number of items in the preliminary scale is required because the next step in the process is development testing that refines the items and identifies the most pertinent items for inclusion in the final scale. Development testing and item refinement require pilot testing of the preliminary scale using samples from the population of interest. This testing requires large numbers of subjects to be used in iterative testing. A rule of thumb for determining the sample size required for development testing is approximately 10 subjects for each item in the scale.[7]

The process of item reduction and selection is often accomplished by examining the "internal consistency" of the preliminary scale, or how well the scale hangs together in assessing the domain of interest. The association between individual items and the total scale variance is often a good indicator for retention or rejection of individual items. If an item shows a high correlation with the total scale, it suggests a commonality of domain assessment, and the item should be retained. If, on the other hand, the item shows a low correlation to the total scale, it suggests a lack of commonality of domain assessment, and the item can be removed from the scale. Additionally, the relationship of individual items to the internal consistence of the scale can be determined, and the items that increase internal consistency when removed can be discarded.

An important check to assess the adequacy of the scaling metric is identification of items with floor or ceiling effects. Floor effects occur when the lowest scaling metric artificially restricts the lowest measurement of the domain element. Ceiling effects are just the opposite, where the highest scaling metric restricts the measurement of the domain. Floor and ceiling effects are measured by the percentage of a given sample scoring at the extreme scaling metric values. If these percentages are disproportionate to the other metric values, removal or modification of the scaling metric values should be considered.

The process of item refinement is an iterative process that includes new development testing with each new version of the scale. After this process is completed (an event that is often difficult to determine), the final scale can be developed. Although the time required to develop a useful rating scale may seem to be burdensome, the final product is something that can be useful, not only to a single investigator, but to the entire field. However, even after completing the steps outlined in this chapter, the rating scale is not finished. The final scale needs to undergo clinimetric examination to assess its reliability and validity. The process of clinimetric examination is presented in Chapter 3 of this volume.

REFERENCES

1. Nunnally JC, Bernstein IH. *Psychometric Theory*. 3rd ed. New York: McGraw-Hill; 1994.
2. Murphy LL, Spies RA, Plake BS, eds. *Tests in Print VII*. Lincoln, Nebraska: Buros Institute for Mental Measurements; 2010.
3. Morgan DL, ed. *Successful Focus Groups: Advancing the State of the Art*. Newbury Park, California: Sage; 1993.
4. Ritchie J, Spencer L. Qualitative data analysis for applied policy research. In: Bryman A, Burgess RG, eds. *Analysing Qualitative Data*. London: Routledge; 1994:305–329.
5. Dalkey NC, Helmer O. An experimental application of the Delphi method to the use of experts. *Manag Sci*. 1963;9:458–467.
6. Lawshe CH. A quantitative approach to content validity. *Personnel Psychol*. 1975;28:563–574.
7. Gorsuch RL. *Factor Analysis*. 2nd ed. Hillsdale, NJ: Erlbaum; 1983.

2

STATISTICS FOR THE SCALE DEVELOPER

Barbara C. Tilley

Summary

When a new scale is developed, as described in Chapter 1, the scale must undergo psychometric testing, including cognitive pretesting, assessments of the internal structure or clinimetrics including test-retest reliability, internal consistency, factor structure, differential item functioning, correlations with scores of the some construct from other instruments, and tests of the ability of the scale to detect change over time. If a scale is modified or administered in a new way, some psychometric testing of the revision is also required.

There is a large body of statistical literature on each of the approaches to psychometric testing, and the presentation of extensive details is beyond the scope of this book. This chapter summarizes the major types of approaches and the focus of each approach, with some basic references to articles and software for those who wish to conduct these analyses.

INTRODUCTION

When a new scale is developed, as described in Chapter 1, the scale must undergo psychometric testing to determine whether we can trust that the scale measures the constructs of interest in a way that is consistent and interpretable. If an existing scale is modified, or administered in a new way, the Food and Drug Administration (FDA) also recommends psychometric testing of the revision.[1] In assessing scales, the concepts of *validity* and *reliability* are often mentioned. Reliability is inversely related to error in the scale, and is necessary but not sufficient for the scale's validity. There are many types of validity, but, in all instances, validity is an attribute of the scale score in the context of the population of interest, rather than a property of the instrument itself.[2] Validity must be determined for each intended interpretation. In general, validity measures "the degree to which evidence and theory support the interpretations of test scores entailed by proposed uses of the test."[3] For example, a sleep scale for subjects with Parkinson's disease may have excellent psychometric properties in this population, and the scores are very useful in interpreting the type and magnitude of the sleep problems encountered by a subject with PD and for measuring disease progression in the sleep domain. Nonetheless, the scores on this sleep scale are unlikely to be interpretable if the same scale is used to measure sleep disorders in infants. For this reason, the term "validity" needs to be applied to populations where the scale has actually been tested successfully.

This chapter presents some aspects of psychometric testing used in scale development, including cognitive pretesting, measurement of test-retest reliability and internal consistency, assessment of the scale's factor structure, correlation with scores from other instruments, ability to assess change over time or differentiate among subgroups with the construct being measured, and ability to function across different populations (differential item functioning). While this overview does not go into extensive detail, it provides a framework for understanding the uses of the various approaches, with references, including some citations to available software.

CONTENT EVIDENCE

Content evidence is a somewhat-subjective assessment of a scale's ability to measure the overall construct it is intended to measure.[2] This evidence may be a description of the scale development process, as described in Chapter 1. Other approaches include factor analysis to identify sub-constructs within the scale, as described below. Factor analysis is usually conducted once revisions to the scale have been completed based on cognitive pretesting and other assessments of reliability. If items in the scale load on multiple factors, this evidence may suggest that the sub-constructs in the scale are not measuring what the researchers intend.

COGNITIVE PRETESTING

Cognitive pretesting is used to assess task difficulty for both examiners and respondents, whether or not the scale is self-administered. In addition, the technique evaluates a respondents or caregiver's interest, attention span, and comfort with all questions. Overall comprehension of both the examiner and respondent are assessed, along with problems of logical structure in questions that could affect understanding.[4] Cognitive pretesting is useful when testing a new scale,[5] converting a generic scale to a disease-specific scale,[6] or developing a subset of items to measure new constructs, such as for an item bank.[7] Cognitive pretesting was used in the initial psychometric testing of the Movement Disorders Society Unified Parkinson's Disease Rating Scale (MDS-UPDRS) and is being used in translating the scale into other languages in order to assure that the translations capture the nuances of that scale.[8]

In general, there is no standard method to modify scales based on the results of cognitive pretesting.[7] The experts who are developing the scale discuss and modify the scale according to the pretesting results (although some authors have suggested additional qualitative or quantitative methods).[5-7] Scale development requires multiple rounds of cognitive pretesting until the scale is ready for the next phases of psychometric testing.

RELIABILITY

A goal of scale development is to produce a scale that has high test-retest and inter-rater reliability across different examiners and subjects, or to at least to understand its reliability in the population where the scale will be used.

Test-retest

Test-retest reliability measures the reproducibility within an individual subject. The same instrument is administered twice to the same person at different times. The times are chosen to be in close enough temporal proximity to decrease the likelihood that the individual has changed in some way. The measure of reliability is usually the correlation of responses—Pearson's, or Spearman's or Phi Coefficients[9]—depending on whether the scale is continuous, ordinal, or binary. All measures are easily calculated in standard statistical software packages. The Phi Coefficient is usually found with the procedures that calculate Chi-square or other tests to compare proportions. An acceptable value would generally be correlations or Phi Coefficients greater than 0.90.[10]

Inter-rater reliability

Inter-rater reliability measures within and across examiner agreement when the same or multiple examiners use the scale on the same individual. Agreement is measured by calculating Cohen's Kappa (for binary or categorical data) and intra-class correlations for continuous data. When scales are binary or categorical, Kappa can be shown to be a special case of the intra-class correlation coefficient.[11,12] Lin's concordance coefficient[13,14] can also be used when the data are ordinal or continuous. Lin's concordance coefficient (LCC) has an advantage over the intra-class correlation coefficient in that the LCC combines two coefficients measuring both precision and accuracy. Precision is measured by Pearson's correlation coefficient, assessing whether pairs of observations fall on a fitted linear line. The coefficient for accuracy assesses how closely the fitted line agrees with a 45-degree line. For Kappa, Landis and Koch give guidelines suggesting 0.75 or greater as an indicator of excellent agreement.[15] For LCC, values of the LCC: <0.9 can be considered poor; 0.9–0.95, moderate; 0.95–0.99, substantial; and >0.99, almost perfect.[16]

As noted above for validity, reliability is a property of the score and not of the scale itself. The same scale administered to different populations of individuals may have different levels of test-retest reliability. The same scale used by different examiners (e.g., trained versus untrained) in different groups of individuals may have different levels of inter-rater reliability.[2]

INTERNAL CONSISTENCY

Items that are used in constructing a scale should be correlated with each other since they are hypothesized to measure the same thing. This is termed "internal consistency." There are multiple ways to measure internal consistency, but the most commonly used is Cronbach's alpha (Cα).[17] Cα should increase as the correlation among items in a scale increases. Cα is influenced both by the correlation among items in a scale and by the number of items in the scale. As the number of items increases, the value of the Cα increases. If the Cα is too large, it may indicate that there are redundant items in the scale.[18]

FACTOR ANALYSIS

A scale generally includes multiple questions chosen to represent some underlying factors (dimensions or latent constructs) of interest where the number of factors is less than the number of questions. As an example, in PD, a scale to measure the overall motoric severity of the illness may have many questions, but logical factors may fall into the cardinal features of the disease: namely, tremor, bradykinesia, rigidity, and gait/balance function. Factor analysis is used in order to identify and confirm these underlying dimensions of a scale. The factor-analysis approach differs from principal-components analysis where each component is a linear combination of all items measured. If there are nine questions (items) in the scale, there will be nine principal components that include all items. As already stressed, in factor analysis the number of factors identified is usually less than the number of items in the scale, and generally there are different items of importance in each factor. For example, Part IV of

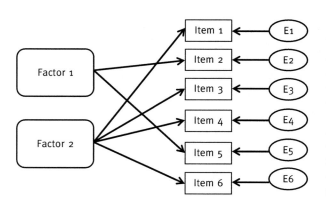

FIGURE 2-1   Common Factor Model. Each observed response (item 1 through item 6) is partially influenced by underlying common factors (factor 1 and factor 2) and partially by underlying unique factors (E1 through E6).[21] This diagram does not show the inherent variability that would exist when the scale is evaluated or used in practice, and the diagram assumes an orthogonal rotation leading to independent factors.

MDS-UPDRS has six questions. Two factors are identified. Four of the six questions represent a factor related to fluctuations and the OFF state, and two questions represent a factor related to dyskinesia. (See Figure 2-1 for a general diagram of a common factor structure.)

Identifying the factors

To determine the number of factors in a scale, the scale must be administered to a group of subjects. The number of subjects studied should be at least five to 10 times the number of questions (items) in the scale.[19] The subjects should represent the population in which the scale would be used, and there should be sufficient across-subject variability to assess the factor structure based on a range of scores on the scale. Using an exploratory factor analysis program such as SAS[19] for continuous item scores or M-Plus[20] for either categorical or continuous item scores, eigenvalues are computed. The eigenvalue for a factor represents the percent of variation explained by the factor.

Choosing the number of factors to retain and the scale items included in the factor

To choose the number of factors, differing approaches are suggested. The simplest to implement is to choose factors with eigenvalues greater than one. Another approach is to order the eigenvalues and choose factors identified as occurring to the left of a bend in a scree plot. Both approaches tend to overestimate the number of factors, with the latter being the most subjective. Another approach is to use a Monte Carlo simulation[21] or parallel analysis.[22] After the factors are chosen, factor-analysis programs can perform various types of rotations used to determine the scale items to be included in each factor. A typical rotation is orthogonal, to develop an independent set of items for each factor. As a rule of thumb, the items that have factor loadings (values representing the correlation between the item and the factor) of 0.4 or more are retained in the factor. If there is reason to believe that the factors are not independent, an oblique or other rotation can be used, although rotations that are not orthogonal may not provide a unique set of items for each factor.[19]

Confirmatory factor analysis

Once the initial factors are identified, a second step is a confirmatory factor analysis to determine how well the factor structure that has been identified fits the scale data. While confirmatory factor analysis can be conducted on data set used in the construction of the scale, ideally there would be a subsequent confirmatory factor analyses in a new data set. Common test statistics assessing the fit of the factor structure are the Confirmative Fit Index (CFI) and root mean-square error (RMSE). Hatcher provides a comprehensive discussion of confirmatory factor analysis and the test statistics that can be used,[19] as does Brown.[23] While the program Hatcher uses, SAS, is for continuous data only, the conceptual approach and interpretation of the test statistics are also applicable to M-Plus. The report on a clinimetric analysis of the new MDS-UPDRS gives examples of both an exploratory and a confirmatory factor analysis.[7]

CORRELATIONS WITH OTHER INSTRUMENTS

Another step in assessing the scale is to compare the scale to other similar instruments, if these exist. For example, the MDS-UPDRS was compared to the UPDRS.[8] Even though the MDS-UPDRS was expected to be more comprehensive than the UPDRS, scale developers believed it was important to determine if the two instruments were similar in their factor structure. In addition to factor analysis, the approaches to assessing correlation, described under comparing measurements between raters, can also be used.

ABILITY TO DIFFERENTIATE AMONG SUB-GROUPS OF INTEREST AND MEASURE CHANGE OVER TIME

Once the scale has been assessed as describe above, the next step would be pilot testing on subjects for whom the scale is intended and who represent a range of scale values. Using standard statistical approaches, the pilot data can be used to determine if the scale can separate different sub-groups, such as those with mild and severe disease. If the scale is to be used as a primary measure in longitudinal clinical research or clinical trials in the future, a longitudinal pilot study to assess the ability of the scale to measure change over time must be conducted. One approach to pilot testing is to incorporate the scale as a secondary measure in an ongoing study. If the scale is to be used as a primary measure in an ongoing study prior to longitudinal pilot testing, enough data should be collected on other previously validated scales that measure some aspects of change over time for comparison to the new scale, in order to assure the new scale is correlated with validated measures of change.

DIFFERENTIAL ITEM FUNCTIONING

If the scale is developed in one population and is to be used in another, differential item functioning (DIF) should be evaluated. DIF occurs when the probability of a score on an item differs between groups even though the actual ability or disease severity or other latent trait in the two groups is the same. For example, there is a potential for DIF when using a scale developed for young adults in a group of older retirees or when using a scale developed in one culture on another culture. There are several approaches to the assessment of DIF. Assessment can be conducted using multiple-indicator, multiple cause structural equation models (MIMIC) models in M-Plus,[24] or using Item Response Theory,[25] or using a simple logistic regression with interaction terms. In the presence of DIF, the item can be excluded to increase the validity of the scale,[26] although the overall score should be interpreted taking this omission into account. Another option would be to modify the item, requiring more psychometric testing. Teresi provides a comparison of the analytical approaches for identifying DIF.[26]

CONCLUSIONS AND FUTURE DIRECTIONS

It should be clear from the two chapters on scale development that changing an existing scale or developing a new scale are not trivial undertakings. Careful thought and extensive efforts are required to achieve scientifically sound and reliable scales that can be used by the scale developer and other investigators. Much of this book is based on materials developed by the Task Force for Parkinson's Disease Rating Scales, sponsored by the Movement Disorder Society. In reviewing scales covering multiple domains of PD disability and impairment, the Task Force has recommended the development of only two new scales; namely, the development of the Movement Disorder Society revision of the Unified Parkinson's Disease Scale (MDS-UPDRS) (see Chapter 7) and a new scale for psychosis (see Chapter 18). For all others, the recommendations have focused on further studies of existing scales, because of the very heavy burden of new scale development. With the advent of new statistical methods, further testing of scales to enhance their accurate detection of disability and impairment allows for a continual evolution of measurement precision.

REFERENCES

1. US Department of Health and Human Services Food and Drug Administration. *Guidance for Industry. Patient-Reported Outcome Measures: Use in Medical Product Development to Support Labeling Claims* (draft guidance). 2006.
2. Cook DA, Beckman TJ. Current concepts in validity and reliability for psychometric instruments: theory and application. *Am J Med.* 2006;119:166e7–166e16.
3. American Educational Research Association, American Psychological Association, National Council on Measurement in Education. *Standards for Educational and Psychological Testing.* Washington, DC: American Educational Research Association; 1999.
4. Willis GB. *Cognitive Interviewing: A Tool for Improving Questionnaire Design.* Thousand Oaks, CA: Sage Publications; 2005.

5. Poole HM, Murphy P, Nurmikko TJ. Development and preliminary validation of the NePIQoL: a quality-of-life measure for neuropathic pain. *J Pain Symptom Manage*. 2009;37(2):231–245.

6. John H, Treharne GJ, Hale ED, Panoulas VF, Carroll D, Kitas GD. Development and initial validation of a heart disease knowledge questionnaire for people with rheumatoid arthritis. *Patient Educ Couns*. 2009;77: 136–143.

7. Christodoulou C, Junghaenel DU, DeWalt DA, Rothrock N, Stone AA. Cognitive interviewing in the evaluation of fatigue items: results from the patient-reported outcomes measurement information system (PROMIS). *Qual Life Res*. 2008;17:1239–1246.

8. Goetz CG, Tilley BC, Shaftman SR, et al. Movement Disorder Society–sponsored revision of the Unified Parkinson's Disease Rating Scale (MDS-UPDRS): scale presentation and clinimetric testing results. *Mov Disord*. 2008;23:2129–2170.

9. Yule GU. On the methods of measuring association between two attributes. *J Roy Stat Soc*. 1912;75:579–652.

10. Downing SM. Reliability: on the reproducibility of assessment data. *Med Educ*. 2004;38:1006–1012.

11. Cohen J. A coefficient of agreement for nominal scales. *Ed and Psychol Measure*. 1960;20:37–46.

12. Cohen J. Weighted kappa: nominal scale agreement with provision for scaled disagreement or partial credit. *Psychol Bull*. 1968;70:213–220.

13. Lin LI. A concordance correlation coefficient to evaluate reproducibility. *Biometrics*. 1989;45:255–268.

14. Lin LI. Assay validation using the concordance correlation coefficient. *Biometrics*. 1992;48:599–604.

15. Landis J, Koch G. The measurement of observer agreement for categorical data. *Biometrics*. 1977;33:159–174.

16. McBride GB. A proposal for strength-of-agreement criteria for Lin's Concordance Correlation Coefficient. *NIWA Client Report: HAM*. 2005;(no volume):2005–2062.

17. Cronbach LJ. Coefficient alpha and the internal structure of tests. *Psychometrika*. 1951;16: 297–334.

18. Streiner DL, Norman GR. *Health Measurement Scales: A Practical Guide to Their Development and Use*. New York: Oxford University Press; 1989:64–65.

19. Hatcher L. *A Step-by-Step Approach to Using the SAS System for Factor Analysis and Structural Equation Modeling*. Cary, NC: SAS Institute, Inc.; 1994.

20. Muthén LK, Muthén BO. *Mplus. Statistical Analysis with Latent Variables. User's Guide*. Available at: http://www.statmodel.com/download/usersguide/Mplus%20Users%20Guide%-20v6.pdf. Accessed on February 23, 2012.

21. DeCoster J. (1998). *Overview of Factor Analysis*. Retrieved 12/30/2011 from http://www.stat-help.com/notes.html.

22. Ledesma RD, Valero-Moca P. Determining the number of factors to retain in EFA: an easy-to-use computer program for carrying out parallel analysis. *Practical Assessment, Research and Evaluation: A peer-reviewed electronic journal*. 2007;12:1–10. Available at: http://pareonline.net/. Assessed on February 23, 2012.

23. Brown TA. *Confirmatory Factor Analysis for Applied Research*. New York: The Guilford Press; 2006.

24. Jones RN. Identification of measurement differences between English and Spanish language versions of the Mini-mental State Examination: detecting differential item functioning using MIMIC modeling. *Med Care*. 2006;11(suppl 3):S124–S133.

25. Thissen DM. *IRTPRO*. Version 2.1. 2011. Available at http://www.ssicentral.com/irt/IRTPRO_by_SSI.pdf.

26. Teresi JA. Different approaches to differential item functioning in health applications. *Med Care*. 2006;11(suppl 3):S152–S170.

3

HOW TO EVALUATE VALIDATION DATA

Pablo Martinez-Martin and Maria João Forjaz

Summary

Symptoms and many human attributes are not directly observable and lack a gold standard or unit with which to compare the results of estimations. However, measurement is absolutely necessary to determine their current state and the change they experienced over time or secondary to interventions. Therefore, instruments for carrying out measurement of those "constructs" (abstract concepts, such as pain, depression, disability, etc.) are widely applied in clinical research and practice. Such instruments (rating scales, questionnaires) require human inference, by a rater, or direct subjective evaluation by patients; therefore, they are exposed to subjective interpretation and potential bias.

One the most important steps in the development of scales is the validation process, which consists of a series of procedures to determine the quality of the instrument as a tool for measurement. A roster of psychometric attributes or properties to be tested exists, and a series of statistical methods is available to perform their pertinent verification.

In the present chapter, based on qualified guidelines, the authors present the definition of each psychometric attribute, the list of the most accepted statistical methods for testing these properties, the criterion values of these statistical tests to be met by the scale attributes, and additional information for making the validation studies consistent. All the mentioned aspects are differentially stated for the two theories currently leading the development and validation of rating scales and questionnaires: the Classical Test Theory and the Latent Trait Theories, specifically Rasch analysis.

INTRODUCTION

Some chapters in this book are aimed at showing that measurement is indispensable for science and that we need special, valid measures to assess abstract concepts (constructs) that are not directly observable. The constructs related to human attributes cover a wide range of domains, such as physical symptoms (for example, pain, fatigue); mental state (for example, intelligence, anxiety); disability; and feelings (for example, euphoria, anger, frustration). Characteristically, these attributes' lack of a unit (or gold standard) may be interpreted in different ways by different people, and they can be measured only indirectly. Considering these characteristics, measurement of these kinds of concepts is a real challenge because the fundamental prerequisites making the physical measures feasible, particularly direct observation and the existence of a gold standard unit, are not present. Nevertheless, the need to evaluate constructs impelled psychologists and sociologists to develop methods for estimating their intensity based on the assessment of aspects closely related to the researched attribute.

Medicine in general, and neurology specifically, joined that strategy, and a multitude of measurement tools has been developed for assessing those constructs of interest in epidemiological and clinical research and practice. Following the classification of measures used in neurology by LaRocca,[1] rating scales and self-report measures are the instruments applied for evaluating those theoretical objects of measurement. Rating scales require human inference, by a rater, to obtain estimates of a construct and its components. Self-reported measures are direct subjective evaluations, by individuals or patients themselves, of a construct and its components. Rating scales and self-evaluations are relatively quick and simple to apply and analyze, furnishing global information over a long time-frame with low investment in resources and low operating costs. However, they are exposed to subjective interpretation and potential bias such as "yea-saying," "end-aversion," etc.[2] Therefore, rating scales and assessment questionnaires (henceforth, "scales") have to demonstrate they posses enough metric quality to be considered measures.

VALIDATION OF A SCALE

The procedure aimed at checking the properties of a scale as a measurement instrument is named *validation*. This is a dynamic, never-ending process in which every new study provides information contributing to the evidence about the validity of the scale and the relations of the construct with other constructs.

Most of the scales have been validated following the principles of the Classical Test Theory (CTT), a psychometric theory establishing that the construct possesses a theoretical value that can be indirectly measured through observable components related to it. A basic assumption of this theory is that individuals are able to distinguish between grades of intensity to which

numeric valuations (scores) are assigned. If these assumptions are valid, the scores of a valid measure should reflect the value of the construct, differing from the true score solely as a consequence of random error.[2-4] CTT is relatively easy to understand, the statistical methods to be applied for testing the measurement attributes are easily available, and it remains the most-used model for development and validation of scales. However, important conceptual and methodological problems arise when the characteristics of instruments designed under the CTT principles are compared with those of the "genuine scientific measures" (physical measures) if the characteristics of a physical measure are considered. Some of those problematic assumptions and facts are: presumption of homogeneous contribution of items to the final score and equivalence of response options among different items; ordinal level of the response options (that are added to produce a total score); confidence intervals too wide for individual use; presumed homogeneous distribution of the error of measurement; sample-dependent reliability or validity; and test-dependency of the assessed health status.[2-7]

The main alternatives to the CTT are the Latent Trait Theories or modern psychometric methods: namely the Item Response Theory (IRT) and the Rasch analysis. They come from the education field and are based on the relationship (probability) between the characteristics (difficulty) of the item and the individual's ability. Assumptions of the scales developed through Latent Trait Theories are unidimensionality (that a single trait underlies all the items in the model) and "local independence" (that the probability of answering any item positively is independent of the probability of answering any other item positively). Scales based on IRT and Rasch analysis are robust, allowing that observed data, which are in interval level of measurement, could be tested against the theoretical model. "Interval level of measurement" is an expression of a concept, which is explained in the parentheses. Interval level of measurement means that data are no categorical or ordinal, but real numbers like with physical measures (meter, kilogram, liter, etc.). Therefore, from a scientific point of view, they are sounder than scales based on the CTT. Their main disadvantages are related to the complexity of the conceptual framework, the need of large samples (up to $n \geq 500$ for some IRT models), and the need of specific statistical packages. In addition, invariance may not hold among different samples, and Latent Trait Theories are not useful to construct clinimetric indices containing causal variables.[2,3,6–11]

Although an increasing number of measures has been developed or revised applying Latent Trait Theories, mainly Rasch analysis, most of the existing rating scales and most of the scales in development in neurology are validated on the basis of the CTT. To determine the quality of a scale, the results from validation studies have to be compared with the standard values accepted for each psychometric attribute. The standard thresholds and ranges used to test validation data by both methods, CTT and Rasch analysis, will be reviewed in this chapter.

ASSESSING THE SCALES: CLASSICAL TEST THEORY APPROACH

Following some publications and recent guidelines, the main psychometric attributes to be tested in a health measure, are reliability, validity, and responsiveness, although really longer list is pertinent (Table 3-1).[2,3,5,11–19] The criteria accepted for that properties will be reviewed below, and some examples about will be shown in boxes.

• **Conceptual and measurement model**: Framework defining the construct to be measured and the target population to which the scale will be applied. The scale variability, level of measurement, and scoring method are also determined in this early phase of scale development.
• **Item scaling**: Testing of item scaling assumptions determines the correct grouping of the items into scales, whether the items are measuring the same construct, and whether the items can be summed without weighting or standardization to produce a score. Exploratory factor analysis helps establish the grouping of items to form subscales. An item is correctly grouped into a scale

Table 3-1. Main Psychometric Attributes of a Scale

1. Conceptual and measurement model
2. Item scaling (scaling assumptions)
3. Feasibility and acceptability
   Computable data (data quality)
   Floor and ceiling effects
   Distribution of scores and skewness
4. Reliability
   Internal consistency
   Reproducibility—Test-retest, Intra-rater
       Inter-rater
5. Validity
   Content and face validity
   Criterion validity
   Construct validity—Structural validity
       Hypothesis testing validity
       Cross-cultural validity
6. Responsiveness
7. Interpretability
8. Respondent and administrative burden
9. Alternative forms

Source: Based on references 2,3,5,11–19

when the correlation with its own scale exceeds the correlation with other scales by at least two standard errors (standard error of a correlation coefficient $= \sqrt{[(1-r^2)/(n-2)]}$). These analyses of item convergent and discriminant validity (multi-trait scaling or multi-trait–multi-item method) identify scaling success and scaling failures (Box 3-1). Items identified as scaling failures or probable scaling failures should be considered for elimination. Equivalence of the items allows that to be summed to produce scores, and this property is demonstrated when they have similar response option frequency distribution, means and standard deviations, and item–total correlations ($r > 0.30$).[11,16,20,21]
• **Feasibility and acceptability**: These properties are related to each other and have been defined as the "extent to which a scale can be used successfully in the intended setting to which it was designed" and "how acceptable is a scale for respondents to complete," respectively. They are determined through the response rate and the

proportion of missing data for each item (and scale) and the distribution of scores in the sample, respectively.

• The acceptable proportion of *missing data* ranges from <5%[16] to <10%.[21–23] For unweighted instruments, missing data can be estimated acceptably from the mean of the available items if the latter represent ≥50% of all items in the scale (simple mean imputation), although more complex methods (e.g., multiple imputation) perform better when missing data are ≥30%.[11,24,25]

• *Floor and ceiling effects* occur when a high proportion of respondents score at the lowest and highest value of the scale, respectively. A proportion higher than 15% indicates the existence of the effect,[12] although some authors allow up to 20%.[20,21]

• *Additional aspects* of acceptability are related to the adequate distribution of scores: (1) the skewness statistic should be between −1 and +1[20,21,26,27]; (2) observed scores should cover the possible score range of the scale[21]; (3) mean scores should be close to the mid-point (median) of the scale.[20,21,28]

An example of acceptability analysis is shown in Box 3-2.

• **Reliability**: It is defined as the degree to which an instrument is free from random error. It includes two attributes: internal consistency and reproducibility.

• *Internal consistency* (or internal reliability) refers to the extent to which all the items in a multi-item scale are measuring the same construct. It is based on the homogeneity (inter-correlations) of the items at one point in time. Exploratory or confirmatory analysis should be performed in order to establish the existence of potential dimensions (subscales) into the tested scale. For scales composed of several subscales, the internal consistency of each one should be calculated separately. The most adequate measure of internal consistency is the Cronbach's alpha index, whose value should be 0.70 to 0.95. Low values are indicative of poor association among the items in the scale, whereas values higher than 0.95 suggest redundancy. For individual comparisons, an alpha 0.90 to 0.95 is required. The Kuder-Richardson formula 20 (KR-20) is appropriate for items with dichotomous response, and its outcome is interpreted as for alpha.[2,3,11,15–18]

• Other methods for assessing the internal consistency include the inter-item correlation (r = 0.30–0.70); item-total corrected correlation (proposed threshold ranges from r > 0.20 to r > 0.40); and item homogeneity (mean of the inter-item correlation, r > 0.30).[2,3,16,29,30]

• The *reproducibility* includes two aspects: (1) inter-rater agreement at one point in time, and (2) intra-rater or test-retest (in self-applied scales) agreement, which refers to the stability of an instrument over time, assuming the concept measured remains stable. The time between first and second assessments should be long enough to avoid recall, but not so long that changes in the condition have occurred. The recommended number of observations, as a global rule, is ≥50,[17] but it may be adjusted using formulas like that by Chiccetti (1976) (minimal sample, $N \geq 2k^2$, where k is the number of ordinal points in the scale).[31] For all these aspects of reproducibility, a high proportion of agreement is desirable, but not sufficient, because agreement by chance is not controlled. For continuous variables, the Pearson correlation coefficient is not useful, because it does not control for systematic differences.

The recommended methods for assessing the reproducibility of a scale are: for binary data, kappa coefficient; for polychotomous ordinal data, weighted kappa (with linear or quadratic weights); for continuous data, the intraclass correlation coefficient (one- or two-way, random effects model, depending on the scenario) or the Lin's concordance correlation coefficient.[32] Interestingly, weighted kappa with quadratic weights is equivalent to the intraclass correlation coefficient, two-way random effects, single measure. When more than two scores should be compared simultaneously, the Kendall's W concordance coefficient may be applied. For all these coefficients, values ≥0.70 are considered satisfactory (0.90–0.95 for individual measurement).[2,11,13–18,32] A method proposed by Bland and Altman is used to obtain the limits of the agreement between two scales that are on the same level of measurement (mean change ± 1.96 x standard deviation of change, for a 95% confidence interval).[33]

The *equivalent-forms reliability* refers to the agreement between scores of different instruments designed to measure the same construct. Usually, one of them is considered the standard or benchmark, and the capacity of the other to predict the standard scores is tested through linear regression. Agreement between two scales is tested with same methods applied for assessing test-retest.[11]

• **Validity**: It is defined as the extent to which a scale measures the concept it is supposed to measure. Its components are: content and face validity, criterion validity, and construct validity.

• *Face validity* is defined as the extent to which a measure gives the impression that it measures what it is intended to measure and is established by judgements and statements about.

• *Content validity* refers to the extent to which a measure covers important parts of the domain to be measured. Empirical estimation of this kind of validity, the Lynn's Content Validity Index, may be obtained from an expert panel.[2,34,35]

• *Criterion validity* refers to the extent to which scores of the instrument are related to an independent measure taken as the criterion or gold standard. The rationale for the choice of the criterion should be clearly stated, and the tested scale has to demonstrate a close relationship with that gold standard (concurrent validity) or the ability to predict the criterion (predictive validity). Comparison criterion-scale (sensitivity, specificity, receiver operating characteristic (ROC) curves, phi coefficient) for diagnostic instruments,[2,15] and agreement or correlation coefficients (standard, r ≥ 0.70)[16–18] for rating scales are usually applied. If distinction among groups characterized by the criterion is intended, multiple regression or discriminant analysis should be used.[1]

• *Construct validity* may be defined as the "evidence supporting a proposed interpretation of scores based on theoretical implications associated with the construct being measured."[15] Three types of construct validity are recognized by the Consensus-based Standards for the selection of health status Measurement Instruments (COSMIN) panel: structural, hypotheses testing, and cross-cultural validity.

The *structure of the scale* is determined by exploratory or confirmatory factor analysis and is related to the scaling assumptions and content validity. The components of a dimension or (sub)scale should be combined adequately, reflecting the same concept (construct or part of the construct), and according to the theoretical model. Interpretation of factor analysis results requires knowledge of the statistical technique and adequate sample size (100 or more subjects). The bases of the multi-trait method were outlined in the "Scaling Assumptions" section.[2,3,11]

Concerning *convergent and divergent validity*, the scale should be tested in relation to *a priori* hypotheses that establish the expected relationships of the scale with other measures and variables: high association with measures assessing the same construct or closely related constructs (convergent validity); low correlation with measures evaluating unrelated constructs (divergent or discriminant validity); mean values significantly different between groups of patients in different situation (known groups, extreme groups, or discriminative validity). There is no consensus on the magnitudes of the correlation coefficients to be considered high, moderate, or low correlation. From a review of the literature, values lower than 0.35 (range: 0.30–0.40) are indicative of weak association; from an average value of 0.35 to values around 0.60 (range: 0.50–0.70) corresponds to moderate correlation; and higher values are considered strong correlation(Figure 3.1).[3,14,36–40] Obviously, the more related the instruments are

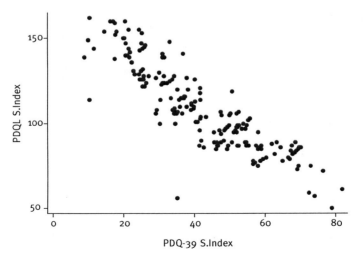

FIGURE 3-1   Scatter Plot Showing the Association (Convergent Validity) Between the Summary Indexes of the PDQ-39 and PDQL Questionnaires (r = 0.91) (Dataset from *Qual Life Res.* 2007;16: 1221–1230).[41]

each other, the more exigent values should be used. The multi-trait–multi-method analysis is adequate for a simultaneous testing of convergent and discriminant validity.

Known-groups validity is determined by comparison of the scale scores among subjects with known differences. Parametric or non-parametric statistics (e.g., unpaired t-test, ANOVA, or Mann-Withney or Kruskal-Wallis tests) are used to determine the known-groups validity.[2,3,11] The magnitude of the differences is the most interesting parameter (*p* value informs only on the statistical significance) to determine whether the scale evaluates different populations according to the grouping by an external criterion. For example, a scale to assess motor impairment in Parkinson's disease (UPDRS-Part 3) should discriminate among patients in different Hoehn and Yahr stages (Box 3-3).

Internal validity refers to the inter-correlation between the subscales of a rating scale. Moderate correlation (r = 0.30–0.70), representing some association between dimensions but not redundancy, is considered satisfactory[20,21] (Box 3-4).

Terwee et al. consider that construct validity is satisfactory when at least 75% of the results support the *a priori* hypotheses, in (sub)groups of at least 50 patients.[17]

- *Cross-cultural validity*: Frequently, a scale should be used in a cultural setting different from the original where it was designed and validated. The procedures for translation and adaptation to a new language and cultural environment are critical when the instrument is to be used in self-assessment. The procedure includes independent translations and back-translations by bilingual persons, each step followed by consensus, comparison with the original measure, amendments, pretesting in a well-characterized sample representative of the target population, and final validation study. Confirmatory factor analysis can identify items having a different sense or function in the new setting.[14,15,19,42]

- **Responsiveness**: A variety of definitions of responsiveness is found in the literature.[43,44] We prefer to consider *responsiveness* as "the ability of an instrument to detect change,"[15] a concept equivalent to Liang's "sensitivity to change."[45] The ability to detect a clinically important change or the ability to detect real changes in the concept being measured, as stated by other definitions, are aspects of the interface between responsiveness and interpretability of outcomes. Responsiveness depends on the existence of floor and ceiling effects, the reliability, and the precision (sensitivity) of the instrument. *Precision* is defined as "the ability of the instrument to detect small differences" (or the number of distinctions an instrument makes). For example, a scale with a scoring range from 0 to 100 will be more precise than a scale scoring from 0 to 20. Precision measures are the standard error of measurement (SEM), the error variance (SEM^2), or the test information (reciprocal of the error variance), all of them susceptible of taking different values at different points along the scale.[15] Precision determines differences in cross-sectional studies, whereas responsiveness refers to change in longitudinal studies.[11]

Box 3-3. UPDRS–Motor Examination Scores Broken Down by Hoehn and Yahr Stage

(*n* = 511; unpublished data)
Stage 1 (*n* = 42): 14.40 ± 10.40
Stage 2 (*n* = 286): 27.20 ± 13.60
Stage 3 (*n* = 121): 36.60 ± 13.30
Stage 4 (*n* = 53): 49.19 ± 13.92
Stage 5 (*n* = 9): 75.78 ± 10.72
Kruskal-Wallis test: chi-squared with ties = 161.25; p = 0.0001

Box 3-4. Internal Validity of the Unified Parkinson's Disease Rating Scale

($n = 511$; unpublished data)

	UPDRS 1	UPDRS 2	UPDRS 3
UPDRS 2	0.66	—	—
UPDRS 3	0.64	0.79	—
UPDRS 4	0.43	0.65	0.49

Methods for estimation of a scale's responsiveness are many, and, unfortunately, they provide non-equivalent results. The most used are the effect size and the standardized response mean, which are calculated as average change from baseline to follow-up divided by the standard deviation at baseline, or the standard deviation of change, respectively. Also, the responsiveness statistic is frequently used, similar to the previous indices in the numerator, but with the standard difference of the change in stable patients in the denominator. For all the three indices, the same thresholds for interpretation have been given: <0.20, negligible; 0.20–0.49, small effect; 0.50–0.79, moderate effect; and ≥0.80, large effect. Such benchmark values are attractive because they make the interpretation of results easy, but they were really proposed with other intentions (calculation of sample size) and are arbitrary.[2,44,46–48] Responsiveness of two scales may be compared by t-test (the larger the t-statistic, the more sensitive the scale) or through the ratio of the t-tests ($[t\text{-statistic}_1/t\text{-statistic}_2]^2$), named "relative efficiency statistics." If parametric tests are not applicable, squared z-values from the Wilcoxon rank test are used instead of t-tests.[44,49–53] With more than two comparisons, as for inter- and intra-groups at baseline and follow-up, the F-statistic from ANOVA (or the chi-squared from the nonparametric Kruskal-Wallis test) can replace the t-statistics.[11,44,51,52,54]

In addition to those statistics, other tests based on the SEM can be applied to demonstrate that the observed change is a true change. Obviously, to be considered a real change the magnitude of the change should be higher than the error of measurement. The SEM value; the upper limit of the 95% confidence interval for SEM (1.96 SEM); the smallest real difference (1.96 × $\sqrt{2}$ x SEM); and the reliable change index (1.96 × $\sqrt{[SEM_1{}^2 + SEM_2{}^2]}$) have been proposed as thresholds.[12,53,55–58] Although their results differ, all of them really determine the "minimally detectable change" (the smallest change that can be detected by the instrument beyond measurement error), a concept to keep separate from the "minimally important change."[43,46,53,59] Deyo and Centor[60] proposed to apply analysis with the receiver operating characteristics (ROC) curve for identifying the cutoff of the change in scoring indicative a true change. Plotting of the sensitivity and specificity of an instrument with its different cutoffs could be the best way to identify the optimal point for a real change,[61] and an area under the curve ≥0.70 may be considered satisfactory.[17]

Standard values accepted as quality criteria for the above reviewed attributes are shown in Table 3-2.

• **Interpretability** is defined as the extent to which qualitative meaning can be assigned to quantitative scores. *Responsiveness* and *interpretability* are related concepts, although the first focuses on the properties of the scale, and the latter on characteristics of the respondents. A variety of methods has been used to check the meaning of a score or whether a change is really important. Variation of scores over time or after an intervention may be relevant or not for the patients. Statistical significance informs about the certainty for rejecting the null hypothesis

Table 3-2. Psychometric Attributes and Standard Criteria

ATTRIBUTE AND METHODS	CRITERION VALUES	REFERENCES
Feasibility		
Missing data	<5%	16
	<10%	21–23
Acceptability		
Floor and ceiling effects	≤15%	12
	<20%	20, 21
Skewness	Between –1 and +1	20, 26
Observed scores	Full score range	21
Internal consistency		
Cronbach's alpha	>0.70 (group)	15, 17
	0.90–0.95 (individual)	
Item-total correlation	r ≥ 0.20	2, 21, 29
	r ≥ 0.40	
Homogeneity coefficient	>0.30	30
Reproducibility		
Kappa, Weighted kappa	≥0.70	2, 14, 17
Intraclass correlation coefficient	≥0.70	2, 16, 17
Content validity		
Lynn's coefficient	≥75% of experts endorsing the item or scale	34, 35
Criterion validity		
Correlation coefficient	≥0.70	16–18
Hypothesis testing validity		
Correlation coefficient	<0.35 – Low correlation	3, 14, 36–40
	0.35–0.60 – Moderate correlation	
	>0.60 – High correlation	
Known-groups validity	Magnitude of the difference	11
Internal validity	r = 0.30–0.70	20, 21
Responsiveness (change)		
Effect size	<0.20, negligible	2, 44, 46–48
Standardized response mean	0.20–0.49, small effect	
Responsiveness statistic	0.50–0.79, moderate effect	
	≥0.80, large effect	
Responsiveness (true change)		
Standard error of measurement	1 SEM, 1.96 SEM	12, 53, 55–58
Smallest real difference	$1.96 \times \sqrt{2} \times SEM$	
Reliable change index	$1.96 \times \sqrt{[SEM_1^2 + SEM_2^2]}$	

but does not inform about the clinical impact of the change.

For interpretation of a score at one point in time, such strategies as the following may be used: comparison (mean and SD) with norms for matched general population, or normative groups, or relevant known-groups expected to differ in scores; correlation with scores from other measures applied simultaneously and easily interpreted; and familiarity derived from results from a large pool of studies that reported findings on the scale.

For interpretation of change, diverse methods have been proposed: comparison (mean and SD) with norms (general population or normative groups); correlation with change in other measures applied simultaneously and easily interpreted; comparison with change of a external benchmark (like the clinician's global judgement or laboratory tests); magnitude of the change (relative change, effect size statistics); comparison of groups (percent of individuals changing upper a threshold value, t-test or ANOVA; number of patients needed to treat), etc.[12,14,15,17,59,62,63]

The *minimal clinically important difference* (MCID) is defined as "the smallest difference in score in the domain of interest which patients perceive as beneficial and would mandate, in the absence of troublesome side effects and excessive cost, a change in the patient's management."[64] More specific for a change, is the term *minimal important change* (MIC), defined as "the smallest change in score in the construct to be measured, which is perceived as important by patients, clinicians, or relevant others," and this is the relevant concept here.[17,65] Various anchor-based and distribution-based methods for determination of the MIC have been proposed.

The anchor-based approaches use an external criterion, either clinical or patient-based, to operationalize the change, assigning the subjects into groups reflecting no change, or different intensities of positive or negative change (small, moderate, or large, for instance). The anchors may be clinical (e.g., clinical ratings, laboratory tests) or patient-based (e.g., a transition question about change). Selection

of anchors is key, and the most useful are those that can identify the individuals with a small but significant change. Appropriateness and estimation of the minimal significant change in the clinical-based anchors; recall bias in patient-based anchors; dependency on baseline values; and characteristics of the sample can introduce uncertainty and variability in determining the MIC. Therefore, it is recommended that there be a recalculation of MIC in each new study until obtaining robust evidence on a reliable value, as well as the use of several anchors simultaneously (triangulation) to offer a range of values, including the real MIC. Once the group experiencing a "minimal" relevant change has been identified by an anchor, the change in the scale score corresponding to this group will be proposed as the MIC.[46,59,64]

Distribution-based approaches are based on statistical characteristics of the sample. In addition to significance tests (e.g., t-test, growth curve analysis), tests based on variation of the sample (e.g., effect size, standardized response mean, Guyatt's responsiveness statistic), and methods based on precision (e.g., SEM, reliable change index) are applied.[44,46,66,67] These methods are used here to determine the ability of the scale to detect a clinically important change, one of the meanings of "responsiveness."[44] In addition, several distribution-based statistics based on reviews of outcomes from various studies have been proposed as global thresholds for a MIC in some settings: 0.5 standard deviation at baseline,[68,69] 1 SEM,[43,69,70] and 10% of the maximal limit of the scale score.[71,72] A change surpassing the most exigent of these values calculated simultaneously could be considered important from a merely statistical point of view.[53,73] Nonetheless, distribution-based methods do not provide direct information on the clinical relevance of the change but simply express the observed change in a standardized manner. Therefore, anchor-based methods are preferred for estimation of the MIC.[17,66,67]

• **Respondent and administrative burdens** are defined as "the time, effort, and other demands placed on those to whom the instrument is administered (respondent burden) or on those who administer the instrument (administrative burden)."[15] The feasibility and acceptability of a scale are directly related to these attributes. On the other hand, the scale reliability and validity may be also influenced by the burdens. Length and number of scales and questionnaires to be applied should be kept as minimal as possible to avoid fatigue or stress and their consequences (missing data, refusal, withdrawal from the study, etc.). Needed resources and costs (e.g., interviewer, telephone, computer, training) are relevant administrative aspects to be taken into account.[12–16]

- **Alternative forms**: Modified versions of a scale in regard to the mode of administration (self-assessment, by proxy, interview, telephone, computer), short or expanded versions, should be tested (validated) to demonstrate the quality of their psychometric attributes before application in clinical studies.

RASCH ANALYSIS APPROACH

When evaluating validation data, it is important to also incorporate the measurement theory perspective. The simplest application of measurement theory is the Rasch model, a one-parameter (difficulty) logistic model.[9] The Rasch model states that the probability of a person's giving a certain answer, or endorsing an item, is a logistical function of the difference between the person's ability (for example, the patient's cognitive function as measured by the SCOPA-COG[74]) and the item's difficulty (in the SCOPA-COG, the level or degree of cognitive function being measured). Therefore, according to the Rasch model, the person's level of the construct being measured, as well as the level of several items on the same construct, may be estimated independently and therefore compared with each other.

For clinicians and researchers working with classic psychometric validations, it is not so difficult to order patients according to the level of the construct measured; for example, Parkinson's disease patients with the most to the least autonomic dysfunction. However, Rasch analysis also allows ordering the items in the same ruler, expressed in logit units. This permits the researcher to identify the items that are the most difficult, representing a higher level of the construct, and also the easiest items. The former corresponds to the ones with the highest probability of being endorsed, whereas the latter are those with the lowest endorsement probability.

With Rasch analysis, ordinal scales scores may be transformed into linear measures. Most rating scales used in neurology as patient-reported outcome measures are derived from dichotomous items or from items rated in Likert-type response scales. These items are actually measured on ordinal scales, meaning that the distance between the points is not equal and therefore only order comparisons are allowed (one patient is better than another, but we do not know if one patient is twice or three times better than the other). However, in most questionnaires, their items are intended to be summed or averaged to provide a total score, of which means and standard deviations, change scores (essential in clinical trial analysis), and other parametric-based calculations are performed. Scales that fit the Rasch model allow the calculation of valid change scores and access to parametric statistics.

There are many examples of the application of Rasch model to scales specifically developed for PD: SCOPA-COG[74]; SCOPA-AUT[75]; PDQ-39[76–78]; PDQ-8[79]; the 26-item Parkinson Disease Dyskinesia Scale (PDYS-26).[80] Similarly, other general scales validated with PD patients have also been analyzed according to the Rasch model: Nottingham Health Profile[77,81,82]; Hospital Anxiety and Depression Scale (HADS)[83]; Impact on Participation and Autonomy questionnaire[84]; Epworth Sleepiness Scale[85]; Functional Assessment of Chronic Illness Therapy-Fatigue Scale (FACIT-F)[86]; and Fatigue Severity Scale.[86]

Rasch analysis is used to construct new scales, to revise existing ones, and to evaluate the psychometric properties of developed scales.[87] It is also used to guide the construction of item banks, the basis for computer adaptive testing.[88] The key importance of Rasch analysis in the development of existing instruments and judging the quality of new ones has been specifically recognized for quality of life instruments[89] and neurology rating scales.[7] There are a few published papers setting guidelines for evaluating Rasch studies[87,90] or offering a tutorial.[91] Although more focused on a classic psychometric perspective, the COSMIN checklist also refers to some of the criteria to evaluate the methodological quality of item response theory and Rasch analysis studies.[19,92–95] The most frequently used software packages for Rasch analysis are Winsteps[96] and Rasch Unidimensional Measurement Models (RUMM2020[97] or RUMM2030.[98])

Rasch analysis follows an iterative process, where several changes to the original item selection are proposed and tested until model fit is achieved. Besides assessing how well the data fit the Rasch model, Rasch analysis provides information about the scale's reliability; unidimensionality; item bias (differential item functioning, DIF) by specific groups such as sociodemographic variables, diagnostic groups and cross-cultural comparisons; if response categories work as expected in the case of items with more than two response categories; item hierarchy and the relationship between the distribution of persons and items (scale targeting); floor and ceiling effects; and local dependency of items. A brief explanation of each of these parameters is provided and illustrated with the Rasch analysis of the Scales for Outcomes in Parkinson's Disease–Psychosocial (SCOPA-PS, Box 3-5),[99] performed with the statistical software RUMM2020.[97] Since Rasch analysis is an iterative process, the presentation order is purely didactical.

- **Choosing a version of the Rasch model:** There are three main versions of the Rasch model, one for dichotomous items, and two versions used for items answered in a response scale with three or more categories (polytomous items). The rating scale model is used when the distance between the thresholds is equal across items.[100] A threshold is the point where the probability of responding in two adjacent categories is the same. The partial credit model, also known as the unconstrained polytomous model,[101] is applied when the response scale structure differs across items, as in the case of the SCOPA-COG.[74] It is also applied when the distance between the thresholds is not the same (Box 3-6). In RUMM, this is specifically tested with the likelihood ratio test.[102]

- **Fit to the Rasch model:** When analyzing a scale according to the Rasch model, the main goal is to find a nonstatistical difference between the data and the Rasch model. This is measured through goodness-of-fit chi-square, and a non-significant p-value is expected. In RUMM, the chi-square value is reported and a Bonferroni correction for the number of items is used. In addition, both item and person-fit residuals should follow a normal distribution with a mean ± standard deviation (M±SD) of 0±1 (Box 3-7a) and the individual item-fit residual should be within the ±2.5 range (Box 3-7b). Item residual values below −2.5 indicate redundancy (under-discrimination), whereas values above 2.5 indicate that the item is measuring a different construct (over-discrimination). Winsteps reports two fit mean square statistics, INFIT and OUTFIT, and values around one (a frequently used criterion is 0.6–1.4) indicate a good fit.[103]

Box 3-5. The SCOPA-PS: Description of the Scale

The SCOPA-PS aims at assessing the effect caused by PD in the patient's psychosocial functioning, in the last month.[99] It is made up of 11 items, answered in a Likert-type response scale from 0 (never) to 3 (very much). The SCOPA-PS sumscore is expressed as a percentage and is obtained by summing the item scores and dividing by 33, the maximum possible. A higher score indicates a great impact by PD.

Box 3-6. Rasch Analysis of the SCOPA-PS: Threshold Ordering (Initial Model) to Decide Which Rasch Model Version to Use

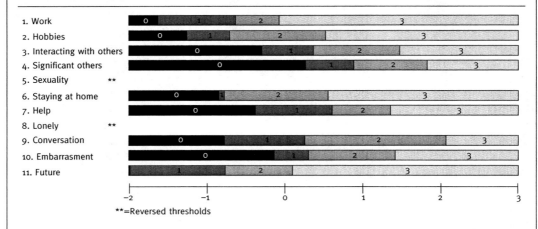

**=Reversed thresholds

Comment: Since the threshold map shows that some items need to be recoded, and the threshold distances vary across the items, the partial credit model should be used.

• **Sample size:** As in most statistical tests, the p-value associated to the goodness-of-fit chi-square is influenced by the sample size. A small sample size generates unstable results, which might jeopardize the generalization of the findings. However, with very large sample sizes, a small deviation from the Rasch model will result in significant chi-square values. A sample size of 250 allows getting accurate estimates of item and person locations regardless of the scale targeting (Box 3-8).[104]

• **Reliability:** Rasch analysis provides an indicator of reliability. In RUMM, this is

Box 3-7a. Rasch Analysis of the SCOPA-PS: Global Fit to the Rasch Model

		STANDARD	INITIAL MODEL	FINAL MODEL
Item fit	M	0	−0.200	−0.269
residual	SD	1	2.523	1.552
Person fit	M	0	−0.238	−0.274
residual	SD	1	1.054	1.020
Item-trait	χ^2 (DF)	Low	140.821 (55)	62.463 (45)
interaction	Prob.	NS	<0.000001	0.043

M: mean; SD: standard deviation; Prob.: probability; NS: Non-significant; DF: Degrees of freedom

Comment: The initial Rasch analysis showed a poor fit to the Rasch model, with a significant difference chi-square at the adjusted p-level of 0.0045 (0.05/11 items). The initial misfit was especially reflected in the relatively large standard deviation of the item residuals (2.523, well above the standard value of 1). The final model, after introducing several modifications to the scale, displayed a satisfactory fit, as expressed by the non-significant chi-square, and M±SD item and person fit residuals close to 0±1.

Box 3-7b. Rasch Analysis of the SCOPA-PS: Individual Item Fit (Final Model)

ITEMS	LOCATION	STANDARD ERROR	FIT RESIDUAL	χ^2 (DF = 5)	PROB- ABILITY
Item 1: Work	−0.771	0.067	−1.679	6.994	0.221
Item 2: Hobbies	−0.474	0.069	−2.265	11.441	0.043
Item 3: Interacting with others	0.520	0.085	−1.562	6.376	0.271
Item 6: Staying at home	−0.346	0.069	−0.066	9.852	0.080
Item 7: Help	0.582	0.088	−0.919	6.438	0.266
Item 8: Lonely	0.281	0.101	1.210	2.323	0.803
Item 9: Conversation	0.531	0.084	−0.600	3.386	0.641
Item 10: Embarrassment	0.571	0.086	1.072	4.473	0.484
Item 11: Future	−0.896	0.069	2.392	11.181	0.048

df: degrees of freedom

Comment: In the initial analysis, item 4 (relationship with partner, family, friends) had showed a low fit residual (−3,286) indicating item redundancy, and was therefore removed. Item 5 (sexuality) was also removed due to DIF and significant misfit, as explained in Box 3-9. In the final model, all items displayed fit residuals within the ±2.5 range, with a non-significant associated chi-square.

provided by the Person Separation Index (PSI). It is equivalent to Cronbach's alpha, but it uses the person estimates in logits instead of the raw scores. Its interpretation is also similar: values of 0.70 or higher are required for group comparisons; and 0.85 or higher for individual use (Box 3-9). Winsteps reports the item separation

ratio, and the criterion values are 1.5 and 2.5 for group or individual use, respectively.[87]

• **Threshold ordering**: In the case of polytomous items, it is important to check whether the thresholds are ordered. Linacre presents eight criteria for rating scale optimization.[107] Disordered thresholds indicate that respondents are not able to discriminate between too many response options, or response options have confusing labels (such as "sometimes" and "frequently"). It is expected that respondents

Box 3-8. Rasch Analysis of the SCOPA-PS: Sample Size and Descriptives

The sample was formed by 387 PD patients. The study design was multi-center, cross-sectional.[105] The main descriptive characteristics are as follows: 54.3% men; M±SD age of 65.86 (range: 31–91) years; 74.7% of patients were in the mild (1 and 2) Hoehn and Yarh stage.

Box 3-9. Rasch Analysis of the SCOPA-PS: Reliability

The PSI for the final, nine-item model was 0.835. This value allows to statistically differentiate among three groups.[106]

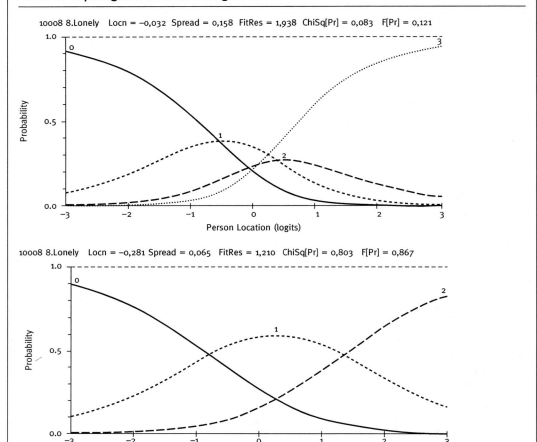

Box 3-10. Rasch Analysis of the SCOPA-PS: Category Probability Curve for Item 8 (Lonely) Showing Disordered (Top), and Ordered (Bottom) Thresholds After Collapsing the Central Categories

10008 8.Lonely   Locn = −0,032 Spread = 0,158 FitRes = 1,938 ChiSq[Pr] = 0,083   F[Pr] = 0,121

10008 8.Lonely   Locn = −0,281 Spread = 0,065 FitRes = 1,210 ChiSq[Pr] = 0,803   F[Pr] = 0,867

Comment: Besides item 5 (sexuality), item 8 (lonely) initially displayed reserved thresholds (top graphic). After collapsing the middle response categories ("a little" and "quite a bit," respectively), the item showed ordered thresholds (bottom graphic).

will use categories in a manner consistent with the metric estimate of the underlying construct. This can be visually inspected through category probability curves (Box 3-10). Disordered thresholds frequently result in item misfit, and can be corrected by collapsing adjacent categories.

• **Local independency:** Item *local independence* means that, once the variance explained by the Rasch factor is removed, the items do not show further associations.[108] This is examined

by the correlations between the residuals, and no correlations higher than 0.30, or noticeably higher than the rest, are expected (Box 3-11). When a group of items is locally dependent, it means that the answers to these items are linked in some way, so that the answer in one item will determine the answer in the others. It would be the case for two items measuring the functional ability to climb one or several flights of stairs, respectively. These locally dependent items may be combined into a single one, a testlet or subtest, working as a super item (climbing stairs, in the example provided).

• **Unidimensionality:** Along with local independency, unidimensionality is a basic Rasch model assumption. Unidimensionality implies that the scale measures only one construct, which allows the items to be summed together to form a scale with only one dimension. A strict test of unidimensionality has been proposed by Smith.[109] In a principal-components analysis of the residuals, after the Rasch factor has been taken into account, two sets of items are defined according to the correlations (positive and negative) between the items and the first residual factor (Box 3-12a). Then the person estimates of these two sets of items are compared through t-tests (Box 3-12b). For a scale to be unidimensional, less than 5% of the t-tests should be significant, or the lower bond of the binomial confidence interval should overlap 5%.[109,110]

• **Differential item functioning (DIF):** DIF occurs when two sample groups with the same level of the construct being measured answer in a different way to an item. For example, for the same level of autonomic symptoms, men and women might differ in the way they respond to the item "sialorrhea."[75] DIF is absent when significant differences are obtained in the analysis of variance (ANOVA) with Bonferroni correction. Uniform DIF, when differences by group are consistent across the construct range, is corrected by splitting the item and providing different estimates for each group. If two or more items present uniform DIF, they may be grouped into a testlet and compared with the remaining items to see if DIF cancels out (Box 3-13).[111,112] Non-uniform DIF usually results in the item's being removed. There are two interesting applications of DIF: one is to test invariance across countries; and the other, across time.

• **Scale targeting:** Scale targeting compares the distribution of the person locations

Box 3-12a. Rasch Analysis of the SCOPA-PS: Principal Component Loadings (Final Model) to Assess Unidimensionality

ITEM	FIRST PRINCIPAL COMPONENT
Item 11: Future	−0.483
Item 10: Embarrassment	−0.455
Item 6: Staying at home	−0.207
Item 8: Lonely	−0.199
Item 9: Conversation	−0.138
Item 3: Interacting with others	−0.077
Item 7: Help	−0.051
Item 2: Hobbies	0.816
Item 1: Work	0.823

Comment: Two sets of items were defined, one with the negative loadings (seven items) and the other with the positive loadings (two items). The person locations of the two sets of items were compared through *t*-tests.

Box 3-12b. Rasch Analysis of the SCOPA-PS: Distribution of t-test Values to Assess Unidimensionality

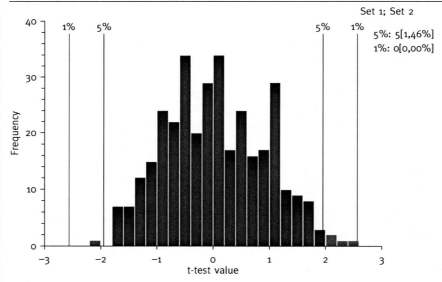

Comment: The distribution of the *t*-test values, comparing the person locations for the two sets of items, indicates that only 1.46% (below the 5% criterion) of the tests was significant. The associated binomial 95% confidence interval was −0.01–0.04. Thus, strict unidimensionality was supported. This indicates that the scale was measuring only one construct, and, therefore, that item scores may be summed.

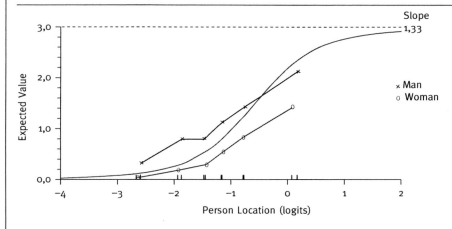

Comment: In the initial analysis, item 5 (sexuality) showed a high fit residual (4.911), indicating that it was measuring a different construct than the rest of the items in the scale. DIF analysis showed a bias by sex: at the same level of the trait, men had a higher probability of endorsing this item than women. DIF was not cancelled out at the sublet level, so item 5 was split into two items, item 5M (sexuality in man) and 5W (sexuality in woman), and locations were calculated independently for men and women. Since item 5M continued to show a high fit residual, item 5 (sexuality) was removed.

In the final model, items 8 (lonely) and 9 (conversation) also displayed uniform DIF by sex, in opposite directions. When these two items were combined into a testlet, and compared with the other items, DIF cancelled out.

with the item difficulties in the same scale, centered in zero logits. In the case of polytomous items, the threshold distribution is taken. It is expected that the item or threshold locations cover the entire range of patients across the construct being measured. On the other hand, for a well-targeted measure (not too easy and not too hard for the population) the M±SD of the person locations should be 0±1 logits. A negative mean value implies that the sample was located at a lower level of the construct than the average of the scale. Item difficulties should be adequately spread along the measure, and the covered range should not be too narrow; for most cases, a range of −4 to 4 logits is usually considered sufficient. The person-item distribution graphic (Box 3-14) also allows for detecting floor and ceiling effects. The PSI becomes less informative in the presence of significant floor and ceiling effects.[113]

• **Raw sumscores to a linear measure.** Once a good fit to the Rasch model is achieved and the assessed parameters are satisfactory, the raw sumscore may be converted into a linear measure. Instead of using a logit ruler centered in zero, the values may be linearly transformed into a convenient value and range: for example, 0–100. The relationship between the ordinal scores and the interval measures is characteristically an ogive, S-shaped, rather than linear (Box 3-15). In the central part, there is a close relationship between the raw ordinal scores and the linear measure. However, the distance becomes wider as we move closer to the extremities of the measurement ruler. Raw scores to linear measure conversion tables are very helpful for clinicians and researchers, since

Box 3-14. Rasch Analysis of the SCOPA-PS: Person Item Threshold Distribution Graph (Final Model) to Assess Scale Targeting

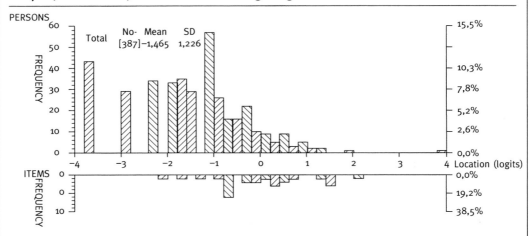

Comment: The SCOPA-PS measure, for the final model, showed a slight floor effect (4.85%). The scale range was restricted, from −2 to 2 logits. More items measuring the lower levels of psychosocial impact could be needed. The M±SD person location was −1.465±1.226, indicating that the patients displayed a lower level of psychosocial impact than the average of the scale. The easiest threshold items were the first thresholds of items 1 (work) and 11 (future), whereas hardest was the third threshold of item 9 (conversation).

it allows obtaining linear estimates without having to perform Rasch analysis on the data. The self-scoring form is also a useful tool for rapidly obtaining results in a linear measure.[114] Table 3-3 summarizes in a checklist the main aspects to take into consideration when evaluating validation data using Rasch analysis.

• **Final comments:** Despite its strengths, Rasch analysis also presents some limitations and disadvantages. First, contrary to the classic psychometric approach, it is necessary to have specific software to run Rasch analysis. Second, some scales might not fit the Rasch model, because it only takes into consideration one parameter, difficulty. There are other logistic models that take into consideration two and three parameters.[8] Third, Rasch analysis results should not be over-generalized into populations very different than the one studied. This is also the case for classic psychometric methods. A measure that is valid and reliable for a specific diagnostic group (for example, PD), does not mean that it will also be so for a different one (such as multiple sclerosis). Fourth, Rasch analysis, as well classic psychometric methods, should be applied for scales following a reflective or effect indicator model.[115,116] Most, but not all,[117] patient-reported outcome scales follow a reflective indicator model. Finally, most researchers and clinicians do not feel familiar with the measurement theory and its specific vocabulary and methods. We hope that this chapter, along with other texts,[54,89,91,103] will contribute to familiarizing researchers and clinicians working with rating scales in PD.

Acknowledgments

We thank Alba Ayala for her contribution to the Rasch analysis of the SCOPA-PS.

Box 3-15. Rasch Analysis of the SCOPA-PS: Raw Sumscore to Linear Measure Conversion Table (Top) and Graphic (Bottom)

RAW SUMSCORE	LINEAR MEASURE (LOGIT SCALE)	LINEAR MEASURE (0–100 SCALE)	RAW SUMSCORE	LINEAR MEASURE (LOGIT SCALE)	LINEAR MEASURE (0–100 SCALE)
0	0.00	−3.67	14	50.33	0.10
1	10.81	−2.86	15	52.47	0.26
2	18.16	−2.31	16	54.61	0.42
3	23.10	−1.94	17	56.88	0.59
4	26.97	−1.65	18	59.28	0.77
5	30.17	−1.41	19	61.82	0.96
6	32.98	−1.20	20	64.49	1.16
7	35.51	−1.01	21	67.56	1.39
8	37.78	−0.84	22	71.16	1.66
9	40.05	−0.67	23	75.43	1.98
10	42.19	−0.51	24	80.91	2.39
11	44.19	−0.36	25	88.65	2.97
12	46.33	−0.20	26	100.00	3.82
13	48.33	−0.05			

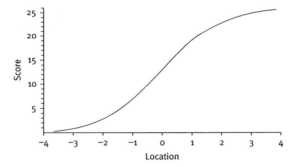

Comment: The raw sumscore to linear measure conversion table provides a way of obtaining a linear measure from the raw scores. This linear measure may be expressed in logits, or rescaled into a more convenient range, in this case 0–100 (table, top part). Since items 4 and 5 were removed, and the response category scheme was changed for item 8, the raw score range is different than for the initial SCOPA-PS. The relationship between the raw score and the linear measure is characteristically ogive-shaped (graphic, bottom part).

Table 3-3. Checklist: Main Aspects to Take into Consideration When Evaluating Validation Data Through Rasch Analysis

1. Indication of the statistical software used (most common: RUMM2020,[97] Winsteps[96])

2. In the case of polytomous items, the version of the Rasch model is specified (rating scale[100] or partial credit model[101])

3. Sample size is adequate (around 250, for most cases[104])

4. Global fit to the Rasch model (RUMM: non-significant chi-square, individual item fit within ±2.5, M±SD item and person fit residual approaching 0 ± 1[87,91]; Winsteps: INFIT and OUTFIT close to 1[103])

5. Satisfactory reliability for group or person comparisons (RUMM: PSI ≥ 0.70 for group and ≥ 0.85 for individual comparisons[87,91]; Winsteps: item separation ratio ≥1.5 and 2.5, respectively[103])

6. For polytomous items, ordered thresholds

7. Local dependency: present (correlation coefficients between residuals below 0.30[108]) or absent; if present, how it was corrected (item removal; sublets)

8. Reasons for item removal: measuring a different construct; redundancy; DIF; etc.

9. DIF: which factors were analyzed (age, gender, etc); presence/absence; uniform/non-uniform; how it was dealt with (item splitting, item removal, testlets to see if it cancels out at the test level)[111,112]

10. Unidimensionality: when testing strict unidimensionality through principal components of residuals, less than 5% of the t-tests are significant, or the lower bond of the binomial confidence interval overlaps 5%[109]

11. Scale targeting: spread of items across the continuum; distribution of person locations with M±SD approaching 0 ± 1; floor/ceiling effect; item (threshold) hierarchy

Source: Based on references 54, 89, 91, 103

References

1. LaRocca NG. Statistical and methodologic considerations in scale construction. In: Munsat TL, ed. *Quantification of Neurological Deficit.* Boston: Butterworth Publishers; 1989:49–67.

2. Streiner DL, Norman GR. *Health Measurement Scales: A Practical Guide to Their Construction and Use.* 4th ed. Oxford: Oxford University Press; 2008.

3. Nunnally JC, Bernstein IH. *Psychometric Theory.* New York: McGraw-Hill; 1994.

4. DeVellis RF. Classical test theory. *Med Care.* 2006;44(suppl 3)(11):S50–S59.

5. McDowell I. *Measuring Health: A Guide to Rating Scales and Questionnaires.* New York: Oxford University Press; 2006.

6. Hobart J. Rating scales for neurologists. *J Neurol Neurosurg Psychiatry.* 2003;74 (suppl 4):iv22–iv26.

7. Hobart JC, Cano SJ, Zajicek JP, Thompson AJ. Rating scales as outcome measures for clinical trials in neurology: problems, solutions, and recommendations. *Lancet Neurol.* 2007;6(12):1094–1105.

8. Birnbaum A. Some latent trait models and their use in inferring an examinee's ability. In: Lord FM, Novick MR, eds. *Statistical Theories of Mental Scores.* Reading, MA: Addison-Wesley; 1966.

9. Rasch G. *Probabilistic Models for Some Intelligence and Attainment Tests.* Expanded edition. Chicago: University of Chicago Press; 1980.

10. Wright BD, Masters GN. *Rating Scale Analysis. Rasch Measurement.* Chicago: MESA; 1982.

11. Fayers PM, Machin D. *Quality of Life: The Assessment, Analysis and Interpretation of Patient-Reported Outcomes.* 2nd ed. Chichester, UK: John Wiley & Sons Ltd.; 2007.

12. McHorney CA, Tarlov AR. Individual-patient monitoring in clinical practice: are available health status surveys adequate? *Qual Life Res.* 1995;4(4):293–307.

13. Fitzpatrick R, Davey C, Buxton MJ, Jones DR. Evaluating patient-based outcome measures for use in clinical trials. *Health Technol Assess.* 1998;2(14):i–74.

14. Chassany C, Sagnier P, Marquis P, Fullerton S, Aaronson N. Patient-reported outcomes:

the example of health-related quality of life: a European guidance document for the improved integration of health-related quality of life assessment in the drug regulatory process. *Drug Information Journal.* 2002;36(1):209–238.

15. Scientific Advisory Committee of the Medical Outcomes Trust. Assessing health status and quality-of-life instruments: attributes and review criteria. *Qual Life Res.* 2002;11(3): 193–205.

16. Smith SC, Lamping DL, Banerjee S, et al. Measurement of health-related quality of life for people with dementia: development of a new instrument (DEMQOL) and an evaluation of current methodology. *Health Technol Assess.* 2005;9(10):15–19.

17. Terwee CB, Bot SD, de Boer MR, et al. Quality criteria were proposed for measurement properties of health status questionnaires. *J Clin Epidemiol.* 2007;60(1):34–42.

18. Mokkink LB, Terwee CB, Stratford PW, et al. Evaluation of the methodological quality of systematic reviews of health status measurement instruments. *Qual Life Res.* 2009;18(3):313–333.

19. Mokkink LB, Terwee CB, Knol DL, et al. The COSMIN checklist for evaluating the methodological quality of studies on measurement properties: a clarification of its content. *BMC Med Res Methodol.* 2010;10:22.

20. Hobart J, Lamping D, Fitzpatrick R, Riazi A, Thompson A. The Multiple Sclerosis Impact Scale (MSIS-29): a new patient-based outcome measure. *Brain.* 2001;124(pt 5):962–973.

21. van der Linden FA, Kragt JJ, Klein M, van der Ploeg HM, Polman CH, Uitdehaag BM. Psychometric evaluation of the Multiple Sclerosis Impact Scale (MSIS-29) for proxy use. *J Neurol Neurosurg Psychiatry.* 2005;76(12):1677–1681.

22. WHOQOL Group. The World Health Organization Quality of Life assessment (WHOQOL): development and general psychometric properties. *Soc Sci Med.* 1998;46(12):1569–1585.

23. Marinus J, Visser M, van Hilten JJ, Lammers GJ, Stiggelbout AM. Assessment of sleep and sleepiness in Parkinson disease. *Sleep.* 2003;26(8):1049–1054.

24. Jenkinson C, Heffernan C, Doll H, Fitzpatrick R. The Parkinson's Disease Questionnaire (PDQ-39): evidence for a method of imputing missing data. *Age Ageing.* 2006;35(5):497–502.

25. Shrive FM, Stuart H, Quan H, Ghali WA. Dealing with missing data in a multi-question depression scale: a comparison of imputation methods. *BMC Med Res Methodol.* 2006;6:57.

26. Hays RD, Anderson R, Revicki D. Psychometric considerations in evaluating health-related quality of life measures. *Qual Life Res.* 1993;2(6):441–449.

27. Holmes W, Bix B, Shea J. SF-20 score and item distributions in a human immunodeficiency virus-seropositive sample. *Med Care.* 1996;34(6):562–569.

28. Martinez-Martin P, Rodriguez-Blazquez C, Abe K, et al. International study on the psychometric attributes of the non-motor symptoms scale in Parkinson disease. *Neurology.* 2009;73(19):1584–1591.

29. Ware JE Jr, Gandek B. Methods for testing data quality, scaling assumptions, and reliability: the IQOLA project approach. International Quality of Life Assessment. *J Clin Epidemiol.* 1998;51(11):945–952.

30. Eisen M, Ware JE Jr, Donald CA, Brook RH. Measuring components of children's health status. *Med Care.* 1979;17(9):902–921.

31. Cicchetti DV. Assessing inter-rater reliability for rating scales: resolving some basic issues. *Br J Psychiatry.* 1976;129(5):452–456.

32. Schuck P. Assessing reproducibility for interval data in health-related quality of life questionnaires: which coefficient should be used? *Qual Life Res.* 2004;13(3):571–586.

33. Bland JM, Altman DG. Statistical methods for assessing agreement between two methods of clinical measurement. *Lancet.* 1986;1(8476):307–310.

34. Lynn MR. Determination and quantification of content validity. *Nurs Res.* 1986;35(6):382–385.

35. Remple VP, Hilton BA, Ratner PA, Burdge DR. Psychometric assessment of the Multidimensional Quality of Life Questionnaire for Persons with HIV/AIDS (MQOL-HIV) in a sample of HIV-infected women. *Qual Life Res.* 2004;13(5):947–957.

36. Juniper EF, Guyatt GH, Jaeschke R. How to develop and validate a new health-related quality of life instrument. In: Spilker B, ed. *Quality of Life and Pharmacoeconomics in Clinical Trials.* 2nd ed. Philadelphia: Lippincott-Raven; 1996:49–56.

37. Luo N, Johnson JA, Shaw JW, Feeny D, Coons SJ. Self-reported health status of the general adult U.S. population as assessed by the EQ-5D and Health Utilities Index. *Med Care.* 2005;43(11):1078–1086.

38. Fisk JD, Brown MG, Sketris IS, Metz LM, Murray TJ, Stadnyk KJ. A comparison of health

utility measures for the evaluation of multiple sclerosis treatments. *J Neurol Neurosurg Psychiatry*. 2005;76(1):58–63.

39. Simon SD. *Statistical Evidence in Medical Trials: What Do the Data Really Tell Us?* Oxford: Oxford University Press; 2006.

40. Bonin-Guillaume S, Sautel L, Demattei C, Jouve E, Blin O. Validation of the Retardation Rating Scale for detecting depression in geriatric inpatients. *Int J Geriatr Psychiatry*. 2007;22(1):68–76.

41. Martinez-Martin P, Serrano-Duenas M, Forjaz MJ, Serrano MS. Two questionnaires for Parkinson's disease: are the PDQ-39 and PDQL equivalent? *Qual Life Res*. 2007;16(7):1221–1230.

42. Bullinger M, Anderson R, Cella D, Aaronson N. Developing and evaluating cross-cultural instruments from minimum requirements to optimal models. *Qual Life Res*. 1993;2(6): 451–459.

43. Beaton DE, Bombardier C, Katz JN, Wright JG. A taxonomy for responsiveness. *J Clin Epidemiol*. 2001;54(12):1204–1217.

44. Terwee CB, Dekker FW, Wiersinga WM, Prummel MF, Bossuyt PM. On assessing responsiveness of health-related quality of life instruments: guidelines for instrument evaluation. *Qual Life Res*. 2003;12(4):349–362.

45. Liang MH. Longitudinal construct validity: establishment of clinical meaning in patient evaluative instruments. *Med Care*. 2000;38(suppl 9):II 84–II 90.

46. Crosby RD, Kolotkin RL, Williams GR. Defining clinically meaningful change in health-related quality of life. *J Clin Epidemiol*. 2003;56(5):395–407.

47. Zou GY. Quantifying responsiveness of quality of life measures without an external criterion. *Qual Life Res*. 2005;14(6):1545–1552.

48. Norman GR, Wyrwich KW, Patrick DL. The mathematical relationship among different forms of responsiveness coefficients. *Qual Life Res*. 2007;16(5):815–822.

49. Liang MH, Larson MG, Cullen KE, Schwartz JA. Comparative measurement efficiency and sensitivity of five health status instruments for arthritis research. *Arthritis Rheum*. 1985;28(5):542–547.

50. Husted JA, Cook RJ, Farewell VT, Gladman DD. Methods for assessing responsiveness: a critical review and recommendations. *J Clin Epidemiol*. 2000;53(5):459–468.

51. Hobart JC, Riazi A, Lamping DL, Fitzpatrick R, Thompson AJ. How responsive is the Multiple Sclerosis Impact Scale (MSIS-29)? A comparison with some other self-report scales. *J Neurol Neurosurg Psychiatry*. 2005;76(11): 1539–1543.

52. Martinez-Martin P, Prieto L, Forjaz MJ. Longitudinal metric properties of disability rating scales for Parkinson's disease. *Value Health*. 2006;9(6):386–393.

53. Martinez-Martin P, Carod-Artal FJ, da Silveira RL, et al. Longitudinal psychometric attributes, responsiveness, and importance of change: an approach using the SCOPA-psychosocial questionnaire. *Mov Disord*. 2008;23(11): 1516–1523.

54. Hobart J, Cano S. Improving the evaluation of therapeutic interventions in multiple sclerosis: the role of new psychometric methods. *Health Technol Assess*. 2009;13(12):iii, ix–iii, 177.

55. Wyrwich KW, Wolinsky FD. Identifying meaningful intra-individual change standards for health-related quality of life measures. *J Eval Clin Pract*. 2000;6(1):39–49.

56. Beckerman H, Roebroeck ME, Lankhorst GJ, Becher JG, Bezemer PD, Verbeek AL. Smallest real difference, a link between reproducibility and responsiveness. *Qual Life Res*. 2001;10(7):571–578.

57. Jacobson NS, Truax P. Clinical significance: a statistical approach to defining meaningful change in psychotherapy research. *J Consult Clin Psychol*. 1991;59(1):12–19.

58. Fitzpatrick R, Norquist JM, Jenkinson C. Distribution-based criteria for change in health-related quality of life in Parkinson's disease. *J Clin Epidemiol*. 2004;57(1):40–44.

59. de Vet HC, Terwee CB, Ostelo RW, Beckerman H, Knol DL, Bouter LM. Minimal changes in health status questionnaires: distinction between minimally detectable change and minimally important change. *Health Qual Life Outcomes*. 2006;4:54.

60. Deyo RA, Centor RM. Assessing the responsiveness of functional scales to clinical change: an analogy to diagnostic test performance. *J Chronic Dis*. 1986;39(11):897–906.

61. Deyo RA, Diehr P, Patrick DL. Reproducibility and responsiveness of health status measures. Statistics and strategies for evaluation. *Control Clin Trials*. 1991;12(suppl 4):142S–158S.

62. Guyatt GH, Juniper EF, Walter SD, Griffith LE, Goldstein RS. Interpreting treatment effects in randomised trials. *BMJ*. 1998;316(7132):690–693.

63. Kazis LE, Anderson JJ, Meenan RF. Effect sizes for interpreting changes in health status. *Med Care*. 1989;27(suppl 3):S178–S189.

64. Jaeschke R, Singer J, Guyatt GH. Measurement of health status. Ascertaining the minimal clinically important difference. *Control Clin Trials*. 1989;10(4):407–415.

65. de Vet HC, Terwee CB. The minimal detectable change should not replace the minimal important difference. *J Clin Epidemiol*. 2010;63(7):804–805.

66. Revicki DA, Cella D, Hays RD, Sloan JA, Lenderking WR, Aaronson NK. Responsiveness and minimal important differences for patient-reported outcomes. *Health Qual Life Outcomes*. 2006;4:70.

67. Revicki D, Hays RD, Cella D, Sloan J. Recommended methods for determining responsiveness and minimally important differences for patient-reported outcomes. *J Clin Epidemiol*. 2008;61(2):102–109.

68. Norman GR, Sloan JA, Wyrwich KW. Interpretation of changes in health-related quality of life: the remarkable universality of half a standard deviation. *Med Care*. 2003;41(5):582–592.

69. Wyrwich KW, Bullinger M, Aaronson N, Hays RD, Patrick DL, Symonds T. Estimating clinically significant differences in quality of life outcomes. *Qual Life Res*. 2005;14(2): 285–295.

70. Wolinsky FD, Wan GJ, Tierney WM. Changes in the SF-36 in 12 months in a clinical sample of disadvantaged older adults. *Med Care*. 1998;36(11):1589–1598.

71. Barrett B, Brown D, Mundt M, Brown R. Sufficiently important difference: expanding the framework of clinical significance. *Med Decis Making*. 2005;25(3):250–261.

72. Ringash J, O'Sullivan B, Bezjak A, Redelmeier DA. Interpreting clinically significant changes in patient-reported outcomes. *Cancer*. 2007;110(1):196–202.

73. Honig H, Antonini A, Martinez-Martin P, et al. Intrajejunal levodopa infusion in Parkinson's disease: a pilot multicenter study of effects on nonmotor symptoms and quality of life. *Mov Disord*. 2009;24(10):1468–1474.

74. Forjaz MJ, Frades-Payo B, Rodriguez-Blazquez C, Ayala A, Martinez-Martin P. Should the SCOPA-COG be modified?: a Rasch analysis perspective. *Eur J Neurol*. 2010;17(2):202–207.

75. Forjaz MJ, Ayala A, Rodriguez-Blazquez C, Frades-Payo B, Martinez-Martin P. Assessing autonomic symptoms of Parkinson's disease with the SCOPA-AUT: a new perspective from Rasch analysis. *Eur J Neurol*. 2010;17(2): 273–279.

76. Hagell P, Nygren C. The 39-item Parkinson's disease questionnaire (PDQ-39) revisited: implications for evidence based medicine. *J Neurol Neurosurg Psychiatry*. 2007;78(11): 1191–1198.

77. Hagell P, Whalley D, McKenna SP, Lindvall O. Health status measurement in Parkinson's disease: validity of the PDQ-39 and Nottingham Health Profile. *Mov Disord*. 2003;18(7):773–783.

78. Nilsson MH, Westergren A, Carlsson G, Hagell P. Uncovering indicators of the international classification of functioning, disability, and health from the 39-item Parkinson's disease questionnaire. *Parkinsons Dis*. 2010;2010:984673.

79. Franchignoni F, Giordano A, Ferriero G. Rasch analysis of the short form 8-item Parkinson's Disease Questionnaire (PDQ-8). *Qual Life Res*. 2008;17(4):541–548.

80. Katzenschlager R, Schrag A, Evans A, et al. Quantifying the impact of dyskinesias in PD: the PDYS-26: a patient-based outcome measure. *Neurology*. 2007;69(6):555–563.

81. Christine WH. Cross-diagnostic validity of the Nottingham Health Profile Index of Distress (NHPD). *Health Qual Life Outcomes*. 2008;6:47.

82. Teixeira-Salmela LF, Magalhaes LC, Souza AC, Lima MC, Lima RC, Goulart F. [Adaptation of the Nottingham Health Profile: a simple measure to assess quality of life]. *Cad Saude Publica*. 2004;20(4):905–914.

83. Forjaz MJ, Rodriguez-Blazquez C, Martinez-Martin P. Rasch analysis of the hospital anxiety and depression scale in Parkinson's disease. *Mov Disord*. 2009;24(4):526–532.

84. Franchignoni F, Ferriero G, Giordano A, Guglielmi V, Picco D. Rasch psychometric validation of the Impact on Participation and Autonomy questionnaire in people with Parkinson's disease. *Eura Medicophys*. 2007;43(4):451–461.

85. Hagell P, Broman JE. Measurement properties and hierarchical item structure of the Epworth Sleepiness Scale in Parkinson's disease. *J Sleep Res*. 2007;16(1):102–109.

86. Hagell P, Hoglund A, Reimer J, et al. Measuring fatigue in Parkinson's disease: a psychometric study of two brief generic fatigue questionnaires. *J Pain Symptom Manage*. 2006;32(5):420–432.

87. Tennant A, Conaghan PG. The Rasch measurement model in rheumatology: what is it and why use it? When should it be applied, and what should one look for in a Rasch paper? *Arthritis Rheum.* 2007;57(8):1358–1362.

88. Gershon RC. Computer adaptive testing. *J Appl Meas.* 2005;6(1):109–127.

89. Tennant A, McKenna SP, Hagell P. Application of Rasch analysis in the development and application of quality of life instruments. *Value Health.* 2004;7(Suppl 1):22–26.

90. Smith RM, Linacre JM, Smith EV. Guidelines for manuscripts. *J Appl Meas.* 2003;4(2): 198–204.

91. Pallant JF, Tennant A. An introduction to the Rasch measurement model: an example using the Hospital Anxiety and Depression Scale (HADS). *Br J Clin Psychol.* 2007;46 (pt 1):1–18.

92. Mokkink LB, Terwee CB, Knol DL, et al. Protocol of the COSMIN study: COnsensus-based Standards for the selection of health Measurement INstruments. *BMC Med Res Methodol.* 2006;6:2.

93. Mokkink LB, Terwee CB, Patrick DL, et al. The COSMIN study reached international consensus on taxonomy, terminology, and definitions of measurement properties for health-related patient-reported outcomes. *J Clin Epidemiol.* 2010;63(7):737–745.

94. Mokkink LB, Terwee CB, Gibbons E, et al. Inter-rater agreement and reliability of the COSMIN (COnsensus-based Standards for the selection of health status Measurement INstruments) checklist. *BMC Med Res Methodol.* 2010;10:82.

95. Mokkink LB, Terwee CB, Patrick DL, et al. The COSMIN checklist for assessing the methodological quality of studies on measurement properties of health status measurement instruments: an international Delphi study. *Qual Life Research.* 2010;19(4):539–549.

96. Linacre JM. *WINSTEPS Rasch measurement computer program.* Chicago: Winsteps com; 2009.

97. Andrich D, Lyne A, Sheridon B, Luo G. *RUMM2020.* Perth, Australia: RUMM Laboratory; 2003.

98. Andrich D, Sheridon B, Luo G. *RUMM2030.* Perth, Australia: RUMM Laboratory; 2009.

99. Marinus J, Visser M, Martinez-Martin P, van Hilten JJ, Stiggelbout AM. A short psychosocial questionnaire for patients with Parkinson's disease: the SCOPA-PS. *J Clin Epidemiol.* 2003;56(1):61–67.

100. Andrich D. A rating formulation for ordered response categories. *Psychometrika.* 1978;43(4):561–573.

101. Masters GN. A Rasch model for partial credit scoring. *Psychometrika.* 1982;47(2):149–174.

102. Rost J. An unconditional likelihood ratio for testing item homogeneity in the Rasch model. *Education Research and Perspectives.* 1982;9(1):7–17.

103. Bond TG, Fox CM. *Applying the Rasch Model: Fundamental Measurement in the Human Sciences.* Mahwah, NJ: Lawrence Erlbaum; 2007.

104. Linacre JM. Sample size and item calibration stability. *Rasch Measurement Transactions.* 1994;7(4):328.

105. Martinez-Martin P, Carroza-Garcia E, Frades-Payo B, Rodriguez-Blazquez C, Forjaz MJ, Pedro-Cuesta J. [Psychometric attributes of the Scales for Outcomes in Parkinson's Disease-Psychosocial (SCOPA-PS): validation in Spain and review]. *Rev Neurol.* 2009;49(1):1–7.

106. Fisher W Jr. Reliability statistics. *Rasch Measurement Transactions.* 1992;6(3):238.

107. Linacre JM. Optimizing rating scale category effectiveness. *J Appl Meas.* 2002;3(1): 85–106.

108. Wright BD. Local dependency, correlations and principal components. *Rasch Measurement Transactions.* 1996;10(3):509–511.

109. Smith EV Jr. Detecting and evaluating the impact of multidimensionality using item fit statistics and principal component analysis of residuals. *J Appl Meas.* 2002;3(2):205–231.

110. Tennant A, Pallant JF. Unidimensionality matters! (a tale of two Smiths?). *Rasch Measurement Transactions.* 2006;20(1): 1048–1051.

111. Wainer H, Kiely GL. Item clusters and computerized adaptive testing: a case for testlets. *Journal of Educational Measurement.* 1987;24(3):185–201.

112. Tennant A, Pallant JF. DIF matters: a practical approach to test if differential item functioning makes a difference. *Rasch Measurement Transactions.* 2007;20(4):1082–1084.

113. Marais I, Andrich D. Effects of varying magnitude and patterns of response dependence in the unidimensional Rasch model. *J Appl Meas.* 2008;9(2):105–124.

114. Linacre JM. Instantaneous measurement and diagnosis. *Physical Medicine and Rehabilitation State-of-the-Art Reviews.* 1997;11(2):315–324.

115. Fayers PM, Hand DJ. Factor analysis, causal indicators and quality of life. *Qual Life Res.* 1997;6(2):139–150.

116. Stenner AJ, Burdick DS, Stone MH. Formative and reflective models: can a Rasch analysis tell the difference. *Rasch Measurement Transactions.* 2008;22(1):1152–1153.

117. Fayers PM, Hand DJ. Factor analysis, causal indicators and quality of life. *Qual Life Res.* 1997;6(2):139–150.

4

THE MINIMAL CLINICALLY RELEVANT CHANGE IN RATING SCALES

Cristina Sampaio, Olivier Rascol, and Anette Schrag

Summary

The main type definitions of "minimal relevant change" (MCRC) or "minimal relevant difference" (MCDR) refers to a change for an individual patient or patient group measured between endpoint and baseline. The concept involved originally two constructs: (1) a minimal amount of patient-reported difference, and (2) something significant enough to change patient management. There are several variations on these main conceptual tenants that we discuss in this chapter, namely the issue of the cross-sectional conceptualization. The core of chapter is dedicated to summarize the different methods that can be used to determine experimentally the MCRC for a rating scale. Methods are divided into anchor-based methods and distribution-based methods (statistically based).

INTRODUCTION

There are different concepts and methods associated with the expression "minimal relevant change" (MCRC) or "minimal relevant difference" (MCDR). In this chapter, we will discuss the methodologies used for the determination of values called MCRC or MCRD as applied to rating scales. To achieve a certain degree of homogeneity in the terminology, we adopt the term "MCRC" to refer to a change for an individual patient or patient group measured between endpoint and baseline. If another term is used with the same meaning, it is because we are quoting a given author, and we will note the fact.

The basic issues of scale clinimetrics have been discussed in previous chapters. Here, we address a topic that is intimately related to the

scale's responsiveness to change. The MCRC or MCRD is critical for the interpretation of studies, particularly when the effect of an intervention is to be judged, not only from a statistical analysis, but also from a clinically pertinent perspective on the impacts of impairment or disability.

The choice of the descriptor *minimal* is potentially ambiguous in English. As an adjective, "minimal" can mean "inconsequential" or "too small to be important." In the context of MCRC, *minimal* operates grammatically as an adverb and modifies *relevant*, meaning the change is the smallest change that still is clinically relevant. In this sense, "minimally" is probably the more correct designation.

Minimal clinically important difference, or MCID, was first defined by Jaeschke et al.[1] in 1989. Their operational definition of a minimal clinically important difference was "the smallest difference in score in the domain of interest which *patients* perceive as beneficial and which would mandate, in the absence of troublesome side effects and excessive cost, a change in the patient's *management*." This definition involved two constructs: (1) a minimal amount of patient-reported difference, and (2) something significant enough to change patient management.

Overall, MCRC and MCID are often used interchangeably, although MCID has sometimes been used to delineate the difference between treatment groups, and the linking of management decisions to MCID is not part of its original definition. The original concept of MCRC (or MCID, as Jaeschke called it) was an individual, longitudinal change from baseline. Guyatt[2] was more concerned with defining an appropriate benchmark of important change against which to assess the responsiveness of an instrument or scale, than in judging the importance of that change in terms of patient valuation.

However, since Jaeschke's landmark paper, which is considered the first to connect the minimal change to a judgement of benefit to practical management consequences, modifications of the definition were published,[3-6] not all of which include a longitudinal concept of MCRC. A few studies have adapted the definition of MCRC to refer to cross-sectional outcomes,[7,8] considering the difference between groups at the study's end instead of a difference at an individual level across time.

Most of the literature related to this concept is connected to the notion of therapeutic intervention and to improvement. However, as the field develops, it is important to understand that there are other visions associated with the concept of MCRC: one of them is deterioration over time in progressive disorders like neurodegenerative diseases. One should not, however, assume that MCRC for deterioration is automatically equivalent to that for improvement.

MCRC is a patient-derived score that reflects changes determined by a clinical intervention or the natural disease progression that are meaningful for the patient. At present, there are many different methods to obtain an MCRC, just as there are many different factors that can influence the MCRC value. *Thus, the MCRC for a rating scale is not a single, unique value.* Each calculation is population- and context-dependent. The values obtained are not absolute values that can be used as standards worldwide. However, in principle, it is possible to establish workable ranges for given situations, with strong evidence that the MCRC is a useful determination to achieve for scales.[9]

Below, we describe the different methods that have been considered to determine the MCRC. Some methods rely on subject-related anchors and are generally linked to the individual's evaluation before and after an intervention. This strategy makes them representative of the concept defined by Jaeschke et al. They determine a change that is relevant and can help patient-management or decision-making. Methods that rely only on a statistical analysis are important for statistical relevance but cannot document even highly significant changes that impact patients. Designing trials with appropriate sample sizes that detect changes in the range of the MCRC allows this integration of statistical and clinically pertinent information.

METHODS TO CALCULATE MCRC

Methods are divided into anchor-based methods and distribution-based methods (statistically based).[10,11]

Anchor-based approaches

Anchor-based approaches compare the change in the target rating scale to another measure of change, considered an *anchor* or *external* criterion. Very rarely, a true objective external criterion is used. Most commonly, studies compare the target rating scale scores to the patients' answers to another subjective assessment, typically a global assessment rating in which the patients rate themselves as to some extent "better," "unchanged," or "worse." The choice of a subjective assessment as an external criterion is not ideal, but reflects to the lack of a satisfying objective assessment. It is debatable how adequate is the use of global ratings is in particular, the possible interference by "recall bias" is a concern.[12] The use of clinician derived global assessment of change such as the clinical global impression change score (CGI-c) has also been proposed as an alternative, but a clinician derived change score may not reflect the patient prespective and is subject to the criticisms that such an approach of using a single-item assessment should be extensively validated, which is not the case for most clinical applications of such CGI. Other anchors have been used, and the use of an external criterion is the common characteristic of all anchor-based approaches.

Four variations may be identified among the anchor-based approaches:

"Within-patients" score change: The patient's retrospective rating of change is assessed using a global transition question (as the "anchor" or "external reference").[13] This strategy has become the most commonly used method for determining the MCRC. The rating scale is assessed prospectively at two time points: at the second assessment, the subject is also asked to think back to the first time point and judge the degree of change in that particular outcome. In this assessment, the patient is offered a series of graded options—often this five-point version: "much worse," "a little worse," "the same/no change," "a little better" and "much better and sometimes with more options." This was the method used by Schrag et al.,[14] who published the first-ever estimate for MCRC of UPDRS. Recently, Hauser et al.,[15] using similar methods, found values that are slightly lower. The possible explanation of these issues resides in a highly technical discussion that we will not expand in this chapter.

"Between-patients" score change: Another method used to determine the MCRC, particularly in the case of health-related quality of life (HRQOL) scales, is to group the rating scale scores by clinical criteria familiar to clinicians, called *clinical anchors*.[16] This technique is sometimes called the "known-groups approach," where "known" is shorthand for "the clinical status of the groups is known."[17] This method implies to that the scores in the scale under study

are related to well-characterized scores or well established scales. It is analogous to converting degrees of Fahrenheit degrees to Celsius. This is an obvious oversimplification, since in converting temperature from Fahrenheit to Celsius, we only convert, measurement units, , keeping the parameter measured the same—temperature—,In the clinical setting, the parameter measured by each of the related scales is not exactly the same. However, the conceptual principle of the method is one of interconversion.

The work of Shulman et al.[18] in the field of Parkinson's disease, is an example of the use of the interconversion method The clinical important differences of UPDRS were estimated using as referentials three established scales: (1) the SF-12; (2) the Schwab and England (SE) Scale; and (3) the Hoehn and Yahr stages.

Sensitivity- and specificity-based approach: Receiver-operator curves are normally used to determine a diagnostic test's ability to detect true cases of disease (in turn defined by a gold-standard method), but have been "imported conceptually" o determine MCRCs. In this approach, the rating scale score replaces the "diagnostic test," and a clinical anchor functions as the gold standard. The anchor distinguishes patients who were significantly improved or deteriorated from subjects who did not significantly changed. Various cut-points on the rating scale(s) are used to classify patients as "improved" or "not improved," and the cutoff point with the optimal ROC characteristics (sensitivity and specificity) is taken as an estimate of the MCRC. The ROC approach has been applied in two ways. Originally, the anchor was a clinical criterion, but increasingly, the anchor is a global transition question.[19]

Social comparison approach: This approach requires patients to judge themselves in relation to others with the same condition (based on between-patient differences), and in some studies has been found to produce similar results to the within-patient change approach and the global transition method discussed above.

Distribution-based approaches

Distribution-based approaches compare the change in rating scale scores to some measure of variability, such as the standard error of measurement, the standard deviation, or the effect size.

STANDARD ERROR OF MEASUREMENT (SEM)

The SEM is the variation in the scores due to the unreliability of the scale or measure used. A change, smaller than the identified SEM, is most likely the result of measurement error, rather than a true observed change. At the least, 1 SEM may be used as the yardstick of true change for individual change scores, and possibly for mean group change scores. The SEM is commonly used as an approximation for the MCRC. The estimation of the SEM does not involve a patient's or proxy's input about whether a change is minimally important in any sense; it has no "anchor" or "external reference point" regarding clinical pertinence. Thus, although the SEM is not really a method for estimating the MCRC, it serves as a convenient proxy.[20]

Associated with the SEM is the minimal (or smallest) detectable change (MDC). The MDC is the smallest change that can be considered above the measurement error, with a given level of confidence (usually 95% confidence level). Clearly, a valid MCRC should be at least as large as the observed MDC.[21]

EFFECT SIZE AND STANDARD DEVIATION

Effect size is a standardized measure of change obtained by dividing the difference in scores from baseline to post-treatment by the SD of the baseline scores. The value of the effect size represents the number of SDs by which the scores have changed from baseline to post-treatment. By convention (as defined originally by Cohen), an effect size of 0.2 is considered small, 0.5 moderate, and 0.8 large.[22] Used in conjunction with an external criterion, effect size ascertains the responsiveness of the external criterion. For instance, the effect size should be small in patients reporting no change and large in patients reporting a great improvement.[23] The change in scores corresponding to the small effect size has been used as a proxy for MCRC.

A number of "rules of thumb" to calculate the MCRC using the SD have been suggested. The most well known is ½SD = MCRC. This is supported by work of Norman et al.[3] They found that the value of 0.5 SD corresponded to the MCRC across a variety of studies. The authors attributed their finding to the fact that ½SD represents the limit of the human mental discriminative capacity, a limit that would appear in most patient-reported outcomes. This hypothesis that the detection ½SD is hardwired in the human brain lacks strong scientific support, however.

Others suggests that to obtain the MCRC, one multiplies the SD of the baseline scores by 0.2 (the small effect size).[24] The effect size (ES), like the SEM, or any of the above-mentioned SD-based calculations, has no external reference point or anchor to clinical pertinence for interpretation. It is a "signal-to-noise ratio": the mean difference (or change) in a rating scale divided by the variability among individuals (SD).

Other methods

There are other statistical calculations used to established what can be considered a reliable change in a scale. These are much less well established than the ones already described. Examples are the *reliable change index*, defined as equal to the individual's score before the intervention minus their score after the intervention, then divided by the standard error of the difference (Sdiff) of the test.[25]

USES OF THE MCRC

The knowledge of MCRC is useful for interpreting the impact of an intervention or the severity of a given rate of progression. It also serves to plan clinical trials.

Two different aspects must be distinguished. The first is establishing what change in the outcome measure represents a clinically relevant change for patients. This is the true meaning of the MCRC, as discussed above. The second is establishing the difference in the magnitude of response between the treatment and the control groups that will be considered large enough to establish the scientific or therapeutic relevance of the results. It is the difference between groups, postulated but unknown before the trial is done, that is used to calculate the sample size required for the clinical trial, and this can involve group differences in either central tendency (e.g., means) or in the proportions of responders (e.g., percentages of patients that obtain a defined response). Such responder analyses require a knowledge of what magnitudes of individual change can be considered clinically important so that patients can be categorized as responders and non-responders. This is a crucial step in understanding and interpreting the results of a clinical trial. Whilst the *a priori* knowledge of the range of MCRC should influence the calculation of the sample size, this is rarely done.

If the difference at endpoint between treated and placebo groups is inferior to the MCRC, it is relevant to understand how many patients achieve a given level of improvement, the so-called responders. Thus, one of the utilities of knowing the range of MCRC is the ability to define, with a sound basis, "responders." From there, the statistical analysis of the trial can be moved from expression of changes in a rating scale, to a binary approach related to who is responding or not responding, according with definition created. Results expressed in terms of rates of responders and non/responders are easier to understand by clinicians and even by lay persons. However, when continuous results, like the ones obtained in a rating scale, are transformed in a binary result, there is a loss of information; thus the trial loses statistical power. Therefore, in order to achieve statistical significance, the sample size must be increased. Secondly, the "responders" defined as described are an arbitrary category, and may not correspond to true biological phenotypes, as there will be "responders" in placebo groups as well. Nevertheless, if there is a higher proportion of responders, defined by the MCRC, in the treated group compared to the placebo group, this suggests some benefit from the intervention.

Conclusions about methodology

Fundamental work done in non-neurological disciplines, mainly in oncology and in rheumatology, can be highly informative for applications to Parkinson's disease and other movement disorders. The basics of the methodology are laid down, but the specifics still need to be worked out. The statistical methods as described above are applicable to all fields, but, with a few exceptions, they lack individual definition for the instruments available in field of PD and other movement disorders. It is clear that the statistical parameters are useful for establishing the limits of a tool. For example, a measurement instrument cannot go beyond its standard error of measurement: that is, it is limited by its minimal detectable difference, and effect sizes will always be limited by the standard deviation, which is dependent on sample characteristics and size. However, beyond these statistical aspects, there is much more to be learned about the clinical interpretation of change, and for this, the anchor-based methods are better suited as MCRC determinants, even if the methodologies for MCRC determination are not yet optimal. Use of these methodologies will help ensure that statistical change in rating scale scores can be translated into meaningful outcomes for patients and clinicians.

REFERENCES

1. Jaeschke R, Singer J, Guyatt GH. Ascertaining the minimal clinically important difference. *Cont Clin Trials*. 1989;10(4):407–415.
2. Guyatt GH, Walter S, Norman G. Measuring change over time: assessing the usefulness of evaluative instruments. *J Chronic Dis*. 1987;40(2):171–178.
3. Beaton DE, Bombardier C, Katz JN, et al. Looking for important change/differences in studies of responsiveness. OMERACT MCID working group. Outcome measures in rheumatology. Minimal clinically important difference. *J Rheumatol*. 2001;28(2):400–405.
4. Norman GR, Sloan JA, Wyrwich WK. Interpretation of changes in health-related quality of life: the remarkable universality of half a standard deviation. *Med Care*. 2003;41(5):582–592.
5. Wyrwich KW, Bullinger M, Aaronson N, et al. Estimating clinically significant differences in quality of life outcomes. *Qual Life Res*. 2005;14(2):285–295.

6. de Vet HC, Terwee CB, Ostelo RW, Beckerman H, Knol DL, Bouter LM. Minimal changes in health status questionnaires: distinction between minimally detectable change and minimally important change. *Health Qual Life Outcomes*. 20064(8):54.

7. Osoba D, King M. Interpreting QOL in individuals and groups: meaningful differences. In: Fayers P, Hays R, eds. *Assessing Quality of Life in Clinical Trials: Methods and Practice*. Oxford, UK: Oxford University Press; 2005:243–257.

8. Wells G, Beaton D, Shea B, et al. Minimal clinically important differences: review of methods. *J Rheumatol*. 2001;28(2):406–412.

9. Dworkin RH, Turk DC, McDermott MP, et al. Interpreting the clinical importance of treatment outcomes in chronic pain clinical trials: IMMPACT recommendations. *J Pain Symptom Manage*. 2008;9(2): 105–121.

10. King M. A point of minimal important difference (MID): a critique of terminology and methods. *Expert Rev Pharmacoeconomics Outcomes Res*. 2011;11(2):171–184.

11. Cook C. Clinimetrics corner: the minimal clinically important change score (MCID): a necessary pretense. *J Manual Manipulative Therapy*. 2001;16(4):82–83.

12. Guyatt GH, Osoba D, Wu A, Wyrwich KW, Norman GR, Clinical Significance Consensus Meeting Group. Methods to explain the clinical significance of health status measures. *Mayo Clin Proc*. 2002;77(4):371–383.

13. Copay AG, Subach BR, Glassman SD, Polly DW, Schuler TC. Understanding the minimum clinically important difference: a review of concepts and methods. *Spine J*. 2007;7: 541–546.

14. Schrag A, Sampaio C, Consuell N, Werner P. Minimal clinically important change on the unified Parkinson's disease rating scale. *Mov Disord*. 2006;21(8):1200–1207.

15. Hauser R, Auinger P; on behalf of Parkinson Study Group. Determination of minimal clinically important change in early and advanced Parkinson's disease. *Mov Disord*. 2011;26(5):813–818.

16. Lydick E, Epstein RS. Interpretation of quality of life changes. *Qual Life Res*. 1993;2(3): 221–226.

17. Aaronson NK, Cull A, Kaasa S, et al. The European Organisation for Research and Treatment of Cancer (EORTC) modular approach to quality of life assessment in oncology: an update. In: Spilker B, ed. *Quality of Life and Pharmacoeconomics in Clinical Trials*. Philadelphia, PA: Lippincott-Raven Publishers; 1996:179–189.

18. Shulman L, Gruber-Baldini A, Anderson K, Fishman P, Reich S, Weiner W. The clinically important difference on the unified Parkinson's disease rating scale. *Arch Neurol*. 2010;67(1):64–70.

19. Kvam AK, Fayers P, Wisloff F. What changes in health-related quality of life matter to multiple myeloma patients? A prospective study. *Eur J Haematol*. 2010;84(4):345–353.

20. Wyrwich KW, Tierney WM, Wolinsky FD. Further evidence supporting an SEM-based criterion for identifying meaningful intra-individual changes in health-related quality of life. *J Clin Epidemiol*. 1999;52(9):861–873.

21. Lauridsen HH, Hartvigsen J, Manniche C, Korsholm L, Grunnet-Nilsson N. Responsiveness and minimal clinically important difference for pain and disability instruments in low back pain patients. *BMC Musculoskelet Disord*. 2006;7(10):82.

22. Cohen J. *Statistical Power Analysis for the Behavioural Sciences*. 2nd ed. Hillsdale, NJ: Lawrence Erlbaum Associates; 1988.

23. Taylor SJ, Taylor AE, Foy MA, Fogg AJB. Responsiveness of common outcome measures for patients with low back pain. *Spine*. 1999;24(17):1805–1812.

24. Samsa G, Edelman D, Rothman ML, Williams GR, Lipscomb J, Matchar D. Determining clinically important differences in health status measures. A general approach with illustration to the health utilities indexes mark II. *Pharmacoeconomics*. 1999;15(2):141–155.

25. Jacobson NS, Truax P. Clinical significance: a statistical approach to defining meaningful change in psychotherapy research. *J Consult Clin Psychol*. 1991;59(1):12–19.

PART TWO

EVALUATION OF PARKINSON DISEASE IMPAIRMENTS AND DISABILITIES: HISTORY, METHODS, AND SCALES

5

A HISTORICAL PERSPECTIVE ON RATING SCALES IN PD: THE PROBLEMS OF EVALUATING IMPAIRMENTS AND DISABILITIES

J. (Han) Marinus and Jacobus J. (Bob) van Hilten

Summary

Rating scales have been used in Parkinson's disease for more than 50 years. During the time that has elapsed since these first initiatives, our views on what makes a good measurement system have changed considerably. This chapter identifies four important developments that have contributed to these changing views: (1) the publication of conceptual models that allow systematic mapping of disease consequences; (2) the progress in the field of clinimetrics; (3) our increased understanding of the spectrum of motor and non-motor features associated with PD; and (4) our better understanding of side effects of medication. The different ways in which these developments have influenced our views on measuring the patient's clinical status in PD research is described, and (expected) future developments are discussed.

A SHORT HISTORY OF RATING SCALES IN PD

Measurement of clinical aspects of Parkinson's disease has a long history. It dates from the end of the nineteenth century, when measurements were mostly performed with mechanical and electronic devices. One of the earliest methods of recording tremor was designed by Charcot and several German neurologists (see review by Boshes et al.[1]). An advantage of these instrumental methods is their potential to produce precise and consistent results by using strict data collection protocols; clear disadvantages, however, are their limited applicability in clinical practice,

due to the often laborious and time-consuming administrative methods, the generally high costs, as well as the fact that usually only a single aspect of a condition is measured.

The need to obtain simple ratings across the full spectrum of motor signs and symptoms characteristic of PD became particularly important with the advent of new treatments that required evaluation of their efficacy. In 1956, England and Schwab published a scale that was used to measure the effect of thalamotomy.[2] This scale used a 10-point scoring system and contained items that evaluated the difficulty in performing daily activities (e.g., dressing, eating, personal hygiene), as well motor items that were assessed by the physician. In the 1960s, the introduction of levodopa in particular stimulated the development of many clinical rating scales, such as the Northwestern University Disability Scale (NUDS, 1961),[3] the Hoehn and Yahr scale (1967),[4] the New York University Rating Scale (NYURS or NYU PDDS; 1968),[5] the Webster scale (1968),[6] the (modified and still currently used) Schwab and England scale (1969),[7] and the Columbia University Rating Scale (1969).[8] As the experience with rating scales in PD increased, the limitations of these instruments became more apparent, leading to the development of many more scales in the following decades (for a review, see Ramaker et al.[9]).

Collectively, the availability of these scales marked an important step forward: it not only represented a form of standardization, but it also allowed the assignment of total scores to patients, based on the severity of their motor features. These scales could be easily administered in the clinic and also allowed monitoring of changes in the severity of the condition over time. Most scales used a more or less similar approach, whereby the presence of motor features characteristic of PD was recorded and their severity was rated, according to anchors provided in the response options. The scores on the separate items were subsequently summed in order to obtain a total score that reflected the severity of the patient's clinical status.

These early scales had a strong focus on the motor aspects of PD and rarely captured other aspects of the disease or side effects of the treatment. The Unified Parkinson's Disease Rating Scale (UPDRS), published in 1987, was an exception: it included sections on non-motor features (i.e., Part 1: Mentation, Behavior, and Mood) and side effects of therapy (Part IV: Complications of Therapy).[10]

Our current views on evaluating and rating PD patients have been influenced by four particularly important developments from the past few decades. The *first* advance was the development of several disease models, such as the International Classification of Impairments, Disabilities and Handicaps (ICIDH),[11] the International Classification of Functioning,

Disability and Health (ICF classification; Figure 5-1),[12] and the model of the "disablement process."[13] These systems, allowing disease aspects to be consistently classified into distinct categories, led to a considerable improvement in conceptual clarity. The *second* development concerns the progress in the field of clinimetrics, with established standards to rate the quality of measurement instruments, including relevant characteristics such as reliability, validity, and responsiveness. The *third* development involves a greater understanding of the disease itself. The increasing awareness that non-motor features (e.g., cognitive impairments, depression, sleep disturbances, autonomic dysfunction) are important aspects of PD that contribute to its overall severity has led to a more comprehensive view of PD, with a resultant appreciation that all important domains must be rated in the full assessment of PD patients.[14] The *fourth* development relates to our increased knowledge of the side effects of dopaminergic medication and the need to monitor these problems in rating the impact of treatments. The side effects can be categorized into motor features (fluctuations, dyskinesias) and non-motor features (compulsive symptoms, psychotic symptoms, daytime sleepiness including sleep attacks, and autonomic symptoms [e.g., orthostatic hypotension]). The different ways these four developments have influenced current views on measuring the patient's clinical status in PD research and clinical practice is described in the following sections, followed by a short discussion of expected future developments.

DEVELOPMENTS IN DISEASE MODELS

The International Classification of Impairments, Disabilities and Handicaps (ICIDH) is one of the older disease models.[11] It consists of a main disease pathway that links several levels of disease consequences: that is, impairments, disabilities, and handicaps. *Impairments* are deficits in structure or function at organ levels, while *disabilities* are difficulties in performing activities; *handicaps* involve the negative social consequences of a disease and concern the difficulty of fully participating in society (e.g., to work, do sports, or perform hobbies). Two important critiques—the negative connotations of the distinguished levels and the absence of potentially modifying (intra-personal and extra-personal) factors—led to the development of ICIDH's successor, the International Classification of Functioning, Disability and Health (ICF classification; Figure 5-1).[12] In this model, the following, more neutrally phrased, levels are distinguished: body structure and function, activity, and participation. In addition, the potential influence of environmental factors (e.g., housing situation, availability of [walking] aids, type of health insurance, presence of partner) and personal factors (e.g., anxiety, depression, locus of control) upon the central disease pathway is acknowledged. Both the ICIDH and the ICF models were developed under the auspices of the World Health Organization. A third model is that of the "disablement process."[13] This approach is quite similar to that of the ICF model; however, within the "activity" level it distinguishes "disabilities" (activities performed in a context, such as dressing) and "functional limitations"

(in context-free situations, such as the "timed up-and-go" test).

The publication of these models, particularly the latter two, enabled a better distinction between various disease consequences, while both acknowledging the mutual interaction between the various levels, as well as the role of potential modifying factors. Most PD rating scales were published before these disease models gained publicity and acceptance (i.e., before 1980), and therefore they often lacked the methodological rigor of some of the newer scales. This time lapse often resulted in a conceptually inappropriate mix of impairments and disabilities in the same scale. For instance, in the original version of the Unified Parkinson's Disease Rating Scale, salivation and sensory complaints were assessed as part of the "Activities of Daily Living" section, which otherwise focused on the patient's ability to perform specific tasks (eating, dressing, hygiene).[10] A similar weakness pertains to the Webster scale (10 items, including nine impairment items and one disability item).

Conscientious application of the conceptual framework and terminology is necessary

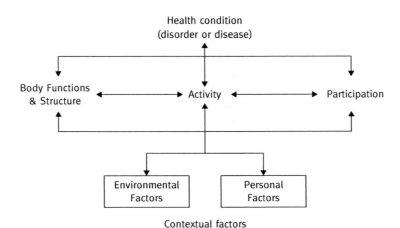

FIGURE 5-1   ICF Model: International Classification of Functioning, Disability and Health (ICF) model. In this model the disease consequences are described at different levels: organ level (body functions and structure), personal level (activities), and societal level (participation). These different levels interact with and influence each other. Patients with the same disease do not all follow the same disease course; there are differences between individuals because environmental (e.g., walking aids, presence of a partner) and personal factors (e.g., coping style, intelligence) modify the course of a disease and its consequences. *Source*: ICF Beginner's Guide (http://www.who.int/classifications/icf/training/icfbeginnersguide.pdf).[34]

in order to construct scales that are appropriately focused and clear. Importantly, items can be measured at different levels; for instance, tremor can be measured at the structure level (frequency, amplitude); the activity level (interference with activities, such as tying shoe laces); or at the participation level (interference with social life, such as feeling embarrassed when eating out in a restaurant). Note that an outcome becomes increasingly less disease-specific and more relevant from the patient's point of view if one moves from left to right in Figure 5-1.[6]

The developments in this field have been important contributions to a more systematic approach in scale development in PD, and they also provide the methodology to evaluate whether instruments are properly structured, conceptually clear, and measure distinct aspects of the disease.

DEVELOPMENTS IN CLINIMETRICS

The science concerned with measurement in clinical medicine is known as *clinimetrics*, a term that was first coined by Alvan Feinstein.[15] Interestingly, the history of clinimetrics in medicine is much younger than that of measurement in other disciplines, such as psychology ("psychometry") and sociology ("sociometry"), where particularly the need to quantify rather abstract constructs such as mood, intelligence, and well-being was felt decades before. Besides Feinstein, there were others who contributed greatly to developments in clinimetrics, such as Kirshner and Guyatt[16]—who published a seminal paper in 1985 describing a methodological framework for assessing health indices—and Streiner and Norman—who published an influential book on the development and use of health measurement scales in 1989.[17] Kirshner and Guyatt stated that, in general, three types of clinical measures can be distinguished: *predictive, discriminative,* and *evaluative* measures.[16] They demonstrated that the required clinimetric properties differed in each of these types of measures. Predictive measures have the objective of making a diagnosis or predicting future developments, making the statistical association with a criterion measure (criterion validity) and reliability important

characteristics; responsiveness, however, is not a relevant attribute for a predictive measure. (The terms *validity, reliability,* and *responsiveness* are not discussed here, as they are described in detail in Part I.) Discriminating measures are used to distinguish among subjects: for instance, with respect to length, weight, cognitive performance, or severity of dyskinesias; construct validity and reliability (large and stable between-subject variation) are therefore particularly important, whereas responsiveness is irrelevant. For evaluative measures that aim to detect clinically relevant changes over time, however, responsiveness is an essential characteristic, in addition to longitudinal construct validity and reliability.[16] In their handbook, Streiner and Norman described the relevant steps in constructing and testing measurement instruments, along with methods to assess these.[17]

Today, researchers and clinicians are increasingly aware that rating scales must display good clinimetric characteristics in order for us to be able to attach any credence to the results that are obtained with them. The demonstration of good clinimetric properties, however, is not enough: a scale will only perform properly if it is used in the "right" setting and in the "right" population. This indicates that the use of a particular scale should enable its users to obtain answers to their specific research questions, which means the content of the scale must closely resemble the construct that is to be measured. It also requires that information be available on the performance of the instrument in the intended population.

Early rating scales in PD were based either on the views of individuals or on consensus among neurologists, with little or no rigorous testing. Furthermore, changes to existing scales were frequently made to suit the needs of an individual researcher, without any additional formal testing. Currently, higher standards for the development and testing of rating scales exist, and it is now considered essential that rating scales be developed with scientific rigor. Therefore, successful testing and demonstration of validity, reliability, and, if applicable, responsiveness are essential steps in modern scale-development and acceptance in research or clinical practice.

In addition to this minimal standard, other points should be considered. If a scale is to be used in different target populations, information must be available on its performance in these separate populations. Another important point concerns independent testing; confidence in the quality of a particular scale will increase considerably if the clinimetric properties have been confirmed by persons other than the developers. Additionally, if the scale is to be used in different countries (e.g., in multinational studies), cross-cultural validity of the scale and official translations that meet the standards of the original scale must first be demonstrated. Another point to take into account is whether the scale has been developed from a clinimetric or psychometric perspective. In the first situation, there usually is a clear notion of what should be measured (e.g., the symptoms of a disease, for instance motor impairments in PD); in this case, internal consistency of the total scale (but not the relevant subscale) is not a necessary property, since the various symptoms of a disease are known in advance, but are not necessarily related to each other.[18] In PD, for instance, tremor has frequently been demonstrated to behave quite independently from the other features of this condition. This situation however, creates problems with the summation of such scores, a difficulty that can be circumvented if a salient factor structure—allowing for the summation of scores on items within such a factor—is identified. In a psychometric approach, there is no clear notion of the constituting components of the construct (e.g., well-being, quality of life), and therefore an initial item pool is created from which items are selected on the basis of predefined criteria (e.g., high item–total correlation, belonging to a factorial structure, stable test-retest characteristics, etc.). To summarize, clinimetrics is content-driven and usually concerned with multidimensional indexes, whereas psychometrics is mainly statistically driven and concerned with unidimensional scales.

Together, the developments in this field have led to a better understanding of how the quality of rating scales in PD should be evaluated, and they have provided standards against which this can be tested.

DEVELOPMENTS IN THE CLINICAL VIEW OF PARKINSON'S DISEASE

Although in his *Essay on the Shaking Palsy* (1817),[19] James Parkinson described some non-motor features of PD in addition to the motor features of this condition, the disease remained mainly characterized by its motor features for more than a century. The introduction of dopaminergic drugs in the 1960s placed further emphasis on the evaluation of motor features and contributed considerably to the tunnel vision of PD as a slowly progressive movement disorder, associated with loss of dopaminergic nigrostriatal neurons. Although effects of the disease on mood and cognition had already been known for many years, there has been a growing awareness, particularly in the last two decades, that the clinical spectrum of PD also encompasses many important non-motor manifestations.[20] These non-motor manifestations include cognitive impairment, autonomic dysfunction, depression, and impairment of olfaction, sleep and sensory function, which matches up with findings from Braak and others showing degeneration of non-dopaminergic transmitter systems in PD.[21] These non-motor disturbances may already be present before the onset of motor problems and could play a particularly prominent role in the middle and late stages of the disease.[22,23] The awareness that non-motor features play an important role in the clinical spectrum of PD has led to many initiatives to improve existing instruments.[24]

Since the advent of dopamine-replacement therapy, it has become clear that this treatment is associated with motor (motor fluctuations and dyskinesias) and psychiatric (psychosis and impulse-control disorders) complications. Pre- and post-synaptic changes in the different pathways of the dopamine system are key in the development of the motor and psychiatric complications; they reflect the consequences of a combination of factors, including the progressive nature of the disease, compensatory mechanisms, gender, and the pulsatile treatment with short-acting dopaminergic drugs. The processes responsible for the development of psychiatric complications probably differ from those involved in the generation of motor complications.[24,25] The complications of dopaminergic therapy become more prevalent as the disease progresses, and they add considerably to the disease burden.[26,27] Consequently, evaluation of these complications has received growing attention, which in its turn has resulted in additional items in dedicated sections of existing scales (e.g. MDS-UPDRS) and newly developed rating scales, entirely dedicated to one domain (e.g., compulsive and psychotic symptoms).[28,29] These scales will be discussed in later chapters.

FUTURE DEVELOPMENTS

The developments described in the previous paragraphs have been acknowledged in several disciplines and have led to initiatives, such as the recent and ongoing initiative by the Movement Disorder Society (MDS), to evaluate the quality of existing measurement instruments in a systematic way and to promote the use of scales that have been found valid, reliable, and responsive. This book is a direct reflection of this effort in the field of PD. Examples of similar steps in other disciplines are the IMMPACT (Initiative on Methods, Measurement, and Pain Assessment in Clinical Trials)[30] and the OMERACT (Outcome Measures in Rheumatoid Arthritis Clinical Trials).[31] Some of these initiatives date back much further (OMERACT has been active since 1992) than the MDS initiative to develop the MDS-UPDRS and to critique existing scales for assessing PD impairments and disabilities. All these initiatives extend their activities beyond the promotion of the use of scientifically sound rating scales: OMERACT, for instance, has published guidelines on reporting requirements for longitudinal observational studies and has provided recommendations to determine the smallest detectable difference in radiological progression.[32,33]

As biomarker research advances in the area of PD, measurement tools to rate disease severity and longitudinal progression may develop and offer rating measures beyond clinical assessments. Other important and allied developments in measurement research are applicable to future PD studies, particularly a focus on particular groups of scale items and the use of more elaborate statistical analysis techniques. As long as a cure for PD is not available, therapies will be aimed at slowing down the progression of clinical decline, and a measurement system to monitor disease progression is important to this effort. Scales or items within scales that are precise enough to detect differences between groups in the rate of progression in a valid and reliable way are particularly important—because these studies focus primarily on early PD, the measurements must allow for the detection of very minor changes and establish their overall significance clinically. This need highlights the fact that fine discrimination is required. In studies of disease progression that enroll patients already on medication, it may be important that scales focus in a reliable and valid manner on clinically pertinent signs and symptoms that are relatively insensitive to symptomatic dopaminergic medication.

Modern psychometric methods such as item response theory and Rasch analysis may be used to develop scales that target interval levels and can consequently be used to construct scales that allow for the justified use of parametric statistics. A second advantage of these methods is their higher efficiency, allowing for reduced sample sizes in comparison to standard analytical approaches. Rasch analysis also provides a method to determine if existing scales can be transformed to approach true interval properties. These new approaches offer a variety of opportunities for testing established scales and for developing new scales to focus on global and specific aspects of PD.

REFERENCES

1. Boshes B, Wachs H, Brumlik J, Mier M, Petrovick M. Studies of tone, tremor and speech in normal persons and parkinsonian patients. *Neurology.* 1960;10:805–813.
2. England AC, Schwab RS. Postoperative evaluation of 26 selected patients with Parkinson's disease. *J Am Geriatr Soc.* 1956;4:1219–1232.
3. Canter GJ, De La Torre R, Mier M. A method for evaluating disability in patients with Parkinson's disease. *J Nerv Ment Dis.* 1961;133:143–147.

4. Hoehn MM, Yahr MD. Parkinsonism: onset, progression and mortality. *Neurology.* 1967;17:427–442.

5. Alba A, Trainor FS, Ritter W, Dacso MM. A clinical disability rating for Parkinson patients. *J Chronic Dis.* 1968;21:507–522.

6. Webster DD. Critical analysis of the disability in Parkinson's disease. *Mod Treat.* 1968;5: 257–282.

7. Schwab RS, England AC. Projection technique for evaluating surgery in Parkinson's disease. In: Gillingham FJ, Donaldson IML, eds. *Third Symposium on Parkinson's Disease.* Edinburgh: E. and S. Livingstone; 1969:152–157.

8. Yahr MD, Duvoisin RC, Schear MJ, Barrett RE, Hoehn MM. Treatment of parkinsonism with levodopa. *Arch Neurol.* 1969;21:343–354.

9. Ramaker C, Marinus J, Stiggelbout AM, van Hilten BJ. Systematic evaluation of rating scales for impairment and disability in Parkinson's disease. *Mov Disord.* 2002;17:867–876.

10. Fahn S, Elton RL. Unified Parkinson's disease rating scale. In: Fahn S, Goldstein M, Marsden D, Calne DB, eds. *Recent Developments in Parkinson's Disease.* Florham Park, New Jersey: MacMillan; 1987:153–163.

11. World Health Organization. *International Classification of Impairments, Disabilities, and Handicaps: A Manual of Classifications Relating to the Consequences of Diseases.* Geneva: World Health Organization; 1980.

12. WHO. International classification of functioning, disability and health homepage. Available at: http://www3.who.int/icf/icftemplate.cfm. Accessed on February 20, 2012.

13. Verbrugge LM, Jette AM. The disablement process. *Soc Sci Med.* 1994;38:1–14.

14. Cheng EM, Tonn S, Swain-Eng R, Factor SA, Weiner WJ, Bever CT Jr. Quality improvement in neurology: AAN Parkinson disease quality measures: report of the Quality Measurement and Reporting Subcommittee of the American Academy of Neurology. *Neurology.* 2010;75:2021–2027.

15. Feinstein AR. *Clinimetrics.* 1st ed. New Haven, CT: Yale University Press; 1987.

16. Kirshner B, Guyatt G. A methodological framework for assessing health indices. *J Chronic Dis.* 1985;38:27–36.

17. Streiner DL, Norman GR. *Health Measurement Scales: A Practical Guide to Their Development and Use.* 2nd ed. Oxford, UK: Oxford Medical Publications; 1995.

18. de Vet HCW, Terwee CB, Bouter LM. Clinimetrics and psychometrics: two sides of the same coin. *J Clin Epidemiol.* 2003;56: 1146–1147.

19. Parkinson J. An essay on the shaking palsy. *J Neuropsychiatry Clin Neurosci.* 2002;14: 223–236.

20. Chaudhuri KR, Healy DG, Schapira AH. Non-motor symptoms of Parkinson's disease: diagnosis and management. *Lancet Neurol.* 2006;5:235–245.

21. Lang AE, Obeso JA. Challenges in Parkinson's disease: restoration of the nigrostriatal dopamine system is not enough. *Lancet Neurol.* 2004;3:309–316.

22. Hely MA, Morris JG, Reid WG, Trafficante R. Sydney multicenter study of Parkinson's disease: non-L-dopa-responsive problems dominate at 15 years. *Mov Disord.* 2005;20:190–199.

23. van Rooden SM, Visser M, Verbaan D, Marinus J, van Hilten JJ. Patterns of motor and non-motor features in Parkinson's disease. *J Neurol Neurosurg Psychiatry.* 2009;80:846–850.

24. Chaudhuri KR, Tolosa E, Schapira A, Poewe W, eds. *Non-Motor Symptoms of Parkinson's Disease.* Oxford, UK: Oxford University Press; 2009.

25. Fabbrini G, Brotchie JM, Grandas F, Nomoto M, Goetz CG. Levodopa-induced dyskinesias. *Mov Disord.* 2007;22:1379–1389.

26. Aarsland D, Marsh L, Schrag A. Neuropsychiatric symptoms in Parkinson's disease. *Mov Disord.* 2009;24:2175–2186.

27. Visser M, van Rooden SM, Verbaan D, Marinus J, Stiggelbout AM, van Hilten JJ. A comprehensive model of health-related quality of life in Parkinson's disease. *J Neurol.* 2008;255:1580–1587.

28. Visser M, Verbaan D, van Rooden SM, Stiggelbout AM, Marinus J, van Hilten JJ. Assessment of psychiatric complications in Parkinson's disease: the SCOPA-PC. *Mov Disord.* 2007;22:2221–2228.

29. Weintraub D, Hoops S, Shea JA, et al. Validation of the questionnaire for impulsive-compulsive disorders in Parkinson's disease. *Mov Disord.* 2009;24:1461–1467.

30. Dworkin RH, Turk DC, Farrar JT, et al. Core outcome measures for chronic pain clinical trials: IMMPACT recommendations. *Pain.* 2005;113:9–19.

31. Tugwell P, Boers M. OMERACT conference on outcome measures in rheumatoid arthritis clinical trials: introduction. *J Rheumatol.* 1993;20:528–530.

32. Lassere M, Boers M, van der Heijde D, et al. Smallest detectable difference in radiological progression. *J Rheumatol.* 1999;26:731–739.

33. Wolfe F, Lassere M, van der Heijde D, et al. Preliminary core set of domains and reporting requirements for longitudinal observational studies in rheumatology. *J Rheumatol.* 1999;26:484–489.

34. World Health Organization. Towards A Common Language for Functioning, Disability, and Health: ICF. Available at: http://www.who.int/classifications/icf/training/icfbeginnersguide.pdf. Accesssed on February 20, 2012.

6

THE MOVEMENT DISORDER SOCIETY RATING SCALES REVIEW METHODOLOGY

Anette Schrag

Summary

This chapter summarizes the general methodology used in the Movement Disorder Society Rating Scales Reviews. Whilst some variability exists due to the nature of each topic and the evidence available, the standardized approach aims at comparability of results to allow an informed choice of instrument in each setting and awareness of deficiencies in available evidence to stimulate further research.

BACKGROUND AND PURPOSE

The number of different scales used to evaluate the motor and non-motor aspects of Parkinson's disease has expanded very considerably over the years. By 2001, the bewildering range of available scales and relative lack of knowledge concerning their strengths and weaknesses prompted an initiative by the Movement Disorder Society to review and assess the full evidence in this area to guide researchers and clinicians and to highlight areas in need of further development. The purpose of this Task Force was threefold: to critique existing scales in a uniform manner; to identify clinical areas not adequately covered by current rating instruments; and to make recommendations on maintaining, modifying, and developing new scales to keep pace with evolving scientific advances.

The initial reviews, covered in this part of the book, were concerned with scales assessing the core features of Parkinson's disease, including the Unified Parkinson's Disease Rating Scale (UPDRS) and the Hoehn and Yahr staging system,[1] and later expanded to scales for assessing motor complications and impact on patients' quality of life. With the increasing knowledge that Parkinson's disease is far more than a motor disorder, the third part of the book reviews scales assessing non-motor features of PD, as described in Part 3.

METHODOLOGY

There are some necessary differences in the methodology used to review these diverse areas, ranging from measurement of wearing-off fluctuations[2] to assessment of apathy[3]; the task force effort was also spread out over several years, leading to some adaptation of the core methods. However, the structure of these reviews uses similar methodological constructs and criteria to allow comparability among them.

Administrative organization and critique process of MDS Rating Scales Task Force reviews

The steering committee of the MDS task force on rating scales for PD invited a chairperson to focus on one aspect of PD and to form a committee to critique existing rating scales for their use in PD, and to place them in a clinical and clinimetric/psychometric context. Whilst not including a comprehensive list of experts in one area, each group included a small number of individuals with diverse backgrounds and complementary expertise in the areas of relevance to the chapter, also aiming for geographical and gender balance. The task force members selected the scales to be included in the review and identified unresolved issues and limitations of the critiqued scales. Each scale was reviewed by at least one task force member, but the completed reviews were assessed by all members to obtain a consensus. A structured assessment of the scales with regard to their descriptive properties, availability, content, use, acceptability, clinimetric properties, and overall impression in patients with PD was undertaken on each topic. The aim of this process was to identify all published scales that (1) could be used as diagnostic screening tools to establish the presence or absence of features of PD, and/or (2) could be used to assess the severity of the problem.

Literature search strategy

Medline on PubMed was systematically searched for relevant papers. Only published peer-reviewed papers were included.

Rating scales classification

The classification used was originally developed for the Appendix of Ancillary Scales to complement the MDS-sponsored revision of the Unified Parkinson's Disease Rating Scale (MDS-UPDRS).[4]

The general definitions used in the task force critiques were the following: a scale was considered "recommended" if it had been applied to PD populations, if there were data on its use in studies beyond the group that developed the scale, and if it had been studied clinimetrically and found to be valid, reliable, and sensitive to change. A scale was considered "suggested" if it had been applied to PD populations, but only one of the other criteria applied. A scale was "listed" if it met only one of the three criteria defined for "recommended" scales. The clinimetric criterion referred to clinimetric testing in any population of patients, but scales tested in PD populations with good clinimetric profiles were favored over those successfully tested in other populations, but not PD. Among recommended scales, this prioritization was discussed in the body of the report and conclusions to allow differentiation between scales where several scales were "recommended".

The final assessments were based on consensus among the task force members, and the steering committee of the overall Task Force on Rating Scales for PD. Each report was submitted and approved by the Scientific Issues Committee of the MDS before submission to *Movement Disorders*, and the chapters in this book are largely book-format adaptations of peer-reviewed manuscripts published previously. As the process is ongoing, some chapters are based on near-final considerations by the topic committee, but have not received the same MDS and journal peer-review. In these cases, a sentence clarifies this point in the individual chapter.

OUTCOME

These reviews are intended to help inform researchers and clinicians about which instrument to use and how to interpret their findings by establishing the strengths, weaknesses, and level of evidence available for each. They are conducted and written by researchers in the areas that are reviewed, and they represent expertise of researchers in neurology, scales development, statistics, and areas relevant to the topic from around the world. Whilst they do not provide new evidence in themselves, they highlight deficiencies and the need for better scales and more evidence. These reviews have also informed the National Institute of Neurological Disorders and Stroke (NINDS) Common Data element exercise. The task force has now almost finished its initial task of providing a comprehensive evidence base for scales of PD. This will, however, inevitably remain a work in progress, and will require updating as new evidence becomes available and more sophisticated scale-development and assessments emerge.

References

1. Goetz CG, Poewe W, Rascol O, et al. Movement Disorder Society Task Force report on the Hoehn and Yahr staging scale: status and recommendations. *Mov Disord.* 2004;19(9):1020–1028.
2. Antonini A, Martinez-Martin P, Chaudhuri RK, et al. Wearing-off scales in Parkinson's disease: critique and recommendations. *Mov Disord.* 2011;26(12):2169–2175.
3. Leentjens AF, Dujardin K, Marsh L, et al. Apathy and anhedonia rating scales in Parkinson's disease: critique and recommendations. *Mov Disord.* 2008;23(14):2004–2014.
4. Goetz CG, Tilley BC, Shaftman SR, et al. Movement Disorder Society–sponsored revision of the Unified Parkinson's Disease Rating Scale (MDS-UPDRS): scale presentation and clinimetric testing results. *Mov Disord.* 2008;23(15):2129–2170.

7

UNIFIED PARKINSON'S DISEASE RATING SCALE (UPDRS) AND MOVEMENT DISORDER SOCIETY REVISION OF THE UPDRS (MDS-UPDRS)

Christopher G. Goetz

Summary

The UPDRS has been the most widely used scale to assess impairment and disability in PD. This scale meets the criteria for (1) specific use in PD; (2) wide usage by multiple groups over many years and in many contexts covering the gamut of PD severities; and (3) sound clinimetric properties, especially for the two primary scale components, Part II (Activities of Daily Living), and Part III (Motor Examination) (*Recommended Scale*). Because some instructions are ambiguous, some items function poorly clinimetrically, and many non-motor elements of PD are not captured in this scale, however, the Movement Disorder Society sponsored a revision of the UDPRS, termed the MDS-UDPRS. This scale, officially released in 2009, is already being used in PD clinical trials, involving multiple groups studying PD at different levels of severity, and prior to its official release, it underwent extensive clinimetric testing, with strong outcomes. The MDS-UPDRS therefore meets the criteria set forth by the Movement Disorder Task Force on PD Rating Scales to be designated as *Recommended*. The scale furthermore is being translated into official non-English language versions, each undergoing clinimetric testing against the English edition.

INTRODUCTION

The Unified Parkinson's Disease Rating Scale (UPDRS) was originally developed in the 1980s[1] and over the next two decades became the most widely used clinical rating scale for Parkinson's disease (PD).[2] In 2001, the Movement Disorder Society (MDS) sponsored a critique of the UPDRS, and this document lauded the strengths of the scale but identified a number of ambiguities, weaknesses, and areas in need of inclusion to reflect current scientific developments.[3] The summary conclusions recommended the development of a new version of the UPDRS that would retain the core four-part structure of the original scale, but resolve problems and especially incorporate a number of clinically pertinent PD-related problems poorly captured in the original version. The effort resulted in a new version of the scale, termed the MDS-Sponsored UPDRS Revision (MDS-UPDRS).[4,5] As in other chapters of this section, the criteria set forth by the Movement Disorder Society Task Force on Rating Scales to designate a given scale as Recommended, Suggested, or Listed have been applied to the UPDRS and MDS-UPDRS.

UNIFIED PARKINSON'S DISEASE RATING SCALE

Scale description

STRUCTURE

The UPDRS is a scale that was developed as an effort to incorporate elements from existing scales to provide a comprehensive but efficient and flexible means to monitor PD-related disability and impairment.[1] Prior to its development, multiple scales, including the Webster,[6] Columbia,[7] King's College,[8] Northwestern University Disability,[9] New York University Parkinson's Disease Scale,[10] and UCLA Rating Scales[11] were used in different centers, making comparative assessments difficult. The development of the UPDRS involved multiple trial versions, and the final published scale is officially known as "UPDRS Version 3.0."[1] The scale itself has four components, largely derived from pre-existing scales that were reviewed and modified by a consortium of movement disorders specialists. The four parts are: Part I, Mentation, Behavior and Mood (four interview items); Part II, Activities of Daily Living (13 interview items); Part III, Motor Examination (14 examination items with 26 total scores to account for different body parts and right/left side assessments); Part IV, Complications (11 items with a mixture of interview assessments as well yes/no responses based on rater judgement).

The UPDRS is exclusively a severity scale of impairment and disability and is not used for the diagnosis of PD. It is heavily weighted toward assessing motor issues, although Part I assesses some elements of cognition and behavior, and Part IV assesses the presence or absence of non-motor elements such as orthostatic dizziness and sleep. The original concept of the scale was to provide a core assessment tool that could be accompanied by additional measures to focus on global impairment or specific elements in more detail (Stanley Fahn, personal communication). For example, whereas the UPDRS is often accompanied by and reported with such scales as the Schwab and England and Hoehn and Yahr scales, these latter scales are not part of the UPDRS per se.[12,13] The full scale takes approximately 30 minutes to complete.[14]

HANDLING COMORBIDITIES

PD is more prevalent in subjects over age 50, and the coexistence of other diseases like diabetes, stroke, and arthritis can confound the evaluation of PD-related impairment and disability. Furthermore, short-term disabilities resulting from a fracture or the exacerbation of rheumatic disease may increase patients' overall disability without altering the severity of the PD itself. Conversely (for example), correction of cataracts may improve overall patient function and facilitate the execution of activities of daily living without directly affecting their PD. Finally, common coexistent disorders like depression can potentially affect the speed of patients' movement, alter their motivation, and enhance their perceptions of disability even when their PD itself is stable. The question of how the UPDRS should accommodate these various issues of comorbidities is not specifically detailed in the scale instructions.[1] Two different prototypical paradigms could be used: the first, a concerted attempt to disregard all components of impairment or disability due to conditions unrelated to PD, using the UPDRS as a scale of PD-related dysfunction in its purest sense; second, a strategy involving a "rate-as-you-see" approach, using the UPDRS to describe a patient's functional impairment regardless of its direct relationship to PD. The first approach has the advantage of focusing on PD itself, but it is highly susceptible to investigator and patient bias. For accurate assessment of Part III, the rater would need to have a list of comorbidities to maximize the appropriate interpretation of signs. The second strategy deals with the reality of the patient's status without interpreting an underlying cause for impairment, but will be likely to inflate ratings that have minimal or no direct relationship to PD. Standardized instructions for rating PD in the context of comorbidities do not exist in the current UPDRS, and the task force members agreed that clarification of data handling for comorbidities would be an important asset of a future scale modification. The "rate-as-you-see" method for Part III (Motor Examination) would probably reduce inter-rater variability, but the inclusion of "open fields" in the margins of the scale document for raters to note the contribution of other medical conditions would be needed for full interpretation. Lang[15] suggested open-field marginal notations to indicate when dyskinesias (D), excessive Parkinsonian tremor (T), or apraxia (A) confound the execution of rated tasks. Similar notations could be included in the margins of the scale for confounding comorbidities that cause weakness, orthopedic problems, or non-Parkinsonian coordination deficits. Although these notations could not be handled in a simple statistical manner, they would be potentially useful in clinical practice.

In contrast, Part II (Activities of Daily Living) has instructions asking patients specifically to rate disability that *they* attribute to PD.[1] The task force members acknowledged that most individual patients are comfortable with this introspective process, although patient bias may be unstable over time and subject to educational efforts and patient experience that clarify the contribution of other illnesses to overall disability.

In clinical trials, the problems related to comorbidities and their impact on UPDRS scores can be minimized by excluding patients with medical conditions that confound interpretation of the primary rating measure. Alternatively, some studies permit comorbid conditions, but only when they are stable and of long duration. If these conditions do not overly elevate the baseline scores and introduce concerns about "ceiling effects," the UPDRS can still measure change from the intervention under study.

ADDITIONAL POINTS

When the UPDRS was developed, score ranges were not identified to categorize the severity of Parkinsonism and thereby provide clinicians with score ranges appropriate to "Slight," "Mild," "Moderate," and "Severe" forms of PD. Although Activity of Daily Living (ADL: Part II) scores, derived from patient datacorrelated with the objective, physician-derived Motor section (Part III) scores,[14] no study has determined score ranges to fit well with clinically pertinent designations of "mild," "moderate," or "severe" PD. Overall ratings such as the Schwab and England scale or the Clinical Global Impression of severity could be used to define "slight," "mild," "moderate" and "severe" PD, and then tested against UPDRS. With this analysis, UPDRS scores could be developed to define numerically these clinical categories, expressed as ranges with 95% confidence intervals.

Rather than consider UPDRS score ranges as indicative of disease severity, another approach has considered constellations of specific items from Part II and Part III to identify patients with predominant tremor and those with predominant bradykinesia, postural reflex compromise, and gait features.[16] The tremor-predominant group, having high scores on historical and objective ratings of tremor, have been shown to have slower overall progression of disability and higher quality of life ratings compared to those whose UPDRS scores documented predominance of mid-line gait and balance difficulties.[17]

Key evaluation issues

USE IN PARKINSON'S DISEASE AND APPLICATION ACROSS THE DISEASE SPECTRUM

Whereas many scales used in the assessment of various aspects of PD are derived from scales developed for other conditions, the UPDRS was specifically designed for PD. Of all available clinical scales for the assessment of Parkinsonian motor impairment and disability, the UPDRS has been the most commonly used.[2,3] Sixty-nine percent of 1994–1998 articles using a PD-rating scale relied on the UPDRS as the standard tool.[2] This wide utilization has been an international one, and the UPDRS has predominated as the primary scale in published studies from both the United States and other geographical regions. It has been applied with equal frequency in studies of early and late PD.[3] The wide usage and global acceptance of the scale has resulted in its use for numerous multi-center studies. Furthermore, the standardized ratings allow for summary scores used to communicate global severity of impairment and disability.

To foster uniform application, early workers with the UPDRS developed a teaching-video-tape that standardized the practical application of the scale and served to provide a certification program to enhance inter-rater reliability.[18] This training tape has been widely used for personal training and self-assessment, and has become a frequently used component of rater training for multi-center studies using the UPDRS as a key outcome measure.

The UPDRS has been used in studies of early, mild, and moderate but stable PD, and severe disease and motor fluctuations.[19,20] Prior studies have demonstrated that the scale favors the assessment of moderate and severe impairments, and may not be ideally configured to assess very mild disease-related signs and symptoms.[21] Although the UPDRS has been extensively applied to clinical trials of early PD to test the concept of neuroprotection or the impact of therapies on reducing the need to start levodopa therapy, "floor" effects potentially limit the scale's utility in the early stages of the illness where impairment is subtle. To address this issue, some studies have permitted the inclusion of 0.5 ratings or other designations based on such anchors as "may be normal for healthy elderly subjects."[22] Modification of the UPDRS with such new wording or rating options, however, has not been validated.[3]

USE BY MULTIPLE AUTHORS

The UPDRS was designed to be administered by neurologists familiar with PD, but it has been utilized in clinical trials by trained study coordinators and non-physician professionals, especially in community-based studies.[23] The motor section of the UPDRS (Part III) has repeatedly been employed in attempts to develop surrogate

markers for disease progression like beta-CIT-SPECT or 18-F-Dopa-PET.[24,25] The UPDRS is also the common reference scale in studies of instrument development for rating specific aspects of PD.[26–28] American and European regulatory agencies rely on the scale for new drug approvals,[29] and the UPDRS has also been used to define the placebo response in PD.[30] Almost all recent trials of surgical interventions for PD, related to both intracerebral transplantation and deep brain surgery, have employed the UPDRS. It is a key component of the Core Assessment Programs for Intracerebral Transplantation and Surgical Interventional Therapies for PD (CAPIT/CAPSIT).[31,32] Although specifically developed to assess PD, the UPDRS has been utilized to rate Parkinsonian features of other conditions, including normal aging, progressive supranuclear palsy, and Lewy body dementia.[23,33,34]

CLINIMETRIC ISSUES

Extensive clinimetric evaluations have been conducted on the UPDRS. In one systematic review of studies assessing clinimetric properties of impairment and disability scales for PD, one third focused primarily on the UPDRS.[2] Clinimetric scale evaluation usually assesses a scale's reliability and validity. Reliability evaluations assess the amount of measurement error in a scale, while validity evaluations assess the degree to which a scale measures what it is purported to measure. Reliability and validity are not independent: a scale cannot be valid if it is not reliable, but it can be reliable without being valid.

Reliability can be divided into two major domains: internal consistency (the degree to which scale items measure similar constructs) and rater consistency or stability (the level of rating agreement across multiple raters or in a single rater across time). The UPDRS has shown excellent internal consistency across multiple studies[14,35,36] and retains this consistency across stages of disease severity as measured by the Hoehn and Yahr staging system.[36,37] This high degree of internal consistency may be artificially inflated due to redundancy in the large number of items in Parts II and III of the UPDRS.

Assessments of rater consistency have examined both inter-rater reliability and intra-rater reliability. Inter-rater reliability appears adequate for the total UPDRS[14,26] as well as the Activities of Daily Living[38] and the Motor Examination[22,39] sections. There are two reports of unacceptably low inter-rater reliability for selected items assessing speech and facial expression on the Motor Examination section of the UPDRS.[22,39] Other studies, however, reported acceptable inter-rater reliability estimates for these items.[3,14] There are numerous published reports examining intra-rater reliability. One study used the UPDRS, and another used a modified version of the scale applied to elderly community subjects without the specific diagnosis of PD.[39,23] Both of these studies showed low to medium intra-rater reliability. Among 400 early-stage PD subjects examined on two occasions, separated by approximately two weeks, the intraclass correlation coefficients were very high: total score 0.92; Mentation 0.74; Activities of Daily Living 0.85; Motor 0.90.[40]

Validity can be divided into three major domains: face or content validity, criterion validity, and construct validity. The UPDRS has adequate face validity and samples important and typical domains associated with PD. In addition, its construction was guided by experts in the field and based on previous scales. Criterion validity has not been established because there is no absolute "goldstandard" that can be used for this assessment. The majority of validation studies have assessed the construct validity of the UPDRS. These studies have generally found satisfactory results regarding convergent validity with other instruments assessing PD, such as the Hoehn and Yahr or Schwab and England scales, or timed motor tests.[28,34,36,37,47] Divergent validity, or the degree to which the scale does not measure domains unrelated to PD, has not been well established. However, one study found a significant correlation between the UPDRS and measures of mental status and depression.[14] This finding may not indicate poor divergent validity, but rather the association of mental status and mood changes with PD.

Multiple studies have examined construct validity of the UPDRS through factor analysis. These studies have found between three and six factors that account for a significant proportion of the total scale variance.[14,26,35-37] The resultant factors form rational groupings of the items, and suggest that the scale has a valid multidimensional assessment format. One factor structure, composed of six factors—axial/gait bradykinesia, right bradykinesia, left bradykinesia, rigidity, rest tremor, and postural tremor—has been shown to be stable across "on" and "off" stages[36,37] and to have a similar factor structure when used in other movement disorders.[33]

Responsiveness has been well established for the UPDRS (see above) and in fact, the European and US regulatory agencies have favored the UPDRS as a vital primary outcome measure for establishing effective PD therapies. Several longitudinal studies of PD have demonstrated that the UPDRS increases over time, and scores are higher at key clinical decision-making points like the need to introduce symptomatic therapy.[19,41-43] Numerous studies indicate that the UPDRS is responsive to therapeutic interventions. Significant improvements in total UPDRS scores, individual subscales (Parts II and III), and averages of subscale scores obtained during "on" and "off" scores among fluctuators have been documented in comparison with placebo.[44] UPDRS improvements have been seen in patients with dose-finding studies of new dopaminergic treatments of advanced disease as well as in studies focusing on mildly disabled patients.[45,46] Published reports using the UPDRS, however, have focused almost exclusively on Caucasians, and the UPDRS characteristics have not been extensively investigated in different racial or ethnic minorities.[48] Furthermore, the effects of gender and age on UPDRS ratings during treatment interventions have not been specifically examined.

Minimal Clinically Relevant Difference (MCRD) or Minimal Clinically Important Change (MCIC) and Minimal Clinically Relevant Incremental Difference (MCRID) are additional clinimetric properties that are particularly important to a scale used to monitor disease progression or therapeutic response. Integral to the strength and utility of a rating scale is the determination of increases or decreases that represent clinically relevant changes in the disease under consideration. Identifying the threshold or smallest difference between two assessments that has an impact on disability or handicap in a disease is known clinimetrically as the Minimal Clinically Relevant Difference (MCRD) or Minimal Clinically Important Change (MCIC). However simple and straightforward the MCRD may be conceptually, very few scales are associated with a well-defined MCRD. Several factors complicate the establishment of an MCRD for the UPDRS. First, PD signs vary throughout the day in Parkinsonian patients, even without motor fluctuations. The natural moment-to-moment or visit-to-visit variation in the UPDRS among patients considered to be stable in overall function has not been extensively studied.[40] Second, because the four subscales of the UPDRS measure different aspects of PD and rely on physician-based and patient-based assessments, a single MCRD may not exist. Third, for a disease like PD, different MCRD values may apply at different disease severities. Specifically, a smaller MCRD may likely apply to groups of patients with mild disease, whereas a larger differential value would be expected for groups with more severe illness. MCRD has been particularly wellstudied for pain-assessment scales and to a lesser degree in assessment measures for asthma and chronic obstructive pulmonary disease.[49-52]

The MCRD concept is applicable in two settings, individual and group. At the individual level, though an MCRD is not statistically enumerated, intervention decisions within each physician–patient relationship are guided by this concept of a minimal change from the prior visit that warrants clinical recognition. For the design of clinical trials involving groups of patients, a uniform MCRD definition is desirable for analyses of both efficacy and futility. In some studies using the UPDRS, a 30% improvement in the Part III score has been applied to define "responders."[46] This empiricallydetermined figure is often used in clinical medicine, based largely on the erroneous assumption that placebo effects occur in 30% of patients, regardless of disease, scale, study duration, or impairment under consideration.[53,54] The 30% UPDRS

change from baseline used in clinical studies has not been experimentally derived, and furthermore, does not specifically presume to represent a minimal change of clinical significance.

One method of establishing an MCRD would be to follow patients with both sequential UPDRS scores and a global estimate of change: for example, the Clinician Interview–based Impression of Change scale[55,56] This scale ranges from 1 ("very much improved") to 4 ("no change") to 7 ("very much worse") relative to either a prior visit or a determined baseline. The key anchors, 3 ("minimally improved") or 2 ("moderately improved"), could potentially be examined relative to the corresponding UPDRS scores to calculate an MCRD expressed as appropriate UPDRS ranges and confidence intervals. If such ratings are obtained from the investigator and patient, these values could be examined against the total UPDRS as well as the specific scale sections. One study examined the MCRD in a large sample of early PD patients before and after starting dopaminergic therapy.[57] The anchor used to identify subjects with a clinically pertinent treatment-related improvement was the Clinical Global Impression-Improvement scale obtained at study end. The group had mild PD with Hoehn and Yahr stages I–III. For the motor section of the UPDRS (Part III), a reduction of 5 points was calculated as the most appropriate cutoff point for a clinically pertinent improvement across all Hoehn and Yahr stages. For the ADL section (Part II), a reduction of two points for Hoehn and Yahr stages I and II subjects and three points for Hoehn and Yahr stage III subjects was calculated as pertinent. In this cohort of mild patients, Parts I and IV contributed very low scores to the total UPDRS, so that the final total UDPRS MCRD or MCIC was estimated as 8 points. Another study examined UPDRS total and motor scores in comparison to Schwab and England Activities of Daily Living Scale (10% rating differences), Hoehn and Yahr stage (one stage differences) and Quality of Life measures (1 standard deviation on the Short Form Health Survey). Motor UPDRS scores changed approximately two points when a minimal clinically important difference occurred, between 4.5 and 6.7 points when the change was considered of moderate clinical importance, and 16 to 18 points for large, clinically important differences.[58]

Allied to the concept of MCRD is the Minimal Clinically Relevant Incremental Difference (MCRID). Rather than comparing two assessments within a patient or group (pre- vs. post-treatment), this terms refers to the difference between two groups at the end of a comparable period. In the case of a clinical trial, the MCRID would determine the relevant expected difference at the end of a treatment between a placebo group and the patients receiving the treatment in question. Knowing the MCRID would allow clinicians to determine the threshold UPDRS value that would *discriminate* the two treatments. So far, there is no experimentally generated or systematically analyzed data on an MCRID for the total or subcomponent scores of the UPDRS. There is, however, limited experience with this concept based on expert opinion or reliance on differences found in previous trials. In these cases, opinions or data widely accepted by the scientific community are used to determine estimates of an end of treatment score associated with clinically important differences in patient function between two interventions and thereby to estimate an MCRID. Among the few examples of an empirically used MCRID based on experience and literature reviews, in one pallidotomy trial that enrolled advanced PD patients with high preoperative UPDRS motor scores, an MCRID for Part III of the UPDRS motor was established at 10 points.[59] In a randomized trial that compared levodopa to pergolide for three years, an *a priori* stopping rule for established superiority of one treatment over the other was set as a between-group difference greater than four points in the Part III UPDRS score at one year.[60]

Strengths and weaknesses: In the context of marked strengths and wide usage of the UPDRS, a number of limitations nonetheless exist. First, as a composite scale, the UPDRS is uneven in the type of information it gathers. For example, Section I is conceptually different from parts II and III, and as a screening assessment for the presence of depression, dementia, or psychosis, it cannot be used as an adequate severity measure of any of these behaviors. In cases of interventions targeting such non-motor problems of PD, specific additional scales are generally used.[61-63] An appendix to the UPDRS with a series of recommended scales for more detailed measurement of all screening questions would enhance consistency of data collection among researchers. At present, such appendices do not exist. Likewise, Section IV is constructed differently than the rest of the UPDRS, with a mixture of five-point options and dichotomous ("yes/no") ratings that are difficult to analyze together. As such, though this portion is sometimes used in clinical trials, most intervention studies for dyskinesias or motor-fluctuations currently rely primarily on other scales. Many additional dyskinesia scales have been proposed to supplement the UPDRS,[64-66] and most studies of patients with motor fluctuations have used self-scoring ON-OFF diaries.[44] Similarly dichotomous, "yes/no" questions for the presence of gastrointestinal complaints, orthostatic hypotension, or sleep problems (part IV, items 40–42) can only be used as screening items to assess the presence or absence of select clinical problems. The task force members considered these items insufficient to assess the severity of impairment or disability related to non-motor domains of PD.

Some items of the motor section have relatively poor inter-rater reliability, including speech, facial expression, posture, body bradykinesia, action tremor, and rigidity.[14,22,67] Although the UPDRS teaching tape for Part III provides visual anchors to improve inter-rater reliability, and a teaching tape was developed to guide raters in the application of Part II, such tapes for the rest of the UDPRS have not been developed.[18,68] A specific example of a key testing problem is the assessment of postural stability in Part III. Because the response of the patient and the assigned rating depend directly on the force of the postural threat, standardized instructions and application of the test are essential for consistent ratings. These instructions are not part of the UPDRS.

Additionally, there is some redundancy of items in both the ADL and motor sections. While duplication of material enhances the internal consistency of the scale, some critics consider such enhancement a spurious inflation.[14] Redundancy also increases the time required to administer the scale. Efforts to reduce redundancy have led to the Short Parkinson's Evaluation Scale (SPES), based directly on the UPDRS, but with fewer items and reduced rating options of 0 to 3.[26] Whereas the elimination of redundancy and the enhancement of inter-rater reliability are overall positive goals for scales, the shrinkage of numerical options clinimetrically diminishes the capacity to discriminate change. The majority of the Task Force considered 0 to 4 ratings preferable to 0 to 3. Allied to the duplication of information is the concern that aspects of Parkinsonian motor impairment in Part III are not necessarily reflective of the impact of each cardinal feature on overall function. For example, bradykinesia-related items are over-represented in terms of the number of assessment items in comparison to tremor and postural stability.

The allocation of items to specific sections of the UPDRS is not altogether consistent, leading to potential ambiguity of interpretation. Part II, Activities of Daily Living, includes a mixture of items that directly relate to daily activities (e.g., dressing, eating), but also examines patient perceptions of primary disease manifestations (e.g., tremor, salivation). Items that overlap these two categories include the gait items that assess primary Parkinsonian features (freezing, falls), but have an impact on walking as an activity of daily living. Renaming Part II "Historical" or "Patient Perceptions" would semantically, but not conceptually, resolve this ambiguity. Items assessing function outside the activities of daily living could alternatively be reassigned to another section of the scale.

The UPDRS Part II is culturally biased, and the anchoring descriptions for some item ratings are not applicable to all ethnic environments. For example, "Dressing" (item 10) describes difficulty with buttons, even though many traditional cultures do not use them; "Cutting Food/Handling Utensils" (item 9) presumes that food is regularly cut for eating and that utensils are used, although some cultures serve food in bite-size portions and some do not use eating utensils. Although the scale was considered applicable to most international urban settings, the UPDRS may be limited by ambiguities when applied in epidemiological research efforts that involve fieldwork in rural and geographically isolated cultures. Even within Western cultures, the UPDRS has been primarily used in studying Caucasians with Parkinson's disease, and it has not been examined extensively in other ethnic or racial groups.[48]

Several key elements of PD are not covered by the UPDRS. When the scale was formulated in the mid-1980s, the developers were well aware of this limitation, but they chose to delete questions on some Parkinsonian impairments, mainly to create a scale that was reasonably simple and short (personal communication, S. Fahn). After over a decade of scale utilization, however, the task force members considered that these initial choices should be reconsidered. In view of the anatomical, neurochemical, physiological, and conceptual evolution in thinking about PD, clinical neuroscientists may now need to have a scale that adequately reflects the multifaceted elements of PD and assesses additional non-motor symptoms and signs that contribute to disability and affect quality of life. The concept that screening questions could cover these topics was favored, but an appendix should be added to the UPDRS and include officially recognized scales to assess each of the screened areas in further depth.[68] Another option would be the development of multiple UPDRS versions of different lengths and different levels of comprehensiveness, leaving the choice of scale to the physician (daily practice, in-depth evaluation, clinical trials). Multiple UPDRS versions, however, would potentially cause reporting ambiguity and undermine the "unified" concept that anchors the UPDRS. The task force members favored the maintenance of a single UPDRS that has sufficient screening questions to capture problems related to all aspects of PD, with official appendices that recommend scales to assess each of the screened areas in further depth when needed.

Final assessment

The UPDRS has been the most widely used scale to assess impairment and disability in PD.

This scale meets the criteria for (1) specific use in PD, (2) wide usage by multiple groups over many years and in many contexts covering the gamut of PD severities, and (3) sound clinimetric properties, especially for the two primary scale components, Part II (Activities of Daily Living) and Part III (Motor Examination). The UDPRS is a *Recommended Scale* for the evaluation of PD severity. It is not diagnostic tool for Parkinsonism or for PD (Table 7-1).

MOVEMENT DISORDER SOCIETY–SPONSORED REVISION OF THE UPDRS [MDS-UPDRS]

Scale description

STRUCTURE

The MDS-UPDRS was designed to retain the strengths of the UPDRS, to resolve ambiguities of the original scale, to provide detailed instructions for uniformity of applications, and to include elements of PD not assessed in the UPDRS.[4] The original four-component design (Parts I–IV) was retained, but the focus of each Part was changed. Part I concerns "non-motor experiences of daily living," Part II concerns "motor experiences of daily living," Part III is retained as the "motor examination," and Part IV concerns "motor complications." Several questions from Part I and all questions from Part II have been designed to be amenable to a patient/caregiver questionnaire format and therefore can be completed without the investigator's input. For the remaining Part I questions that deal with complex behaviors, and all questions in Part IV that deal with motor fluctuations and dyskinesias, the investigator is required to conduct the interview. Part III retains the objective assessments of Parkinsonism, but all tasks now have specific instructions. Rater-involvement time for administering the MDS-UPDRS is estimated to require less than 10 minutes for the interview items of Part I, 15 minutes for Part III, and five minutes for Part IV, resulting in arater-time investment equivalent to the original scale's and meeting the 30-minute goal. The remaining questionnaire items are answered by the patient or caregiver and, other than supervision, do not involve rater time. Whereas the detailed assessments still prioritize the motor aspects of PD, the screening questions on non-motor elements are designed to capture both the presence and the severity of clinically pertinent problems in this domain.

Each question is anchored uniformly with five responses that are linked to commonly accepted clinical terms: 0 = normal, 1 = slight, 2 = mild, 3 = moderate, and 4 = severe. After each clinical descriptor, a short text follows that describes the criteria for each response. While each response is tailored to the question, the progression of disability or impairment is based on a consistent infrastructure. *Slight* (1) refers to symptoms or signs with low enough frequency or intensity to cause no impact on function; *mild* (2) refers to symptoms or signs of frequency or intensity sufficient to cause a modest impact on function; *moderate* (3) refers to symptoms or signs sufficiently frequent or intense to impact considerably, but not prevent, function; *severe* (4) refers to symptoms or signs that prevent function.

The full MDS-UPDRS contains questions and evaluations, divided across Part I (13), Part II (13), Part III (33 scores based on 18, several with right, left, or other body-distribution

Table 7-1. Ratings of UPDRS and MDS-UPDRS

	APPLIED IN PD	USED BY MULTIPLE AUTHORS	GOOD CLINIMETRIC PROFILE	FINAL DESIGNATION
UPDRS	YES	YES	YES	Recommended
MDS-UPDRS	YES	YES	YES	Recommended

The designation of Recommended has been established by the Movement Disorder Society Task Force on Parkinson's Disease Rating Scales (see earlier chapters). When all three criteria are met, the scale is Recommended; when two are met, the scale is Suggested; and when only one is met, the scale is Listed.

scores), and Part IV (6). The total number of ratings on the MDS-UPDRS is 65, in comparison to the 55 rating items on the original UPDRS.

Several new items in the MDS-UPDRS were not captured in any form on the original UPDRS (Table 7-2): anxious mood, dopamine dysregulation syndrome, urinary problems, constipation, fatigue, doing hobbies, getting in and out of bed, toe tapping, and freezing (objective rating). Lightheadedness was assessed in the original UPDRS as "present" or "absent," but in the MDS-UPDRS, the symptom is assessed with the 0 to 4 rating system. Nighttime sleep problems and daytime sleepiness are assessed in the MDS-UPDRS and replace the yes/no sleep disturbances option from the original UPDRS. The question on complexity of motor fluctuations in the MDS-UPDRS merges the three yes/no questions related to predictable, unpredictable, and sudden OFF period from the UPDRS. In regards to tremor, the original action/postural

tremor question has been divided into two questions focusing on each component of tremor separately. For rest tremor, whereas the UPDRS combined amplitude and constancy of tremor into its descriptors, on the MDS-UPDRS, the severity ratings for each body part concern only amplitude, and a separate question rates constancy.

Direct item-to-item mapping from the original UPDRS to the MDS-UPDRS was not envisioned to be possible, because the two scales were not conceptually identical. Nonetheless, because the new version was directly based on the original scale, several parallels and guidelines were utilized in the construction of the MDS-UPDRS. For some questions, the insertion of slight/mild/moderate/severe was sufficient to realign the rating options. In some cases, however, because the original scale often used "mild/moderate/severe/marked," the former rating of 1 (mild) now could be separated into two choices (slight 1 or mild 2) in the MDS-UPDRS. In such cases, the former moderate scores (2) advanced to 3 in the MDS-UPDRS and the former severe (3) and marked (4) were collapsed into one option (severe, 4) in the MDS-UPDRS. In other cases, adjustments in the midranges (2 and 3) were felt to be necessary in order to maintain a consistent conceptual framework of slight/mild/moderate/severe in the MDS-UPDRS. This decision to shift from mild/moderate/severe/marked to slight/mild/moderate/severe as the scale's clinical construct was anchored in two concepts: first, that many clinical trials focus on early PD where change among scores of normal, slight, and mild problems are important to document; and second, that at the high range of impairment or disability (formerly "severe" and "marked"), functional differences may not be clinically relevant. Another conceptual anchor of the MDS-UPDRS, especially apparent in Parts I, II, and IV of the MDS-UPDRS, was the progressing disability from none (0) to a perception of the problem without interference (slight, 1), to interference with isolated activity (mild, 2), to interference with normal activity (moderate, 3), to preclusion of normal activity (severe, 4). This process was not utilized consistently in the original UPDRS, although parallels could be

Table 7-2. Items Covered by the MDS-UPDRS That Were Not Covered, or Incompletely Covered, in the UDPRS

Anxious mood

Fatigue

Dopamine dysregulation syndrome

Urinary problems

Constipation

Doing hobbies

Getting in and out of bed

Toe tapping

Freezing (objective rating)

Lightheadedness (assessed with 0–4 ratings)

Nighttime sleep problems

Daytime sleepiness

Postural tremor (rated separately from kinetic tremor)

Kinetic tremor (rated separately from postural tremor)

Rest tremor amplitude (rated separately from tremor constancy)

Rest tremor constancy (rated separately from tremor amplitude)

constructed between the two versions in many cases. Yes/no questions from the original Part IV were reformatted and refined to fit the 0 to 4 rating format of the rest of the scale in the MDS-UPDRS, so that a partial parallelism between the two versions could be mapped. New items that assessed features not assessed in the original UPDRS could not have been mapped from the original scale. With these caveats, general mapping patterns between the two scales were outlined to allow a guide to raters making the transition between the UPDRS and the MDS-UPDRS, but were not constructed with the aim of allowing automatic substitution (Table 7-3). As part of the clinimetric plan, however, a review of score ranges for each part of the MDS-UPDRS was planned to be tested against the original version (see below).

Table 7-3. Conceptual Mapping of Items and Scores from the Original UPDRS to the MDS-UPDRS

MDS-UPDRS ITEM	ORIGINAL UPDRS ITEM	GENERAL CONCEPTS FOR MAPPING RATINGS FROM THE ORIGINAL UPDRS TO MDS-UPDRS (UPDRS→MDS-UPDRS)
Part I		In the MDS-UPDRS, the conceptual construct focuses on the impact rather than the presence of symptoms, and whereas there is a general parallel between UPDRS and MDS-UPDRS, this emphasis needs to be considered at all times by the rater and/or patient.
Cognitive impairment	Intellectual impairment	General conceptual comparison, although the emphasis is different in the two versions: 0→0; 1→2 (option 1 on MDS-UPDRS new and not captured in original scale); 2→3; 3→4; 4→4
Hallucinations and psychosis	Thought disorder	0→0; 1→0 (vivid dreams not part of this question in MDS-UPDRS); 2→1 or 2; 3→3; 4→4.
Depressed mood	Depression	General conceptual comparison, although the emphasis is different in the two versions:0→0; 1→1; 2→2; 3→3; 4→4
Anxious mood		New item: No comparison
Apathy	Motivation/ initiative	General conceptual comparison, although the emphasis is different in the two versions:0→0; 1→1; 2→2; 3→3; 4→4
Features of dopamine dysregulation syndrome		New item: No comparison
Nighttime sleep problems	Sleep disturbances	0→0; 1 on UPDRS could be 0 (if the patient had only daytime sleepiness) or any of the available ratings on the MDS-UPDRS.
Daytime sleepiness	Sleep disturbances	0→0; 1 on UPDRS could be 0 (if the patient had only nighttime sleep problems) or any of the available ratings on the MDS-UPDRS
Pain and other sensations	Sensory complaints related to Parkinsonism	General conceptual comparison, although the emphasis is different in the two versions: 0→0; 1→1; 2→2; 3→3; 4→4

(continued)

Table 7-3. (continued)

MDS-UPDRS ITEM	ORIGINAL UPDRS ITEM	GENERAL CONCEPTS FOR MAPPING RATINGS FROM THE ORIGINAL UPDRS TO MDS-UPDRS (UPDRS→MDS-UPDRS)
Urinary problems		New item: No comparison
Constipation		New item: No comparison
Lightheadedness on standing	Symptomatic orthostasis	0→0; 1→1,2,3, or 4, depending on severity
Fatigue		New item: no comparison
Part II		*As in Part I, for the MDS-UPDRS, the conceptual construct focuses on the impact rather than the presence of symptoms, and whereas there is a general parallel between UPDRS and MDS-UPDRS, this emphasis needs to be considered at all times by the rater and/or patient.*
Speech	Speech	0→0; 1→1; 2→2, 3→3, 4→4
Salivation and drooling	Salivation	0→0; 1→2 (option 1 on MDS-UPDRS new and not captured in original scale); 2→3; 3→3; 4→4
Chewing and swallowing	Swallowing	General conceptual comparison, although the emphasis is different in the two versions: 0→0; 1→3; (options 1 and 2 on MDS-UPDRS are new and not captured well by the original scale) 2→3; 3→2; 4→4
Eating tasks	Cutting food and handling utensils	0→0; 1→1; 2→2; 3→3; 4→4
Dressing	Dressing	0→0; 1→1; 2→2; 3→3; 4→4
Hygiene	Hygiene	Although MDS-UPDRS focuses on all tasks and does not limit questions to tasks mentioned in UPDRS, general parallelism exists for the two:0→0; 1→1; 2→2; 3→3; 4→4
Handwriting	Handwriting	The MDS-UPDRS emphasizes clarity of writing, not size, but a general parallelism exists for the two scales:0→0; 1→1; 2→1; 3→2 or 3; 4→4
Doing hobbies and other activities		New item: No comparison
Turning in bed	Turning in bed and adjusting bedclothes	The MDS-UPDRS emphasizes regularity of help needed, but a general parallelism exists for the two scales: 0→0; 1→1; 2→2 or 3; 3→3 or 4; 4→4
Tremor	Tremor	The MDS-UPDRS emphasizes interference from tremor, but a general parallelism exists for the two scales: 0→0; 1→1; 2→2; 3→3; 4→4
Getting out of bed, car, or deep chair		New item: No comparison

(*continued*)

Table 7-3. (continued)

MDS-UPDRS ITEM	ORIGINAL UPDRS ITEM	GENERAL CONCEPTS FOR MAPPING RATINGS FROM THE ORIGINAL UPDRS TO MDS-UPDRS (UPDRS→MDS-UPDRS)
Walking and balance	Walking	0→0; 1→1; 2→1 or 2; 3→3 or 4; 4→4
Freezing	Freezing when walking	Conceptually, the focus of the MDS-UPDRS is different from the UPDRS because the need for assistance is emphasized in the MDS-UPDRS rather than the consequence (falls) that will depend on availability of help. Only partial parallelism can be drawn on this question: 0→0; 1→1; 2→2,3,or 4; 2→2, 3, or 4; 4→2, 3, or 4.
	Falls	This item is not part of the MDS-UPDRS because it is not a normal "experience of daily living." Falling is assessed in Part III.
Part III		
Speech	Speech	0→0; 1→1; 2→2; 3→3 or 4; 4→4
Facial expression	Facial expression	0→0; 1→1; 2→2; 3→3; 4→4
Rigidity	Rigidity	Conceptually, the focus of the question has been changed to emphasize resistance to passive movement with greater clarity. Partial parallelism can be suggested: 0→0; 1→1; 2→2; 3→2; 4→3; 4 rating on MDS-UPDRS is not captured by the original scale
Finger taps	Finger taps	The original UPDRS had descriptors (mild, moderate, severe), that fit better with the current designations of slight, mild, and moderate, creating difficulties with a direct parallelism, but the task descriptions allow parallelism: 0→0; 1→1 or 2; 2→2 or 3; 3→3; 4→4
Hand movements	Hand movements	See "Finger taps" for explanation:0→0; 1→1 or 2; 2→2 or 3; 3→3; 4→4
Pronation/supination	Pronation/ supination	See "Finger taps" for explanation:0→0; 1→1 or 2; 2→2 or 3; 3→3; 4→4
Leg agility	Leg agility	See "Finger taps" for explanation:0→0; 1→1 or 2; 2→2 or 3; 3→3; 4→4
Toe taps		New item; no comparison
Arising from chair	Arising from chair	0→0; 1→1; 2→2; 3→3; 4→4
Gait	Gait	0→0; 1→1; 2→2; 3→3 or 4; 4→4
Freezing of gait		New item: no comparison ("Freezing" was in Part II of the original and has been moved to Part III in the MDS-UPDRS)

(continued)

Table 7-3. (continued)

MDS-UPDRS ITEM	ORIGINAL UPDRS ITEM	GENERAL CONCEPTS FOR MAPPING RATINGS FROM THE ORIGINAL UPDRS TO MDS-UPDRS (UPDRS→MDS-UPDRS)
Postural stability	Postural stability	0→0; 1→1 or 2; 2→3; 3→4; 4→4
Posture	Posture	0→0; 1→1; 2→2 or 3; 3→4; 4→4
Global spontaneity of movement	Body bradykinesia	0→0; 1→1; 2→2; 3→3; 4→4
Rest tremor		The MDS-UPDRS separates two features of rest tremor (amplitude and consistency), so there is no parallelism between the original and new versions.
Postural tremor Kinetic tremor	Action/postural tremor Action/postural tremor	The MDS-UPDRS separates these two forms of tremor and focuses only on amplitude, so there is no parallelism between the original and new versions.
Constancy of rest tremor		New item: no comparison. Tremor consistency was considered in original UPDRS but combined with amplitude, making the assessment ambiguous.
Part IV		
Time spend with dyskinesia	Dyskinesia duration	0→0; 1→1; 2→2; 3→3; 4→4
Functional impact of dyskinesias		MDS-UPDRS provides written anchors, whereas the MDS uses only "mild, moderate, severe, marked." 0→0; 1→2 (option 1 on MDS-UPDRS new and not captured in original scale; 2→3; 3→4; 4→4
Time spent in the OFF state	OFF duration	0→0; 1→1; 2→2; 3→3; 4→4
Functional impact of fluctuations		New item: no comparison. Written to run in parallel with Function impact of dyskinesias.
Complexity of motor fluctuations	OFFs predictable (yes/no) OFFs unpredictable (yes/no) OFFs sudden (yes/no)	MDS-UPDRS consolidates concepts covered by several yes/no questions on UPDRS. There is no simple mapping for this reason.
Painful OFF-state dystonia	Presence of early-morning dystonia (yes/no)	0→0; 1→1, 2, 3, or 4

NOTE: Many items have shifted emphasis with the MDS-UPDRS, but this guide shows the general concept behind the two scoring systems and can be used as a reference. The mapping table is a guide and not recommended as an automatic transfer for scores from one scale to the other.

HANDLING COMORBIDITIES

The MDS-UPDRS is specifically structured to "rate what you see," and does not presume that the rater or patient can separate impairment and disability strictly due to Parkinsonism from other comorbidities. This point is carefully outlined in the instructions to raters and patients. The decision to rate impairment and disability without direct relationship to Parkinsonism was made because the scale will be used by people of different levels of education and experience, and a uniformity of application across cultures is desired.[4]

ADDITIONAL POINTS

ON and OFF definitions are provided to ensure uniformity among raters, and the score sheet documents the ON/OFF status associated with the Part III assessment. For Parts I and II, the official scale will not separate ON from OFF, but for special studies, the same questions can be asked separately for ON or OFF periods. Throughout the MDS-UPDRS, specific instructions are provided in order to enhance a uniform application. Finally, questions have been written to be culturally sensitive and applicable to patients of different ethnic and social backgrounds.

As an ongoing process, at the end of the MDS-UPDRS, clinicians and researchers are directed to the Appendix of Additional Scales. This portion of the UDPRS is not considered a static document, but instead will be updated as deemed appropriate by the MDS Task Force of Rating Scales for Parkinson's Disease and posted on the Movement Disorder Society website (see www.movementdisorders.org). This appendix is designed to direct clinicians and research investigators to scales that cover in greater detail the components of the MDS-UPDRS that are only assessed with single items. The task force has previously published assessments of scales for several areas of focus, including depression and psychosis, anxiety, apathy, and dysautonomia.[69-73] These assessments use a standard set of criteria to establish "recommended" and "suggested" scales in an effort to encourage reporting in a consistent manner and to facilitate comparisons among different reports. For items that have not had official task force reports, the subcommittee of the MDS-UPDRS dedicated to the appendix has reviewed scales using the same criteria (Cristina Sampaio, chairperson).

Key evaluation issues

USE IN PARKINSON'S DISEASE AND APPLICATION ACROSS THE DISEASE SPECTRUM

The MDS-UPDRS has been tested in over 800 subjects with PD across the full clinical spectrum of the disease (Hoehn and Yahr stages 1–5) and in different ethnic and racial groups among English speakers. It is also the focus of cross-cultural assessments, and is currently being tested in large populations in several non-English languages (see below).

USE BY MULTIPLE AUTHORS

Although introduced only in 2009, the MDS-UPDRS has already been used in clinical trials involving leadership other than the scale developers. These range from studies of new therapeutic interventions, to responsivity testing (see below), to biomarker research on disease progression.[74-76]

CLINIMETRIC ISSUES

Unlike the UPDRS, the MDS-UPDRS underwent formal cognitive pretesting prior to its full clinimetric assessment. In this phase, versions were tested for rater and patient comfort and understanding. This process led to modifications of wording and the deletion of technical phrases in several questions. Based on successful preliminary testing,[4] the MDS-UPDRS validation program was designed to test the scale's intrinsic attributes, including internal consistency, factor structure, differential item functioning, and its comparability with the original UPDRS.

In the MDS-sponsored clinimetric program, movement disorder specialists and experienced study coordinators examined PD patients with both the UPDRS and the MDS-UPDRS. Special attention was focused on recruitment of diverse race and ethnicity representations. Native English speakers (both raters and patients) participated.

The relationships between the MDS-UPDRS and UPDRS were determined with Spearman's rank order correlations between the two scales for total score and for each Part.[5] Correlations were computed to assess the relationships among the Parts of the MDS-UPDRS. As a measure of internal consistency (reliability), Cronbach's alpha was calculated for each Part. Furthermore, floor and ceiling effects were examined by calculating the percentage of lowest and highest possible scores for each Part. Mplus v. 4.21[77] was used for the factor analysis using polychoric correlations due to the ordinal nature of the data. A factor analysis was run in two parts. An exploratory factor analysis (EFA), informed by eigenvalues and scree plots, was used to determine the number of factors that best represents the data. A cutoff of 0.40 was used to determine the items to retain in a factor. As a second step, a confirmatory factor analysis (CFA) was used in the assessment of dimensionality, with a comparative fit index (CFI) $\geq$ 0.90 defined as an "acceptable fit." If the CFI was less than 0.90, each factor was examined to identify poorly behaved items—that is, those with high loadings on more than one factor.[78] Based on the review of the items and the model fit statistics, additional EFAs and CFAs were run. The process was repeated until the most parsimonious model was found with a CFI $\geq$0.90. We assessed the entire scale as a single factor structure, each Part as a separate set of factors, and all combinations of Parts.

The patient sample included 877 native English-speaking PD patients, 560 men and 317 women.[5] There were 682 non-Latino Caucasians and 195 (22%) of other races or ethnicities, specifically 49 African-Americans, 87 Latinos, 1 native Hawaiian, 43 Asians, and 15 with other races or ethnicities. All Hoehn and Yahr stages were represented, with the majority of patients being Stage II (Stage I = 63, Stage II = 467, Stage III = 174, Stage IV = 109, Stage V = 53, missing 11). The mean age of the cohort was 68.2 years (SD 10.8, range 31–98), and the mean

PD duration was 8.3 years (SD 6.7, range 0–40 years). Fifty-seven patients were not treated with anti-Parkinsonian medications. A total of 685 patients were treated with levodopa in combination with another symptomatic treatment for PD, 115 patients were on symptomatic therapy without levodopa, 5 patients were on levodopa alone, and 15 had missing treatment information. Motor fluctuations were observed in 483 patients, and 304 patients had dyskinesia. A total of 723 were examined in the ON state and 99 in the OFF state, while ON/OFF information was not recorded for 55 patients.

There were 69 raters from 39 English-speaking treatment centers (USA 32, Canada 2, UK 5) who evaluated patients with the original and MDS-UPDRS instruments. All raters were physicians or nurse coordinators regularly working with PD patients, regularly using the UPDRS for clinical care or research purposes, and all were recruited through the MDS. Raters were instructed to perform the UPDRS in their standard manner and to use the MDS-UPDRS following the instructions embedded in the new scale for each item.

Reliability: Internal consistency was computed for each of the MDS-UPDRS Parts—Part I (13 items) alpha = 0.79, Part II (13 items) alpha = 0.90, Part III (29 items) alpha = 0.93, and Part IV (6 items) alpha = 0.79.[5] Mean scores (SD) for each Part were Part I: 11.5 (7.0); Part II: 16.0 (10.0); Part III: 36.8 (18.4); Part IV: 4.0 (4.2).

Validity: The distributions of the total scores in the MDS-UPDRS and original UPDRS were similar: UPDRS mean 61.0 (SD 30.3), covering 55 items; MDS-UPDRS mean 68.4 (SD 32.8), covering 65 items. The MDS-UPDRS showed strong concurrent validity based on high correlations between the two scales (total score r = 0.96), as well as between the individual Parts of the two scales: (Part I, r = 0.76; Part II, r = 0.92; Part III, r = 0.96; Part IV [sum of items 32–39 covering dyskinesias and motor fluctuations on the UDPRS vs. total Part IV from the MDS-UPDRS], r = 0.89). As a measure of internal validity, correlations among the MDS-UPDRS Parts were examined. These analyses confirmed that each Part assesses a different aspect of PD, with most parts, except Parts I and

II, having relatively low correlations (Parts I and II, r = 0.67; Parts I and III, r = 0.43; Parts I and IV, r = 0.39; Parts II and IV, r = 0.44; Parts III and IV, r = 0.22). As anticipated, Parts II and III,which covered patient perceptions of motor function and the objective examination, were more highly correlated (r = 0.66). Our analysis for possible floor and ceiling effects demonstrated a low percentage of lowest and highest scores for Parts I, II, and III: Part I, lowest 0.1%/highest 0.8%; Part II, lowest 0.1%/highest 0.7%; Part III, lowest 0.1%/highest 0.2%. In the case of Part IV, covering the presence and severity of motor complications, there was an expected floor effect, but no ceiling effect: lowest 36.7%/highest 0.1%.[5]

In the factor analysis, exploratory testing of the combined four Parts of the MDS-UPDRS did not identify a single factor structure that could be confirmed (CFI = 0.74). A factor structure combining Parts II and III was explored, but could not be confirmed. Several items had salient loadings on more than one factor, and some items did not load on any factor. A factor structure was also explored for the combination of Parts II, III, and IV. A factor structure with 12 factors was identified by the EFA; however, the CFI was <0.90,too low to provide confirmation. As seen before, several items had salient loadings on more than one factor, and some items did not load on any factor. These combined results allow the conclusion that each Part's summary score is a valid reflection of a target domain relevant to PD; however, because these summary scores for Parts I, II, III, and IV capture different elements of PD and different primary sources (patient vs. rater), it is not possible to use a total MDS-UPDRS score or a score based on combinations of Parts to summarize an overall PD severity measure.[5]

When the MDS-UPDRS Parts were considered individually, both the exploratory and confirmatory analyses identified a factor structure that was statistically consistent (CFI for each Part >0.90) and clinically meaningful for all Parts.[4] For Part I (CFI = 0.94), two factors were identified: one covering depression, anxiety, and apathy, and one covering the other non-motor functions (shared variance = 42.5%). For Part II (CFI = 0.95), three factors were identified: one covering several fine motor functions, one covering tremor and eating tasks, and one focusing on several large motor functions (shared variance = 69.4%). For Part III (CFI = 0.91), seven factors were identified: midline function, rest tremor, rigidity, bradykinesia right upper extremity, bradykinesia left upper extremity, postural and kinetic tremors, and lower limb bradykinesia (shared variance 77.1%). For Part IV (CFI = 1.0), two factors were identified, one focusing on fluctuations including off-state dystonia and the other on dyskinesias (shared variance = 79.2%). Inter-correlations among factors for each Part ranged from 0.04 to 0.71, indicating both unique and shared information provided by the different factors.[5]

Responsiveness: The MDS-UPDRS has undergone responsiveness assessment in relationship to acute levodopa challenges in one study. PD patients received carbidopa/levodopa 25/250 orally, and the change from baseline to peak effect was measured with the MDS-UPDRS.[75] Responsiveness to dopaminergic therapy in chronic trials remains to be officially demonstrated.

MCRD and MCRID: Conceptually, because each item is anchored in a clinical term of "slight" (1), "mild" (2), "moderate" (3), and "severe" (4), archetypal scores for a patient with consistent slight impairment and disability would have scores of 13 for Part I, 13 for Part II, 33 for Part III, and 6 for Part IV, each item receiving a prototypical score of 1. Likewise, for *mild* disease, scores would be double, for *moderate* triple, and for *severe* quadruple these values. Ranges around these prototypical anchors could serve as testable models for a MCRD calculation for differences among clinically pertinent categories of slight, mild, moderate, and severe PD. To date, one study has examined 313 PD patients with wide representation of Clinical Global Impression-Severity (CGI-s) ratings, including mildly ill (n = 94), moderately ill (n = 153), markedly ill (n = 43) and severely ill (n = 20).[79] Discrete and non-overlapping means (95th CI of the means) for the total MDS-UPDRS Part III scores were found for each clinical category. Furthermore, examination of the seven factors composing Part III revealed significantly progressive increases in five factors: axial function, rigidity, right upper bradykinesia, left upper bradykinesia, and leg bradykinesia. Tremor factors (rest and kinetic + posture), however, did not demonstrate progressive increases with increasing CGI-S scores.

To estimate the score change in MDS-UPDRS between two visits associated with a clinically pertinent improvement (MCID), one single-rater study examined 70 PD patients with the MDS-UPDRS and Clinical Global Impression Change Scale (CGI-c).[80] The analysis focused on 234 sequences of two patient visits, divided among those that did not change in terms of their overall Parkinsonism (CGI-c score of 4 or no change) vs. those who had a minimally pertinent clinical improvement (CGI-c score of 3). MDS-UPDRS Part III change score for CGI-C 4 (no clinical change) was 0.46 (95th CI = −0.05; 0.96) and varied slightly by PD severity (mild = 0.47; moderate = 0.25; severe = 0.80). MDS-UPDRS Part III change score for CGI-C 3 (minimal clinically improvement) was −2.41 (95th CI = −3.17; −1.65) and varied slightly across PD severity (mild = −2.73; moderate = −2.07; severe = −1.70). The results allow a functional translation of a numerical change into a clinically pertinent change, and larger samples collected from multiple investigators in different centers with patients across the full spectrum of PD severity are likely to allow clear definition of MCID for the MDS-UPDRS.

Strengths and weaknesses: additional considerations

A strong component of the MDS-sponsored program includes the development of official non-English versions of the MDS-UPDRS. Teams representing over 12 languages are involved in this program, which has three phases: translation/backtranslation; cognitive pretesting; and full clinimetric testing in 350 native-speaking patients and raters. Pre-specified criteria for each MDS-UPRDS Part relative to the English original have been set, and the versions meeting the criteria will receive the designation of "an official MDS version." As of March 1, 2011, the Italian version of the MDS-UPDRS has received this designation, and other language teams are actively in the process of reaching this goal as well.

The effort to revise the original UPDRS into the MDS-UPDRS poses certain practical issues for raters whose use of the UPDRS is well-entrenched and time-honored. There is no specific conversion algorithm established, and regulatory agencies have long respected the UPDRS as a "gold standard." Whereas the developers of the scale and the MDS consider the new scale the natural replacement for the original one, this evolution is likely to take at least a few years for international adoption.

Whereas the MDS-UPDRS item ratings are consistently anchored in the construct of the progression from normal function to minimal, mild, moderate, and severe impairment or disability, the issue of the linearity of the scale has not been statistically tested. This process is a complex one, but the original data set of over 800 PD subjects used for the clinimetric testing will allow this eventual determination.

Final assessment

The MDS-UPDRS, although relatively new, has been used sufficiently outside of its developers, has been applied widely across the spectrum of PD, and has strong clinimetric properties. It therefore can be designated as *Recommended* for the evaluation of PD severity (Table 7-1). The Movement Disorder Society has invested considerable resources in providing training and exposure of the scale for both research and clinical applications. No new treatment, however, has been approved by official regulatory agencies with the MDS-UPDRS improvement as the primary outcome measure.

FUTURE PERSPECTIVES

With two Recommended scales for assessing the severity of PD, what will be the future applications and prioritizations for research and clinical monitoring? Clearly, the MDS-UPDRS has the advantages of capturing very mild disease impairments and disabilities, as well as capturing estimates of many non-motor elements of PD and its treatment. On the other hand, the UPDRS is wellentrenched historically, and investigators interested in longitudinal studies that began with the UDPRS do not have an automatic algorithm for switching to the new scale. It is therefore likely that the two scales will coexist for several years, with the MDS-UPDRS eventually replacing the earlier scale. In this period, several important projects can be envisioned for the MDS-UPDRS, including the ongoing official translation programs into non-English languages, an analysis of differential item function for all items to detect if certain questions are potentially problematic font or certain groups of patients (gender, racial, ethnic, educational background). An important milestone will be met for the MDS-UPDRS when a major regulatory agency approves a new treatment for PD based on data from the MDS-UPDRS as the primary outcome measure.

RECOMMENDED SCALES
UPDRS
MDS-UPDRS

References

1. Fahn S, Elton RL, UPDRS program members. Unified Parkinson's Disease Rating Scale. In: Fahn S, Marsden CD, Goldstein M, Calne DB, eds. *Recent Developments in Parkinson's Disease.* Vol. 2. Florham Park, NJ: Macmillan Healthcare Information; 1987:153–163, 293–304.
2. Ramaker C, Marinus J, Stiggelbout AM, van Hilten BJ. Systematic evaluation of rating scales for impairment and disability in Parkinson's disease. *Mov Disord.* 2002;17:867–876.
3. Movement Disorder Society Task Force on rating scales for Parkinson's disease. UPDRS: status and recommendations. *Mov Disord.* 2003;18:738–750.
4. Goetz CG, Fahn S, Martinez-Martin P, et al. Movement Disorder Society–sponsored revision of the Unified Parkinson's Disease Rating Scale (MDS-UPDRS): process, format, and clinimetric testing plan. *Mov Disord.* 2007;22:41–47.
5. Goetz CG, Tilley BC, Shaftman SR, et al; on behalf of Movement Disorder Society UPDRS Revision Task Force. Movement Disorder Society–sponsored revision of the Unified Parkinson's Disease Rating Scale (MDS-UPDRS): scale presentation and clinimetric testing results. *Mov Disord.* 2008;23: 2129–2170.
6. Webster DD. Critical analysis of the disability in Parkinson's disease. *ModTreat.* 1968;5: 257–258.
7. Duvoisin RC. The evaluation of extrapyramidal disease. In: de Ajuriaguerra J, Gauthier G, eds. *Monoamines noyaux gris centraux et syndrome de Parkinson.* Paris: Masson; 1971.
8. Parkes JD, Zilka KJ, Calver DM, Knill-Jones RP. Controlled trial of amantadine hydrochloride in Parkinson's disease. *Lancet.*1970;1:259–262.
9. Canter CJ, de la Torre R, Mier M. A method of evaluating disability in patients with Parkinson's disease. *J Nerv Ment Dis.* 1961;133:143–147.
10. Lieberman A, Le Brun Y, Boal D. The use of a dopaminergic receptor stimulating agent (Piribendil ET-495) in Parkinson's disease. In: Usdin E, ed. *Advances in Biochemical Psychopharmacology.* Vol.12. New York: Raven Press; 1973:415–425.
11. Diamond SG, Markham CH, Treciokas LJ. A double-blind comparison of levodopa, madopar and Sinemet in Parkinson's disease. *Ann Neurol.* 1978;3:267–272.
12. SchwabJF, England AC. Projection technique for evaluating surgery in Parkinson's disease. In: Billingham FH, Donaldson MC, eds. *Third Symposium on Parkinson's Disease.*Edinburgh, UK: Livingstone; 1968:152–157.
13. Hoehn MM, Yahr MD. Parkinsonism: onset, progression and mortality. *Neurology.*1967;17:427–442.
14. Martinez-Martin P, Gil-Nagel A, Gracia LM, et al. Unified Parkinson's Disease Rating Scale characteristics and structure. The Cooperative Multicentric Group. *Mov Disord.* 1994;9: 76–83.
15. Lang AE. Comments on teaching tape for the motor section of the Unified Parkinson's Disease Rating Scale. *Mov Disord.* 1996;11:344–345.
16. Jankovic J, McDermott M, Carter J, et al. Variable expression of Parkinson's disease. *Neurology.* 1990;40:1529–1534.
17. Marras C, McDermott MP, Rochon PA, Tanner CM, Naglie G, Lang AE. Predictors of deterioration in health-related quality of life in Parkinson's disease. *MovDisord.* 2008;23: 653–659.

18. Goetz CG, Stebbins GT, Chmura TA, et al. Teaching tape for the motor section of the Unified Parkinson's Disease Rating Scale. *Mov Disord*. 1995;10:263–266.

19. Parkinson Study Group. Effects of tocopherol and deprenyl on the progression of disability in early Parkinson's disease. *N Engl J Med*. 1993;328:176–183.

20. Lieberman A, Ranhosky A, Korts D. Clinical evaluation of pramipexole in advanced PD. *Neurology*.1997;49:162–168.

21. Vieregge P, Stolze H, Klein C, Heberlein I. Gait quantification in Parkinson's disease—locomotor disability and correlation to clinical rating scales. *J Neural Transm*.1997;104:237–248.

22. Richards M, Marder K, Cote L, et al. Interrater reliability of the Unified Parkinson's Disease Rating Scale motor examination. *Mov Disord*. 1994;9:89–91.

23. Bennett DA, Shannon KM, Beckett LA, Goetz CG, Wilson RS. Metric properties of nurses' ratings of Parkinsonian signs with a modified UPDRS. *Neurology*. 1997;49:1580–1587.

24. Morrish PK, Sawle GV, Brooks DJ. An [18F] dopa-PET and clinical study of the rate of progression in Parkinson's disease. *Brain*. 1996;119:585–591.

25. Seibyl JP, Marek KL, Quinlan D, et al. Decreased single-photon emission computed tomographic [123I]beta-CIT striatal uptake correlates with symptom severity in Parkinson's disease. *Ann Neurol*. 1995;38:589–598.

26. Rabey JM, Bass H, Bonuccelli U, et al. Evaluation of the short Parkinson's evaluation scale: a new friendly scale for the evaluation of Parkinson's disease in clinical drug trials. *Clin Neuropharm*. 1997;20:322–337.

27. Hogan T, Grimaldi R, Dingemanse J, et al. The Parkinson's symptom inventory (PDSI): a comprehensive and sensitive instrument to measure disease symptoms and treatment side-effects. *Parkinsonism Relat Disord*. 999;5:93–98.

28. Martinez-Martin P, Garcia Urra D, delSerQuijano T, et al. A new clinical tool for gait evaluation in Parkinson's disease. *Clin Neuropharmacol*. 1997;20:183–194.

29. Committee for proprietary medicinal products. Guidance on clinical investigation of medicinal products in the treatment of Parkinson's disease. 1998. Available at: www.pharmacontract.ch/support/pdf_support/056395EN

30. Goetz CG, Leurgans S, Raman R, et al. Placebo-associated improvements in motor function: comparison of subjective and objective sections of the UPDRS in early Parkinson's disease. *Mov Disord*. 2002;17:283–288.

31. Langston JW, Widner H, Goetz CG, et al. Core assessment program for intracerebral transplantations (CAPIT). *Mov Disord*. 1992;7:2–13.

32. Defer GL, Widner H, Marie RM, et al. Core assessment program for surgical interventional therapies in Parkinson's disease (CAPSIT-PD). *Mov Disord*. 1999;14:572–584.

33. Cubo E, Stebbins GT, Golbe LI, et al. Application of the Unified Parkinson's Disease Rating Scale in progressive supranuclear palsy: factor analysis of the motor scale.*Mov Disord*. 2000;15:276–279.

34. Ballard C, McKeith I, Burn D, et al. The UPDRS scale as a means of identifying extrapyramidal signs in patients suffering with dementia with Lewy bodies. *Acta Neurol Scand*.1997;96:366–371.

35. Van Hilten JJ, van der Zwan AD, Zwinderman AH, et al. Rating impairment and disability in Parkinson's disease: evaluation of the Unified Parkinson's Disease Rating Scale. *Mov Disord*. 1994;9:84–88.

36. Stebbins GT, Goetz CG. Factor structure of the Unified Parkinson's Disease Rating Scale: motor examination section. *Mov Disord*. 1998;13:633–636.

37. Stebbins GT, Goetz CG, Lang AE, et al. Factor analysis of the motor section of the Unified Parkinson's Disease Rating Scale during the off-state. *Mov Disord*. 1999;14:585–589.

38. Louis ED, Lynch T, Marder K, et al. Reliability of patient completion of the historical section of the Unified Parkinson's Disease Rating Scale. *MovDisord*. 1996;11:185–192.

39. Camicioli R, Grossmann SJ, Spencer PS, et al. Discriminating mild Parkinsonism: methods for epidemiological research. *Mov Disord*. 2001;16:33–40.

40. Siderowf A, McDermott M, Kieburtz K, et al. Test-retest reliability of the UPDRS in patients with early Parkinson's disease: results of a multicenter clinical trial. *Mov Disord*. 2002;17:758–763.

41. McDermott MP, Jankovic J, Carter J, et al. Factors predictive of the need for levodopa therapy in early, untreated Parkinson's disease. *Arch Neurol*. 1995;52:565–570.

42. Poewe WH, Wenning GK. The natural history of Parkinson's disease. *Neurology*. 1996;47(suppl 3):S146–S152.

43. Oakes D, Parkinson Study Group. Progression of early Parkinson's disease until levodopa therapy is required. *Neurology.* 1990;40 (suppl 1):370.

44. Rascol O, Goetz C, Koller W, et al. Treatment interventions for Parkinson's disease: an evidence based assessment. *Lancet.* 2002;359:1589–1598.

45. Lieberman A, Ranhosky A, Korts D. Clinical evaluation of pramipexole in advanced PD. *Neurology.* 1997;49:162–168.

46. Adler CH, Sethi KD, Hauser RA, et al. Ropinirole for the treatment of early PD. *Neurology.* 1997;49:393–399.

47. Song J, Fisher BE, Petzinger G, Wu A, Gordon J, Salem GJ. The relationship between the UPDRS and lower extremity functional performance in persons with early stage Parkinson's disease. *Neurorehabil Neural Repair.* 2009;2009: 657–661.

48. Tanner CM, Parkinson Study Group. Pramipexole in ethnic minority with Parkinson's disease. *Mov Disord.* 1999; 14(suppl 5):901.

49. Todd KH, Funk KG, Funk JP, et al. Clinical significance of reported changes in pain severity. *Ann Emerg Med.* 1996;27:485–489.

50. Gallagher EJ, Liebman M, Bijur PE. Prospective validation of clinically important changes in pain severity measured on a visual analog scale. *Ann Emerg Med.* 2001;38:633–638.

51. Bird SB, Dickson EW. Clinically significant changes in pain along the visual analog scale. *Ann Emerg Med.* 2001;38:639–643.

52. Jones PW. Interpreting thresholds for a clinically significant change in health status in asthma and COPD. *Eur Respir J.* 2002;19: 398–404.

53. Price DD, Milling LS, Kirsch I, et al. An analysis of factors that contribute to the magnitude of placebo analgesia in an experimental paradigm. *Pain.* 1999;83:147–156.

54. Mattocks KM, Horwitz RI. Placebos, active control groups, and the unpredictability paradox. *Biol Psychiatry.* 2000;47:693–698.

55. Oremus M, Perrault A, Demers L, et al. Review of outcome measurement instruments in Alzheimer's disease drug trials: psychometric properties of global scales. *J Geriatr Psychiatry Neurol.* 2000;13:197–205.

56. Knopman DS, Knapp MJ, Gracon SI, et al. The clinician interview-based impression. *Neurology.* 1994;44:2315–2321.

57. Schrag A, Sampaio C, Counsell N, Poewe W. Minimal clinically important change on the Unified Parkinson's Disease Rating Scale. *Mov Disord.* 2006;21:1200–1207.

58. Shulman LM, Graber-Baldini AI, Anderson KE, Fishman PS, Reich SG, Weiner WJ. The clinically important difference on the UPDRS. *Arch Neurol.* 2010;67:64–70.

59. de Bie RMA, de Haan RJ, Nijssen PCG, et al. Unilateral pallidotomy in Parkinson's disease: a randomized, single-blind, multicentre trial. *Lancet.* 1999;354:1665–1669.

60. Oertel WH, Wolters E, Sampaio C, et al. Pergolide versus levodopa monotherapy in early Parkinson's disease patients: the PELMOPET study. *Mov Disord.* 2006;21:343–353.

61. Parkinson Study Group. Low-dose clozapine for the treatment of drug-induced psychosis in Parkinson's disease. *N Engl J Med.* 1999;340:757–763.

62. Goetz CG, Blasucci LM, Leurgans S, et al. Olanzapine and clozapine: comparative effects on motor function in hallucinating PD patients. *Neurology.* 2000;55:789–794.

63. Giladi N, Shabtai H, Gurevich T, Benbunan B, Anca M, Korczyn AD. Rivastigmine (Exelon) for dementia in patients with Parkinson's disease. *Acta Neurol Scand.* 2003;108:368–373.

64. Luquin MR, Scipioni O, Vaamonde J, et al. Levodopa-induced dyskinesias in Parkinson's disease: clinical and pharmacological classification. *Mov Disord.* 1992;7:117–124.

65. Marconi R, Lefebvre-Caparros D, Bonnet AM, et al. Levodopa-induced dyskinesias in Parkinson's disease, phenomenology and pathophysiology. *Mov Disord.* 1994;9:2–12.

66. Goetz CG. Rating scales for dyskinesias in Parkinson's disease. *Mov Disord.* 1999;14: 48–53.

67. Prochazka A, Bennett DJ, Stephens MJ, et al. Measurement of rigidity in Parkinson's disease. *Mov Disord.* 1997;12:24–32.

68. Goetz CG, LeWitt PA, Weidenman M. Standardized training tools for the UPDRS activities of daily living scale: newly available teaching program. *Mov Disord.* 2003;18: 1455–1458.

69. Schrag A, Barone P, Brown RG, et al. Depression rating scales in Parkinson's disease: critique and recommendations. *Mov Disord.* 2007;22:1077–1092.

70. Fernandez HH, Aarsland D, Fénelon G, et al. Scales to assess psychosis in Parkinson's disease: critique and recommendations. *Mov Disord.* 2008;23:484–500.

71. Leentjens AF, Dujardin K, Marsh L, et al. Anxiety rating scales in Parkinson's disease:

critique and recommendations. *Mov Disord.* 2008;23:2015–2025.

72. Leentjens AF, Dujardin K, Marsh L, et al. Apathy and anhedonia rating scales in Parkinson's disease: critique and recommendations. *Mov Disord.* 2008;23:2004–2014.

73. Evatt ML, Chaudhuri KR, Chou KL, et al. Dysautonomia rating scales in Parkinson's disease: sialorrhea, dysphagia, and constipation—critique and recommendations by movement disorders task force on rating scales for Parkinson's disease. *Mov Disord.* 2009;24:635–646.

74. Stocchi F, Ferreira J, Theewes A, et al. Treatment of dyskinesia in advanced Parkinson's disease: a pilot study with pardoprunox (submitted for publication).

75. Merello M, Gerschcovich E, Ballesteros D, Cerquetti D. Correlation between the Movement Disorder Society Unified Parkinson's Disease Rating Scale

(MDS-UPDRS) and the Unified Parkinson's Disease Rating Scale (UPDRS) during L-dopa acute challenge. *Parkinsonism Relat Disord.* 2011 [epub ahead of print].

76. Parkinson's progression markers initiative: principal investigator Kenneth Marek. Available at:http://www.michaeljfox.org/living_PPMI., 2011.

77. Muthén LK, Muthén BO. *Mplus Users' Guide.* Los Angeles: Muthèn and Muthèn; 1998.

78. Brown T. *Confirmatory Factor Analysis for Applied Research.* New York: Guilford Press; 2006.

79. Goetz CG, Stebbins GT, Simkus V. Severity ranges on the MDS-UPDRS motor examination: comparison to CGI-severity scores. *Mov Disord.* 2009;24(suppl 1):S434.

80. Stebbins GT, Goetz CG, Simkus V. Minimal clinically important change and the MDS-UPDRS motor examination. *Mov Disord.* 2009;24(suppl 1):S436.

8

DYSKINESIA RATING SCALES
IN PARKINSON'S DISEASE

Carlo Colosimo

Summary

Drug-induced dyskinesia is a common phenomenon in Parkinson's disease and may be socially as well as physically disabling for patients. Because of the impact of dyskinesia on activities of daily living, quality of life, and consequent global disability of PD patients, the Movement Disorder Society (MDS) organized a systematic review of the clinimetric properties of the scales used to measure dyskinesia in this disease. This chapter is mainly based on the published review,[1] but includes also part of the supplementary materials produced by the task force and initially published online on the Movement Disorders journal website. A scale was designated "Recommended" if the scale had been used in clinical studies beyond the group that developed it, had been specifically used in PD reports, and if clinimetric studies had established that it was valid, reliable, and sensitive. "Suggested" scales met two of the above criteria; and those meeting one were "Listed." Eight rating scales for dyskinesia that have either been validated or used in PD were identified: Abnormal Involuntary Movement Scale (AIMS), the Unified Parkinson's Disease Rating Scale (UPDRS) part IV, the Obeso Dyskinesia Rating Scale, the Rush Dyskinesia Rating Scale, the Clinical Dyskinesia Rating Scale (CDRS), the Lang-Fahn Activities of Daily Living Dyskinesia Scale, the Parkinson Disease Dyskinesia Scale (PDYS-26), and the Unified Dyskinesia Rating Scale (UDysRS). Based on this review and rating system, four of the reviewed dyskinesia scales (AIMS, Rush Dyskinesia Rating Scale, PDYS-26, and the UDysRS) can be recommended for use in PD populations; all of the remaining met criteria to be suggested. However, some of the recommended scales have significant weaknesses (AIMS does not allow differentiation among the different forms of dyskinesia, and the Rush scale "actual" intra- and inter-rater reliability is not really known). Conversely, the two most recent scales (PDYS-26 and UDysRS) have excellent clinimetric properties and appear to provide a reliable and valid assessment tool of dyskinesia in PD. Since further testing of these newer scales in PD is warranted, no new scales are needed until the available scales are fully analyzed clinimetrically.

INTRODUCTION

Drug-induced dyskinesia is common in Parkinson's disease (PD) and is frequently associated with social and physical disabilities.[2] Prevalence in cross-sectional studies ranges from 20% to 56%, and recognized risk factors are young age at disease-onset, long disease duration, and high total dosage of levodopa and other dopaminergic drugs.[3–5] Studies performed in patients chronically receiving levodopa or after acute dopaminergic challenge suggest that dyskinesia initially appears on the side of the body most affected by Parkinsonian symptoms.[4] In a minority of patients with asymmetric Parkinsonism, dyskinesia can also begin bilaterally or in the cranial region.[5] As PD progresses, dyskinesia inevitably spreads to the other limbs and may also involve the trunk and the cranial region. Dyskinesia in PD can further disable and impair health-related quality of life for those with this chronic disease. The mechanisms responsible for drug-induced dyskinesia are unclear, though several experimental studies suggest a role for the changes within the motor cortico-basal ganglia circuitry provoked by the progressive nigrostriatal degeneration and pulsatile dopamine-replacing treatments.[3]

Several rating scales have been used in clinical practice since the 1970s for assessing dyskinesia in PD. Some were part of global scales that measure motor disability in PD, while others were specifically developed for dyskinesia in PD. Other scales were originally developed for use in other neurological syndromes with dyskinesia, but later adapted to score PD dyskinesia.[6] In the last decade, new pharmacological and surgical treatments for advanced PD have been developed and tested.[7] These efforts are still limited by the lack of a single, validated, and widely accepted clinical rating instrument for dyskinesia.[8] The development of a good clinical rating instrument has been made difficult by inherent features of dyskinesia, such as the great variability of involuntary movements in relationship to the point in time of observation and to the activity carried out by the patient during the evaluation; furthermore, the discrimination among the different subtypes of drug-induced dyskinesia and between dyskinesia and Parkinsonian tremor may not be easily captured in a standard rating scale.

Because of the impact of dyskinesia on activities of daily living, quality of life, and consequent global disability of patients with PD, the Movement Disorder Society organized a systematic review of the clinimetric properties of the scales used to measure dyskinesia in this disease.[1] MDS-sponsored reviews of scales for assessing other clinical aspects of PD have also been previously published,[9–11] and the review of the scales used to measure dyskinesia followed a very similar methodology. This chapter is mainly based on the published review,[1] but it also includes part of the supplementary materials produced by the task force and published online on the Movement Disorders journal website.

METHODS

Task force organization and critique process

The organization of the MDS Task Force on Rating Scales for PD Dyskinesia and the complete methodology for scales identification, selection, and appraisal may be found on the original review produced by the task force[1] and Chapter 6. This chapter is an adaptation of a peer-reviewed manuscript published previously.[1]

Identified scales and their utilization in clinical practice and research

Eight published rating scales for dyskinesia in PD were identified (Table 8-1). These were the Abnormal Involuntary Movement Scale (AIMS),[13] the Unified Parkinson's Disease Rating Scale (UPDRS) part IV,[14] with its recent revision by the MDS,[12] the Obeso Dyskinesia Rating Scale,[15,16] the Rush Dyskinesia Rating Scale,[17] the Clinical Dyskinesia Rating Scale,[18] the Lang-Fahn Activities of Daily Living Dyskinesia Scale,[19] the Parkinson Disease Dyskinesia Scale (PDYS-26),[20] and the Unified Dyskinesia Rating Scale (UdysRS).[21] Home diaries for patients' self-assessment of dyskinesias have been developed,[22] but these rating instruments are primarily focused on motor fluctuations. Given that a chapter reviewing the scales on motor fluctuations is also included in the present book, motor fluctuation diaries that include dyskinesia are not considered in this chapter.

SCALES FOR DYSKINESIA IN PD

A summary review of each identified scale is given here. The complete reviews are available online at the Movement Disorders journal website.

Table 8-1. Descriptive Characteristics of the Scales

SCALE	TIME TO COMPLETE (MINUTES)	PATIENT HISTORICAL RATING	CLINICAL EXAMINATION	ADMINISTRATION BURDEN#
AIMS	15	No	Yes	+
UPDRS	20*	Yes	Yes	+
MDS-UPDRS	20*	Yes	Yes	+
Obeso (CAPIT)	2	Yes	Yes	+
Rush Dyskinesia Rating Scale	5	No	Yes	+
CDRS	10	No	Yes	+
Lang-Fahn	5	Yes	No	+
PDYS-26	10	Yes	No	+
UDysRS	15	Yes	Yes	+

AIMS, Abnormal Involuntary Movement Scale; *UPDRS*, Unified Parkinson's Disease Rating Scale; *MDS-UPDRS,* revised version of the *UPDRS; CDRS,* Clinical Dyskinesia Rating Scale; *PDYS-26,* Parkinson Disease Dyskinesia Scale; *UDysRS;* Unified Dyskinesia Rating Scale
#Administration burden was rated as: "+" (easy, e.g., summing up of the items), "±" (moderate, e.g., visual analogue scale [VAS] or simple formula), "-" (difficult, e.g., VAS in combination with formula, or complex formula), "?" (no information found on rating method).
*Time necessary to complete the whole scale.

AIMS: Abnormal Involuntary Movement Scale

SCALE DESCRIPTION

The AIMS is a clinician-rated instrument to assess the severity of abnormal movements in different parts of the body.[13] The AIMS consists of 10 items organized in a five-point Likert model. Each item is scored on a scale from 0 to 4 (*absent, minimal, mild, moderate, severe*), with higher scores indicating severer abnormal movements. Items 1 to 4 rate the presence and severity of abnormal movements in the face and mouth; items 5 and 6 rate the presence and severity of abnormal movements in the limbs; item 7 rates the presence and severity of abnormal movements in the trunk. The last three items rate, respectively, the global severity of the abnormal movements, the disability derived from the abnormal movements, and patient's awareness of the abnormal movement. The maximum score is 40. Two final points refer to dental hygiene and wearing of dentures.

The scale includes specific instructions to standardize the evaluation and requires the examiner to observe the patient sitting quietly at rest and again while carrying out selected motor tasks. The greatest severity of the abnormal movements is rated. If movements only occur upon activation procedures such as opening and closing of the mouth, finger tapping, standing and sitting, but are not seen spontaneously, the severity rating is ranked as one level lower than if the same intensity is seen spontaneously. The scale does not provide word-anchors to explain the ratings. The scale was originally developed for rating tardive dyskinesia in psychiatric patients (and this is the reason why AIMS is weighted on abnormal movements in the facial-oral-lingual area), but has been subsequently used for rating Huntington's disease– and PD-related dyskinesia. Modifications that exclude the one-point reduction caveat for movements seen only with activation, and exclude the dental questions, have also been used.

KEY EVALUATION ISSUES

AIMS has been used in several studies in PD patients to assess the benefit of medical[23] and surgical[24] procedures in the treatment of dyskinesia, and appears appropriate for responsiveness to an intervention. It therefore fits the criteria of wide usage by multiple authors. AIMS is an objective scale with 10 items, easily administered in about 10–15 minutes. Clinimetric data for AIMS rely mainly on inter- and intra-rater coefficients. In non-PD patients, the scale showed high inter-rater and test-retest reliability for tardive dyskinesia.[25,26] Others substantial clinimetric data (such as floor and ceiling effects, or concurrent validity) are not available. Only the original version of the scale has been assessed, but none of the modified versions of the scale have gone through validation procedures. It is only partially appropriate for dyskinesia in PD. The scale does not capture the phenomenology (dystonia versus other dyskinesia) of the involuntary movements. The clinimetric properties of the scale have been only partly tested in PD. In one study, the mean correlation coefficient (R) between two raters for total score was 0.81 (p < 0.01).[20] Internal consistency, concurrent validity, discrimination validity, and content validity have not been examined in this condition. A partial correlation was found between a modified AIMS version and accelerometric parameters of dyskinesia in PD[27]; however, there is no firm evidence that AIMS is able to detect change in dyskinesia severity across different stages of PD.

STRENGTHS AND WEAKNESSES

AIMS has been extensively used for many years to screen and rate the severity of abnormal involuntary movements in psychiatric patients. The scale is particularly valid for determining an overview of the anatomy of the involuntary movements. The scale also provides a total score for the presence of abnormal movements in the entire body. AIMS is a simple scale, sensitive to changes across patients. The administration of the scale is quick, and repetitive scores can be easily obtained.

AIMS does not capture the specific phenomenology of the movement that is observed, since all movements are merged during the rating. Furthermore, as AIMS was originally developed for the rating of tardive dyskinesia, it emphasizes ratings for movements in the facial-oral-lingual areas, and less for movements in the limbs and trunk, which are more frequently encountered in PD-related dyskinesia.[8] The motor-activation procedures do not reflect the activities of daily living, and it is difficult to determine the impact of the abnormal movement on the subject's life. This scale also does not give an estimate of the duration of dyskinesia during the day and of their patterns (peak-dose or diphasic). In addition, as AIMS was originally developed for the assessment of tardive dyskinesia, a number of modifications of the scale have been introduced by different authors for its use in PD. This has raised problems in the general clinimetric evaluation of the scale.

FINAL ASSESSMENT

AIMS formally fulfils the criteria for a "Recommended" scale (it has been applied to PD populations, there are data on its use beyond the group that developed the scale to rate dyskinesia in PD patients, and minimally sufficient clinimetric studies have been performed). In granting this rating, however, the MDS task force recognized that there have been a number of AIMS versions, and not all have been independently studied or assessed in this report. The designation of "recommended" is tempered by this caution, that different clinimetric properties may have been established with different versions. In addition, the most of the clinimetric data on AIMS come from other disorders than PD, and the overall structure of the scale has been designed to score other types of dyskinesia. Furthermore, although AIMS is also able to measure changes during treatment procedures, it does not allow for phenomenological differentiation between chorea, dystonia, and other forms of dyskinesia. As a final point, it does not allow the impact of dyskinesia on the quality of life of PD patients to be measured.

The Unified Parkinson's Disease Rating Scale (UPDRS)

SCALE DESCRIPTION

The UPDRS was developed by incorporating elements from previous PD scales to provide a comprehensive assessment of disability and impairment in this disease. The development of this scale involved multiple trial versions, and the final published scale is officially known as UPDRS Version 3.0.[14] The UPDRS is the most widely used rating scale for PD, in routine clinical practice and clinical trials.

UPDRS is clinician-rated and seeks to accurately measure the spectrum of PD severity. The scale consists of four subscales: (1) Part I, mental status, behavior, and mood; (2) Part II, activities of daily living, which may be scored in "on" or "off" states; (3) Part III, motor examination (this section produces 27 scores due to assessment of several signs in different parts of the body); and (4) Part IV, complications. Complications should be evaluated in the past week only. Part IV is further divided in three segments: a first segment (a) comprising four items for dyskinesia, including off dystonia, a second one (b) comprising four items for fluctuations, and a final one (c) comprising three items for other complications. Part IV(a) assesses historical information on dyskinesia duration (dividing the waking day into four segments, item 32) and an overall assessment of intensity (item 33). Items 34 and 35 look at the amount of painful dyskinesia and at the presence of early morning dystonia, respectively. UPDRS subscales are used at different frequencies, with those most often used being sections II and III.[6] Scoring of items in parts I, II, and III ranges from 0 to 4 (0 = normal, 4 = severe), while scoring of Part IV is irregular (with some items scoring from 0 to 4, while in others 0 = no and 1 = yes). Total subscale scores are 16 for Section I, 52 for Section II, 108 for Section III, and 23 for Section IV. Total scale score is 199.

KEY EVALUATION ISSUES

The UPDRS has been widely used by multiple authors. Of all the available PD rating scales, the UPDRS is the most thoroughly tested instrument from a clinimetric point of view, with most of the work dealing with parts II and III of the scale. In addition, a teaching videotape is available, standardizing the practical application of the scale and serving as an important tool to enhance inter-rater reliability.[28] Very little

clinimetric work has been specifically performed on the items dealing with dyskinesia.

STRENGTHS AND WEAKNESSES

The main strength of the Part IV of the scale is that it can be performed in the office, and the time required is very short. The UPDRS as a full scale includes good inter- and intra-rater reliability, but the individual or collective items covering dyskinesia have not been independently studied from a clinimetric perspective. The questions, however, capture symptoms over a defined period of time ("the past week") through historical questions that are clearly anchored. On the other hand, being based on just a few items, the scale provides a relatively limited or only a general assessment of the functional impact of dyskinesia. In addition, the impact of dyskinesia on specific abilities (working and social life) is not addressed.

FINAL ASSESSMENT

The UPDRS is "Suggested" as a rating scale for dyskinesia. Two out of three of the criteria are met (use in PD, and use by several investigators). Clinimetric studies are insufficient to meet the third criterion. Despite the identified weaknesses, the original UPDRS, specifically the items covering the disability due to dyskinesia and the amount of the waking day when dyskinesia is present, has been the primary outcome measure in recent clinical trials for anti-dyskinetic agents.[23]

The Movement Disorder Society revised Unified Parkinson's Disease Rating Scale (MDS-UPDRS)

SCALE DESCRIPTION

Because of relevant limitations present in the original UPDRS scale,[29] an ad hoc Task Force of the Movement Disorder Society (MDS) developed a revision of the UPDRS, termed the MDS-UPDRS. Its clinimetric assessment has been published, and the process of translation and validation from English to other languages is currently in an advanced stage.[12]

KEY EVALUATION ISSUES

The task force responsible for the new version of the UPDRS (The MDS-UDPRS) revised and expanded the scale using recommendations from the published critique, maintaining the same four-part structure as the original UPDRS: in particular, dyskinesias are still scored in Section IV, in two items only, 41 and 42. The first item is related to time spent with dyskinesia and is similar to item 32 in the old UPDRS, whereas for item 42 (functional impact of dyskinesia), MDS-UPDRS now provides written anchors in contrast to item 33 of the old UPDRS, which used only *"mild, moderate, severe,* and *marked"* definitions. In the factor structure analysis, involving over 800 cases, both MDS-UDPRS dyskinesia items are grouped as an independent factor in Part IV. Although utilized in PD and having strong clinimetric strengths, the dyskinesia component of the MDS-UPDRS has not yet been used in studies led by authors outside of the original developers.

STRENGTHS AND WEAKNESSES

The main strengths and weaknesses of Part IV of the new scale are similar to those mentioned for the original scale. However, the MDS-UPDRS is more clearly written, and the dyskinesia items comprise an established factor structure. Other clinimetric assessments have not been conducted on the dyskinesia section.

FINAL ASSESSMENT

At the current time, the MDS-UPDRS is also "Suggested." It meets two of the three criteria (use in PD and strong clinimetric testing); because it is new, it has not been used by groups other than the development team. In the near future, the designation is likely to be changed to "Recommended." In any case, MDS-UPDRS will be suitable for dyskinesia treatment trials only as a screening tool or as a secondary endpoint in combination with other, more specific and informative scales.

Obeso Dyskinesia Rating Scale (CAPIT)

SCALE DESCRIPTION

This is the first scale specifically developed to measure the severity of and screen for dyskinesia in PD. This scale combines the patient's historical assessments and the examiner's objective rating of dyskinesia. Disability is assessed using two categories of information: severity (0–5) and duration (0–5). These scores are combined to provide a single score based on the mean of the two subscores. The intensity score combines two clinical issues; namely, patient awareness of movements and the actual observed intensity of such movements. The duration score, similar to the UPDRS Part IV query on duration, divides the waking day into four segments.

KEY EVALUATION ISSUES

After its development, this scale was later included in the widely used Core Assessment Program for Intracerebral Transplantations (CAPIT) protocol for evaluation of patients undergoing neurosurgical interventions for PD.[15,16] This scale has not been subsequently explored from a clinimetric point of view. In the original description of the scale, there is no mention of training required, and only the English version is available.

STRENGTHS AND WEAKNESSES

The main strength of the scale is that it very easy to apply, being the arithmetic mean of just two numbers. Instructions to the rater are simple and clear, apart from the lack of indications about the time frame of dyskinesia evaluation. This short scale is probably suitable just for dyskinesia screening and prevalence studies and not for treatment trials.

FINAL ASSESSMENT

Obeso Dyskinesia Rating Scale has been applied to PD populations, and as a component of the CAPIT protocol it has been extensively used in the evaluation of dyskinesia. The scale lacks validation, however, and needs a careful assessment of its clinimetric properties. Therefore, it is designated as a "Suggested" scale.

Rush Dyskinesia Rating Scale

SCALE DESCRIPTION

The Rush dyskinesia scale[17] contains items derived from the Obeso Dyskinesia Rating Scale.[15,16] The scale assesses the disability severity of dyskinesia based on interference with three standardized motor tasks. The rater observes the patient walking, drinking from a cup, and putting on and buttoning a coat. The greatest degree to which dyskinesia interferes with function is rated on a 0 to 4 scale that includes descriptors (0, absent; 1, minimal severity, no interference with voluntary motor acts; 2, dyskinesia may impair voluntary movements but patient is normally capable of undertaking most motor acts; 3, intense interference with movement control, and daily life activities are greatly limited; 4, violent dyskinesia, incompatible with any normal motor task.) In addition, the rater indicates which types of dyskinesia (chorea, dystonia, other) are present, and which single type is most disabling.

In the original version, three activities were observed, and the highest rating of disability from any of the activities was entered as the score. Modifications have included separate scores for the three activities, and in the more recent Unified Dyskinesia Rating Scale (see below), which incorporates the Rush dyskinesia scale, communication has been added as a fourth task.

KEY EVALUATION ISSUES

This scale is specifically designed for PD and has been applied in many clinical trials beyond the original authors.[23,30] A videotape accompanies the original publication and demonstrates different degrees of severity, examples of chorea without dystonia, dystonia without chorea, and mixed dyskinesia. It included groups of 20 patients rated by 13 physicians and 15 study

coordinators.[17] After responses were returned, each rater evaluated a second tape with 70% repeat cases from the first tape and 30% new cases. Combined physician and coordinator ratings exhibited significant inter-rater and intra-rater reliability for severity of dyskinesia. Inter-rater reliability was higher for physicians than coordinators, but the difference was insignificant. Intra-rater consistency was high for the combined group ($r_{s+} = 0.855$, $p < 0.01$), and physicians were significantly more consistent than coordinators.

The scale also has been rated highly for its ease of application, appropriateness of tasks for reflecting disability, and overall utility. Clinimetric testing revealed relatively high inter- and intra-rater reliability.

STRENGTHS AND WEAKNESSES

The main strength of the scale is that it assesses functional disability of dyskinesia. The evaluation can be performed in the office and the time required is short (approximately five minutes).

In terms of weaknesses, assessments are performed at single time points, and the evaluation time point may or may not reflect the rest of the day. In addition, there is a lack of clear standardization of objects used in testing (cup, coat), and the assessment is usually performed in the office, where the patient may exhibit more or less dyskinesia than he normally does at home. The assessment is confined to an observer who rates motor disability during specified tasks and may not capture disability related to other tasks that are important to the patient. Furthermore, there is no consideration made for pain or discomfort the patient may experience from dyskinesia.

Another shortcoming is that the rater has to consider all types of dyskinesia when assessing interference with function. However, chorea is commonly a peak-dose phenomenon, whereas dystonia is often a wearing-off or "off" phenomenon. It is likely that if a patient has both types of dyskinesia, worsening of the less-disabling type of dyskinesia would not be captured when only the most disabling dyskinesia is rated. This may be particularly relevant in that an anti-dyskinesia medication might improve chorea, but worsen Parkinsonism and dystonia. Conversely, an anti-Parkinsonian medication might improve Parkinsonism and dystonia, but worsen chorea.

Although this scale exhibited good inter- and intra-rater reliability, based on raters viewing the same videotape segments, consistency might be much less during an actual on-site assessment, as raters might not evaluate the patient at exactly the same time, patients may feel more or less comfortable in a particular environment, and the objects that are used during the evaluation may differ in their ability to be manipulated. Thus the actual inter- and intra-rater reliability is not known. Furthermore, it was noted that the ratings were not compared to other scales, nor were they compared to patient self-ratings. Feedback from the coordinators and physicians seemed to indicate that it may not be easy to identify types of dyskinesia and the most disabling dyskinesia.

FINAL ASSESSMENT

Because the scale has been applied to PD populations, utilized extensively in clinical trials, and undergone some clinimetric testing, the Rush dyskinesia rating scale meets the criterion for a rating of "Recommended." It is a scale that assesses only disability and not impairment or patient perceptions, but within these limitations, it fulfils the task force criteria.

CLINICAL DYSKINESIA RATING SCALE (CDRS)

Scale description

Developed by the Swedish group in Lund, CDRS was first published in English in 1999.[18] The scale is in the public domain and was specifically developed for use in PD patients. CDRS independently evaluates hyperkinesia and dystonic posture, scored for each body region (face, neck, trunk, right and left upper extremities, right and left lower extremities). Scores range from 0 (none observed), to 4 (extreme), with use of 0.5-scoring intervals permitted for six items. The maximum total score for each subscale (dyskinesia and dystonia) is 28. Ratings are based on

patient observation at rest and during activation. Separate ratings exist for different body parts, including lateralization, as well as for dystonia and hyperkinesia; no estimate of disability is made, however. The scale was validated by different health care workers, several of whom lacked experience in formal clinical dyskinesia rating, and none of whom was familiar with the scale. Analyses of these ratings are discussed below. The scale is proposed as a screening tool and to measure dyskinesia severity during acute levodopa challenge testing, applicable during "on" and "off" conditions. The scale is appropriate for multiple assessments during a drug cycle. It appears easy to administer while performing standardized PD motor tests and is appropriate for use in the clinical setting or bedside. No instructions on its use are described.

KEY EVALUATION ISSUES

This scale is designed specifically for PD, but has not been used outside its developers. Clinimetrically, inter-rater reliability in PD patients was explored for different groups of raters (neurologists, neurosurgeons, and nurses who specialized in PD); several of them were inexperienced with formal dyskinesia rating, and none of the raters were familiar with the scale until they agreed to perform the ratings for this study. Authors wished to test the scale under conditions representative of the actual situation when a center is engaged in a multi-center clinical trial. CDRS proved excellent for hyperkinesia ($W = 0.88$) and moderate for dystonia ($W = 0.44$). Overall test-retest reliability was satisfactory (Kendall's tau = 0.74). Dystonia ratings had less concordance (with some Kendall tau coefficients as low as 0.31). It is valid across all disease stages, but the scale's sensitivity to change (over time or to treatment) has not been demonstrated.

Several scale properties were not evaluated in the original publication or subsequent studies. Content or criterion validity was not evaluated against a gold standard, nor was construct validity compared to that of other scales. No information on its use across different populations, or on potential differences between genders, was reported, nor was scale utility evaluated in PD patients suffering from dementia. Its properties in dyskinesia occurring in patients other than those with PD was not evaluated. The scale has not been translated and validated in languages other than English.

STRENGTHS AND WEAKNESSES

The CDRS shows an overall high level of reliability, both for individual raters, as well as between different raters assessing the same videotaped patient sequences. The CDRS is a useful tool for clinical evaluation of dyskinesia severity in PD. It also has an appropriate length for its use in clinical settings, and bedside. Nonetheless, it provides limited information, and relevant clinimetric properties remain unexplored.

FINAL ASSESSMENT

Based on the data as outlined above, the CDRS meets the following criteria: it has been used in PD and has some clinimetric testing, but it has not been subsequently used outside of the developing group. It is therefore classified as Suggested.

Lang-Fahn Activities of Daily Living Dyskinesia Scale

SCALE DESCRIPTION

The Lang-Fahn Activities of Daily Living Dyskinesia Scale is an attempt to capture disability that is often not manifested during a routine medical visit. An ordinal scale similar to the UPDRS is the basis for assessing five activities of daily living potentially impacted by dyskinesia at their maximum severity over the most recent few days (handwriting or drawing, cutting food and handling utensils, dressing, hygiene, and walking). Therefore, 0 is assigned for the absence of dyskinesia during the activity. Four is scored for the inability to perform the task independently or even with assistance, when the task is exceedingly difficult or impossible because of the dyskinesia.

The scale is completed by the physician based on historical information provided by the patient. Patients are asked to recall their functioning over the last few days and respond based on the worst interference by dyskinesia. Further information regarding the dyskinesia pattern such as diphasic, peak dose, or dystonia is not captured by the scale. Like other scales based on patients' declarations, it does not take into account that many patients will defer activities until dyskinesia resolves and, therefore, might state that dyskinesia is not disabling.

KEY EVALUATION ISSUES

This scale is specific for PD, but it has not been used widely in publications unrelated to the original authors. One study attempted validation of this scale.[19] Based on the clinical trial in which it was piloted, the Lang-Fahn ADL Dyskinesia Scale did not correlate with the modified Goetz Dyskinesia Rating Scale, had moderate correlation with the patient diary completed one week prior to the visit, and moderate correlation with the clinic assessment by patient and clinician using a Clinician's Global Impression and the Patient's Global Impression. The scale was used in two other studies, but further attempts to validate the scale, including test-retest reliability, have not occurred. The Lang-Fahn ADL Dyskinesia Scale as not been validated in other language, nor is it available in other languages. Therefore, some relevant clinimetric properties remain unexplored for this scale.[6]

STRENGTHS AND WEAKNESSES

The scale is quickly administered and training is not needed for its use. It is constructed on the logical idea of assessing five routine activities potentially influenced by dyskinesia. However, the scale is based on retrospective recall by the patient over the "last few days, the worst interference by dyskinesia," which may be rather vague. Also vague are qualitative words such as *substantial impairment* versus *definitely interfere with*—although there is a statement regarding getting help from others (scores 3 or higher). Furthermore, the scale may not be used to differentiate off and on dyskinesia, and no quality of life assessment of the impact of dyskinesia is provided.

FINAL ASSESSMENT

Despite the weaknesses as outlined above, the Lang-Fahn Activities of Daily Living Scale was applied in PD patients, and some clinimetric studies have been carried out. However, since it has not been used extensively by other groups outside the Parkinson Study Group in North America,[31,32] the Lang-Fahn Scale should be classified as "Suggested" (but weakly so, because of the relatively limited clinimetric data).

Parkinson Disease Dyskinesia Scale (PDYS-26)

SCALE DESCRIPTION

The Parkinson Disease Dyskinesia Scale (PDYS-26)[20] is a 26-item, patient-based measure "for quantifying the impact of dyskinesia on activities of daily living" in PD. Items include basic, instrumental, and social daily activities. The question for each item is about interference by involuntary movements (when they are at their worst) with those activities. Time frame is based on patient recall, and is relatively short (one week) but appropriate. There are five response options per item, scored from 0 (*Not at all*) to 4 (*Activity impossible*). A total score is calculated through the sum of the items' scores (0 to 104).

In the instructions, *dyskinesia* is equaled to "involuntary movements," but some abnormal movements (tremor, dystonia) are excluded. Therefore, the scale assesses choreic dyskinesia.

KEY EVALUATION ISSUES

This scale is specifically designed to assess PD. As a relatively new scale, it has not been widely used, but it may well be incorporated into assessments in the near future. The scale was developed following item response theory (Rasch analysis) principles and methodology. Later, it was validated by means of Rasch analysis, again, and also

applying classical test theory methods. There is only one study (for the original article, see endnote 20) on the psychometric properties of the scale. PDYS-26 has satisfactory acceptability, with no floor or ceiling effect (although neither standard nor observed values are given) and an appropriate distribution of scores. The internal consistency was very high (alpha = 0.97), perhaps related to redundancy, and the item homogeneity coefficient resulted satisfactory (0.59). The test-retest reliability was excellent (for the total score, ICC = 0.92). Concerning the convergent construct validity, PDYS-26 showed strong correlation with the UPDRS[14] items 32 through 34 (R = 0.56–0.71; for the total of these items, R = 0.78). Correlation was moderate to high with items of the Rush Dyskinesia Rating Scale (R = 0.36–0.78) and variable with the components of the AIMS (R = 0.20–0.84). Factor analysis identified a single factor, explaining 58% of the variance.

STRENGTHS AND WEAKNESSES

It is a specific scale for PD patients with dyskinesia. The clinimetric properties of the scale are satisfactory by both methodological approaches.[20] Therefore, the scale is considered a consistent, reliable, and valid measure for assessing the perceived impact of dyskinesia on the ability to carry out daily activities. PDYS-26 is easy to complete, its instructions to patients are concise and clear, and it possesses good acceptability. A particular advantage is its relatively short administration time. One disadvantage is the potential redundancy of some items addressing similar modalities of dyskinesia activation. In addition, the impact of dyskinesia on functional ability for working and hobbies is not specifically addressed. Also, there is no information about PDYS-26 responsiveness and minimal clinically important change at the present time. The task force originally classified the PDYS-26 as "Suggested," since this new scale had not been studied by other groups independent of the investigators who participated in its development. The scale has been used in an additional study by a team led by investigators other than the original developers.[21] The situation has further evolved, since PDYS-26 has been utilized as a functional scale in a multi-center study recently completed, but not yet published (A. Evans and R. Katzenschlager, personal communication). This is a phase II Santhera study with fipamezole, an adrenergic antagonist, as an oromucosal fast-dissolving formulation in combination with levodopa (Study ID Number: SNT-II-004).

FINAL ASSESSMENT

PDYS-26 is "recommended" as a measure for assessing the patient's perception of functional impact from dyskinesia in PD. It has been used in PD and is clinimetrically valid and reliable. Sensitivity to change has not been studied.

The Unified Dyskinesia Rating Scale (UDysRS)

SCALE DESCRIPTION

The Unified Dyskinesia Rating Scale (UDysRS) is a newest rating scale developed specifically for the assessment of dyskinesia in PD.[22] The UDysRS contains both self-evaluation questions (by the patient alone or with their caregivers) and items that are assessed directly by the physician, to objectively rate the abnormal movements associated with PD. The time frame for rating of dyskinesia refers to the prior week (including the day on which the examination is performed). The UDysRS consists of two primary sections ("Historical" and "Objective"); each section is divided into two parts. All parts consist of several items, and each item is scored on a scale from 0 to 4 in a Likert model (0 = normal, to 4 = severe). The total score of the UDysRS ranges form 0 to 104. These are Part I: Historical Disability or patients' perception of On-dyskinesia impact (11 items, maximum score 44); Part II: Historical Disability or patients' perception of Off-dystonia impact (4 items, maximum score 16). In both historical parts, one item (number 1 in Part I and 12 in Part II) is obtained by the rater assisting the patient/caregiver in giving the answer. The second primary section consists of Part III:

Objective Impairment with rating of dyskinesia severity, type of movement (dyskinetic or dystonic), anatomical distribution over seven body regions; the objective evaluation is based on the observation of patients performing four motor tasks: communication, drinking from a cup, dressing, ambulation (7 items, maximum score 28); and Part IV: Disability Scale. The rating is based on the activities performed by the patient in part III (4 items, maximum score 16). The highest value for each body part reflects the impact of dyskinesia on whichever function is rated. The scale provides specific instructions for all questions and comes with a teaching DVD including a certification exercise.[33] This training program, based on various examples of dyskinesia and anchored in scores generated by experts, is aimed at increasing homogeneity of ratings among and within raters and centers.

KEY EVALUATION ISSUES

This scale is designed specifically for PD-associated dyskinesia. Although new, it is already a part of numerous clinical trials of new, putative anti-dyskinesia agents. Internal consistency, factor structure, and reproducibility of the scale were determined in 70 PD patients. Twenty international movement disorder experts participated in the study (for complete methodology see Goetz et al., endnote 22). Inter- and intra-rater reliability scores were calculated for all parts and sections of the scale. In summary, the inter-rater reliability for impairment and disability ranged from fair (kappa 0.4 to 0.59) to very good (kappa ≥ 0.8). The inter-rater reliability for the total score was very good (kappa 0.89). Intra-rater reliability also ranged from fair (kappa 0.4 to 0.59) to very good (kappa > 0.8) for both impairment and disability. The intra-rater reliability for the total score was also very good (kappa 0.90). The UDysRS showed high internal consistency for both the subjective (Cronbach's alpha = 0.92) and objective rating sections (Cronbach's alpha = 0.97). At the moment the scale is available only in English and has not been translated into other languages.

STRENGTHS AND WEAKNESSES

The UdysRS is a comprehensive rating tool that captures patient perceptions, time factor of dyskinesia, anatomical distribution, phenomenology (dystonia versus other dyskinesias), objective impairment, severity, and disability of dyskinesia and dystonia in PD. The tested clinimetric properties of the scale range are excellent. The objective components of the scale, which could be used for frequent ratings during studies involving treatment, also have very good inter- and intra-rater reliability. The motor activation procedures reflect the activities of daily living and provide a global score to reflect the impact of the abnormal movement on the subject's life. The scale has not been evaluated for responsiveness, and has not been used by other groups beside the researchers involved in its development. Convergent validity, discrimination validity, and content validity have not been examined either.

The task force originally classified the UdysRS as "Suggested," since this new scale had not been studied by other groups independent of investigators who participated in its development. The situation has now evolved, since a phase II study investigating the antidyskinetic efficacy of safinamide, a drug with both monoamine oxidase B–inhibiting and anti-glutamatergic properties (sponsored by Merck-Serono), has used this scale, though the results are not yet published (F. Stocchi, personal communication). In addition, two other ongoing studies—a trial with pardoprunox, a new partial dopamine agonist, as an adjunct therapy to levodopa in the treatment of patients with advanced PD and dyskinesia (sponsored by Solvay), and the phase I/II ProSavin* study investigating the use of a new gene-based treatment in advanced PD using a viral vector (sponsored by Oxford Biomedica)— are also using the scale.

FINAL ASSESSMENT

The newest scale to be developed, the UdysRS may now be changed from the suggested status to recommended to rate dyskinesia in PD patients. It has been applied to PD populations, studied clinimetrically as both a consistent and reliable measure, and used by a few international groups. The scale has not however been fully tested to measure its sensitivity to changes.

CONCLUSIONS AND RECOMMENDATIONS

There are several critical problems in developing valid scales to score drug-induced dyskinesia in PD. Firstly, assessment of dyskinesia in PD may be based on objective scoring by the physician or on subjective evaluation (based on patient or caregiver interview), and both the choices have some critical limitations. Objective assessment is limited to a specific point in time when the patient is assessed by the examiner. On the other hand, subjective scoring (based on patient interview) is based on the patient's personal impression and therefore more reflective of the overall dyskinesia burden during the day, but is prone to bias (related to the mood and cognitive status of the patients). A selective reduction of awareness of dyskinesia appearing during the on state is also well-described.[34] In addition, it may be difficult to distinguish dyskinesia from Parkinsonian tremor for the inexperienced examiner, and this is even more of a challenge for the patient. This common mistake may significantly affect the score and the overall evaluation of the disability related to dyskinesia.

An ideal scale for dyskinesia should capture patient perceptions, time factors of dyskinesia, anatomical distribution, objective impairment, and disability. At present four of the reviewed dyskinesia scales (AIMS, Rush Dyskinesia Rating Scale, PDYS-26, and UDysRS) can be recommended for use (Table 8-2). Notwithstanding, in all cases there are specific limitations already mentioned in the description of the scales. Basic clinimetric information is missing for some of the remaining scales. The two more recent scales (PDYS-26 and UDysRS), which have been specifically developed and applied to PD populations with dyskinesia, both have excellent clinimetric properties and appear to provide a reliable and valid assessment of dyskinesia in PD. The wide use of PDYS-26 and UDysRS in future clinical trials will better tell us whether they are reliable and

Table 8-2. Overview of the Scales Assessed and their Classification

SCALE	APPLIED IN PD	APPLIED BEYOND ORIGINAL AUTHORS	SUCCESSFUL CLINIMETRIC TESTING	QUALIFICATION
AIMS	X	X	X*	Recommended
UPDRS	X	X	0**	Suggested
Obeso (CAPIT)	X	X	0	Suggested
Rush Dyskinesia Rating Scale	X	X	X	Recommended
CDRS	X	0	X	Suggested
Lang-Fahn	X	0	X	Suggested
PDYS-26	X	X	X	Suggested
UDysRS	X	X	X	Recommended

For an explanation of the qualification groups: see text.

AIMS, Abnormal Involuntary Movement Scale; *UPDRS*, Unified Parkinson's Disease Rating Scale; *CDRS*, Clinical Dyskinesia Rating Scale; *PDYS-26*, Parkinson Disease Dyskinesia Scale; *UDysRS*; Unified Dyskinesia Rating Scale

*AIMS has several modified versions and it is not entirely clear whether clinimetric analyses are uniform across all versions.

** Clinimetric testing not performed specifically on the part IV.

easy-to-use rating instruments in routine clinical research. As a matter of fact, the PDYS-26, which is a patient-derived scale generating linear measurements, could well complement dyskinesia measures, mainly (even if not exclusively) clinician-based, such as the UDysRS. Since further testing of these scales in PD is warranted, no new scales are needed until PDYS-26 and UDysRS are fully tested clinimetrically.

RECOMMENDED SCALES
AIMS
RUSH DYSKINESIA RATING SCALE
PDYS-26
UDysRS

Acknowledgments

The author would like to thank the following members of the MDS Task force on scales to assess dyskinesia in Parkinson's disease: Pablo Martínez-Martín, MD (Madrid, Spain); Giovanni Fabbrini, MD (Rome, Italy); Robert A. Hauser, MD (Tampa, FL, USA); Marcelo Merello, MD, PhD (Buenos Aires, Argentina); Janis Miyasaki, MD (Toronto, Canada); Werner Poewe, MD (Innsbruck, Austria); Cristina Sampaio, MD (Lisbon, Portugal); Olivier Rascol, MD (Toulouse, France); Glenn T. Stebbins, PhD (Chicago, IL, USA); Anette Schrag, MD, PhD (London, UK); and Christopher G. Goetz, MD (Chicago. IL, USA).

References

1. Colosimo C, Martínez-Martín P, Fabbrini G, et al. Task force report on scales to assess dyskinesia in Parkinson's disease: critique and recommendations. *Mov Disord.* 2010;25:1131–1142.
2. Marsden CD, Parkes JD, Quinn N. Fluctuations and disability in Parkinson's disease: clinical aspects. In: Marsden CD, Fahn S, eds. *Movement Disorders.* vol. 2. London: Butterworth; 1982:96–105.
3. Fabbrini G, Brotchie JM, Grandas F, Nomoto M, Goetz CG. Levodopa-induced dyskinesias. *Mov Disord.* 2007;22:1379–1389.
4. Mones RJ, Elizan TS, Siegel GJ. Analysis of L-dopa induced dyskinesias in 51 patients with Parkinsonism. *J Neurol Neurosurg Psychiatry.* 1971;34:668–673.
5. Fabbrini G, Defazio G, Colosimo C, Suppa A, Bloise M, Berardelli A. Onset and spread of

dyskinesias and motor symptoms in Parkinson's disease. *Mov Disord.* 2009;24:2091–2096.

6. Martinez-Martin P, Cubo E. Scales to measure Parkinsonism. *Handb Clin Neurol.* 2007;83:289–327.

7. Colosimo C, Fabbrini G, Berardelli A. Drug insight: new drugs in development for Parkinson's disease. *Nat Clin Pract Neurol.* 2006;2:600–610.

8. Goetz CG. Rating scales for dyskinesias in Parkinson's disease. *Mov Disord.* 1999;14 (suppl 1):48–53.

9. Schrag A, Barone P, Brown RG, et al. Depression rating scales in Parkinson's disease: critique and recommendations. *Mov Disord.* 2007;22:1077–1092.

10. Fernandez HH, Aarsland D, Fenelon G, et al. Scales to assess psychosis in Parkinson's disease: critique and recommendations. *Mov Disord.* 2008;23:484–500.

11. Leentjens AFG, Dujardin K, Marsh L, et al. Anxiety rating scales in Parkinson's disease: critique and recommendations. *Mov Disord.* 2008;23:2015–2023.

12. Goetz CG, Tilley BC, Shaftman SR, et al. Movement Disorder Society-sponsored revision of the Unified Parkinson's Disease Rating Scale (MDS-UPDRS): scale presentation and clinimetric testing results. *Mov Disord.* 2008;23:2129–2170.

13. Guy W. *Abnormal Involuntary Movement Scale. ECDEU Assessment Manual for Psychopharmacology.* Washington, DC: US Government Printing Office; 1976:534–537.

14. Fahn S, Elton RL, Members of the UPDRS Development Committee. Unified Parkinson's Disease Rating Scale. In: Fahn S, Marsden CD, Calne DB, Goldstein M, eds. *Recent Development in Parkinson's Disease.* vol. 2. Florham Park, NJ: MacMillan Healthcare Information; 1987:153–163.

15. Langston JW, Widner H, Goetz CG, et al. Core assessment program for intracerebral transplantation (CAPIT). In: Lindvall O, Bjorkland A, Widner H, eds. *Intracerebral Transplantation in Movement Disorders.* Amsterdam, The Netherlands: Elsevier; 1991:227–241.

16. Langston JW, Widner H, Goetz CG, Brooks D, Fahn S, Freeman T. Core assessment program for intracerebral transplantations (CAPIT). *Mov Disord.* 1992;7:2–13.

17. Goetz CG, Stebbins GT, Shale HM, et al. Utility of an objective dyskinesia rating scale for Parkinson's disease: inter- and intrarater reliability assessment. *Mov Disord.* 1994;9:390–394.

18. Hagell P, Widner H. Clinical rating of dyskinesias in Parkinson's disease: utility and reliability of a new rating scale. *Mov Disord.* 1999;14:448–455.

19. Parkinson Study Group. Evaluation of dyskinesias in a pilot, randomized, placebo-controlled trial of remacemide in advanced Parkinson's disease. *Arch Neurol.* 2001;58:1660–1668.

20. Katzenschlager R, Schrag A, Evans A, et al. Quantifying the impact of dyskinesias in PD. The PDYS-26: a patient-based outcome measure. *Neurology.* 2007;69:555–563.

21. Carroll CB, Bain PG, Teare L, et al. Cannabis for dyskinesia in Parkinson's disease: a randomized double-blind crossover study. *Neurology.* 2004;63:1245–1250.

22. Goetz CG, Nutt JG, Stebbins GT. The unified dyskinesias rating scale: presentation and clinimetric profile. *Mov Disord.* 2008;23:2398–2403.

23. Hauser RA, Deckers F, Lehert P. Parkinson's disease home diary: further validation and implications for clinical trials. *Mov Disord.* 2004;19:1409–1413.

24. Goetz CG, Damier P, Hicking C, et al. Sarizotan as a treatment for dyskinesias in Parkinson's disease: a double-blind placebo-controlled trial. *Mov Disord.* 2007;22:179–186.

25. Rodrigues JP, Walters SE, Watson P, Stell R, Mastaglia FL. Globus pallidus stimulation improves both motor and nonmotor aspects of quality of life in advanced Parkinson's disease. *Mov Disord.* 2007;22:1866–1870.

26. Whall AL, Engle V, Edward A, Bobel L, Haberland C. Development of a screening program for tardive dyskinesias: feasibility issue. *Nurs Res.* 1983;32:151–156.

27. Sweet RA, DeSensi EG, Zubenko GS. Reliability and applicability of movement disorders rating scales in the elderly. *J Neuropsychiatry Clin Neurosci.* 1993;5:56–60.

28. Hoff JI, van den Plas AA, Wagemans EAH, van Hilten JJ. Accelerometric assessment of levodopa-induced dyskinesias in Parkinson's disease. *Mov Disord.* 2001;16:58–61.

29. Goetz CG, Stebbins GT, Chmura TA, et al. Teaching tape for the motor section of the Unified Parkinson's Disease Rating Scale. *Mov Disord.* 1995;10:263–266.

30. Movement Disorder Society Task Force on Rating Scales for Parkinson's Disease. The Unified Parkinson's Disease Rating Scale

(UPDRS): status and recommendations. *Mov Disord.* 2003;18:738–750.

31. Fahn S, Oakes D, Shoulson I, et al. Levodopa and the progression of Parkinson's disease. *N Engl J Med.* 2004;351:2498–2508.

32. Holloway RG, Shoulson I, Fahn S, et al. Pramipexole vs levodopa as initial treatment for Parkinson disease: a 4-year randomized controlled trial. *Arch Neurol.* 2004;61:1044–1053.

33. Goetz CG, Nutt JG, Stebbins GT, Chmura TA. Teaching program for the Unified Dyskinesia Rating Scale. *Mov Disord.* 2009;24:1296–1298.

34. Amanzio M, Monteverdi S, Giordano A, Soliveri P, Filippi P, Geminiani G. Impaired awareness of movement disorders in Parkinson's disease. *Brain Cogn.* 2010;72: 337–346.

9

EVALUATION OF MOTOR COMPLICATIONS: MOTOR FLUCTUATIONS

Marcelo Merello and Angelo Antonini

Summary

With disease progression and higher L-dopa dose requirements, the vast majority of patients start to experience reduced and variable responses to medication, known as *motor fluctuations*. A series of scales has been identified in the medical literature that are designed to measure motor fluctuations. Unfortunately, clinimetric properties of the majority of these scales, questionnaires, and diaries have not been analyzed in depth, or have achieved poor results. In this chapter, we will describe scales, questionnaires, and diaries evaluating motor fluctuations and review their validity, pros, cons, and recommendations for use. Following the guidelines set by the Movement Disorder Task Force on PD Rating Scales, "Recommended" scales are the Wearing OFF-19 and Wearing OFF-9 questionnaires and the Hauser Parkinson's Disease Diary and the CAPSIT-PD ON-OFF Diary. Whereas the MDS-UPDRS shows promise, it has not been sufficiently used in published studies to reach this designation; it will probably be recommended in the future.

INTRODUCTION

With disease progression and higher L-dopa dose requirement, the vast majority of patients start to experience reduced and variable responses to medication; these responses are termed *motor fluctuations*. The most common fluctuations to emerge in advanced PD are a relatively shortened response to a given dose of medication, with waning of benefit near the end of a dose cycle, termed "wearing off." Also, a slow onset of action can occur, so that a patient takes a dose of medication, but a prolonged period of time elapses before benefit occurs. Occasionally, sudden changes in function occur over minutes or even seconds, and in these cases, patients change from a high-functioning state to a sudden poor response of bradykinesia, rigidity, tremor, and gait abnormalities.[2] Motor fluctuations can also occur spontaneously as part of the disease and not necessarily be related to long-term levodopa therapy. There is often diurnal variation in symptoms, with improvement in the morning and deterioration through the day.[3] Table 9-1 displays the most common forms of motor fluctuations.

Measuring motor fluctuations is challenging because of the number of potentially important aspects involved: frequency, intensity, predictability, phenomenology, and impact on the quality of life. Measurement usually relies to at least some degree on a patient's understanding and awareness of these phenomena, because many measurement tools are anchored in self-report. Also, because they are transient and often cannot be observed directly by the health professional, they may frequently go unrecognized by physicians during their early stages.

Instrumental methods to identify and measure motor fluctuations have been attempted, but results to date have been disappointing.[4] There are three general classes of instruments: rating scales that are anchored in the physician's interview of the patient, questionnaires that are self-report forms, and home-based diaries that track a patient's status throughout the day, usually in 30-minute intervals.

A large number of scales designed to measure Parkinsonian impairment and disabilities have been published in the medical literature, including: three impairment scales (Webster, Columbia University Rating Scale [CURS] and Parkinson's Disease Impairment Scale); four disability scales (Schwab and England, Northwestern University Disability Scale [NUDS], Intermediate Scale for Assessment of PD [ISAPD], and Extensive Disability Scale); six scales evaluating both impairment and disability (New York University ;University of California–Los Angeles Larsen Scale or Assessment of Parkinson's Disease Scale [APDS]); Unified Parkinson's Disease Rating Scale [UPDRS]; Short Parkinson Evaluation Scale; SCOPA MOTOR and MDS-UPDRS. Of these, the

Table 9-1. Motor Fluctuations

1. Early morning akinesia.
2. Wearing-off.
3. ON-OFF.
4. Beginning of dose motor deterioration.
5. End of dose motor deterioration.
6. Sleep benefit.
7. Diurnal fluctuations.
8. Paradoxical kinesis.
7. Yo-yoing.

APDS,[5] ISAPD,[6] UPDRS,[7] MDS-UPDRS,[8] and SPES-SCOPA[9] are the only ones specifically evaluating motor fluctuations. These scales rely on historical information based on the physician's interpretation of patient recall and understanding of terminology.

A number of questionnaires that focus on motor fluctuation detection have also been published, and although they were not designed to rank severity and only identify the presence of motor fluctuation symptoms, they are widely used. These include the 32-item Stacy questionnaire, termed the WOQ-32[10] and the abbreviated forms, the QUICK or WOQ-19,[10] and WOQ-9[11] questionnaires.

Finally, one of the most frequently used tools for monitoring motor fluctuations both in clinical practice and in research is a self-report home diary that is completed by patients or caregivers over a 24-hour period.[12] Home diaries have taken a number of different formats and are anchored in various educational techniques to train patients before application. These scales offer a quantification of the hours in a given day when the patient's medications are working well and Parkinsonism is under good control (ON) and when the patient's medications are not working well (OFF). Dyskinesias (see Chapter 8) are also assessed with this type of tool. This chapter focuses on scales, questionnaires, and diaries available for motor fluctuations evaluation, reviewing their validity, pros, cons, and recommendations for use.

From the outset, it is important to clarify that the primary focus of most motor fluctuation evaluations is "wearing off," which is only one form of motor fluctuation. Whereas sudden ON/OFF, delayed onset of medication effects, and other forms of motor fluctuation occur, they are less frequent. Where appropriate, the discussion will highlight the major aspects of motor fluctuations that have been the studied with each assessment tool. A further important point is that motor fluctuations often occur in the context of involuntary movements, termed *dyskinesias*, both choreic and dystonic. A separate chapter (Chapter 8) will examine the utility of scales for detecting dyskinesia, and this discussion deals with motor fluctuations only.

METHODOLOGY

The core work related to this chapter followed the program to rate scales developed by the Movement Disorder Task Force on PD Rating Scales.[13] In this effort, teams were organized with specialization in a given area of PD disability or impairment, and the literature was searched by electronic search engines and with the knowledge base of the task force members. There are two official definitions for the final conclusions on a given scale. It is "Recommended" if it has been applied to PD populations, if there are data on its use in studies beyond the group that developed the scale, and if it has been studied clinimetrically with at least minimally adequate studies on validity, reliability, and sensitivity to change. A scale is considered "Suggested" if it has been applied to PD populations, but only one of the other criteria applies.

SCALES (SEE TABLES 9-2 TO 9-4)

Assessment of Parkinson's Disease Scale

STRUCTURE

This was the first scale developed to deal with motor complications arising as a result of therapy. It was developed with the aim of assessing a patient's condition over an extended period of time, taking into account motor condition and dyskinesia fluctuation.[5]

The scale assesses daily activities, dyskinesias, wearing off, and on-off (considered together) and confusion. Daily activities (dressing, feeding, hygiene, turning in bed, and walking) are ranked based on two conditions, patient best and patient worst performance scale (0, *normal*) (4, *completely unable*). Wearing off and on-off conditions are not evaluated separately,

Table 9-2. Key Evaluation Points of the Scales

SCALE	APPLIED IN PD	APPLIED BEYOND ORIGINAL AUTHORS	SUCCESSFUL CLINIMETRIC TESTING	QUALIFICATION
APDS	x			Listed
ISAPD	x			Listed
UPDRS	x	x		Suggested
S-MS	x		x	Suggested
MDS-UPDRS	x		x	Suggested
TRS	x			Listed
WOQ-32	x	x		Suggested
WOQ-19, QQ-WOQ	x	x	x	Recommended
WOQ-9	x	x	x	Recommended
Hauser Diary	x	x	x	Recommended
CAPSIT-PD Diary	x	x	x	Recommended

APDS: Assessment of Parkinson's Disease Scale. ISAPD: Intermediate Scale for Assessment of PD. UPDRS: Unified Parkinson's Disease Rating Scale. S-MS: SCOPA Motor Scale. MDS-UPDRS: Movement Disorders Society version of the Unified Parkinson's Disease Scale. WOQ-32: Wearing-off Questionnaire 32. WOQ-19 or QQ-WOQ: QUICK questionnaire for wearing off detection. WOQ-9: Wearing-off Questionnaire 9 questions. Hauser Diary is the Parkinson's Disease Diary. CAPSIT-PD Diary is the Core Assessment Program for Surgical Interventional Therapies in Parkinson's Disease ON-OFF Diary. TRS: the Treatment Response Scale;.

Table 9-3. Main Characteristics of Scales Evaluating Motor Fluctuations*

	APDS	ISAPD	UPDRS	S-MS	MDS-UPDRS	TRS
Structure	0–4/1–4/open	0–4	0–4/yes-no	0–3	0–4	0–3/0–5
Comorbidities	Affected	NE	NE	NE	NE	NE
Use in unselected populations	No	No	Yes	NE	NE	NE
Used by multiple authors	No	Yes	Yes	Yes	No	No
Reliability	NE	Good	NE	High	Highest	NE
Validity	NE	Good	NE	High	Highest	NE
Responsiveness	NE	NE	NE	NE	NE	NE
MCRD/MCRID	NE	Good	NE	NE	NE	NE

APDS: Assessment of Parkinson's Disease Scale. ISAPD: Intermediate Scale for Assessment of PD. UPDRS: Unified Parkinson's Disease Rating Scale. S-MS: SCOPA Motor Scale. TRS: the Treatment Response Scale. MDS-UPDRS: Movement Disorders Society version of the Unified Parkinson's Disease Scale. MCRD/MCRID: Minimal clinical relevant difference and minimal clinical relevant incremental difference. NE: not evaluated.

but ranked on a 1 to 4 scale for frequency and for duration. For frequency, 1 is once a day, and 4 is more than 10 a day. With respect to attack duration, 1 means between 0 and 30 minutes, and 4 means more than 2 hours.

KEY EVALUATION ISSUES

The scale was designed to evaluate patient status over a reasonably long period of time, between seven and 14 days. It can be administered by nurses and physicians, and the assessment can be completed in ten minutes. Clinimetric properties of the scale have not been evaluated, and its use by authors other than the developers has been limited. There is no information on the clinimetric behavior of the scale in unselected PD populations, nor on the minimal clinical relevant difference or the minimal clinical relevant incremental difference.

Table 9-4. Strengths and Weaknesses of Scales Evaluating Motor Fluctuations

	STRENGTH	WEAKNESS
APDS	First attempt to evaluate motor fluctuations.	Serious problems with the structure.
ISAPD	Good structure.	Not in generalized use.
UPDRS	Generalized use.	Structure of Section IV is different from the rest of the scale.
S-MS	Good structure.	Ceiling and floor effects of motor complication section.
MDS-UPDRS	Planned under a strict revision of previous version to address the shortcomings of the predecessors.	New, not in generalized use yet.
TRS	Simple to use.	Not designed to assess specifically wearing-off but rather to grade changes in motor conditions.

APDS: Assessment of Parkinson's disease scale. ISAPD: Intermediate Scale for Assessment of PD. UPDRS: Unified Parkinson's Disease Rating Scale. S-MS: SCOPA Motor Scale. MDS-UPDRS: Movement Disorders Society version of the Unified Parkinson's Disease Scale. TRS: the Treatment Response Scale.

STRENGTHS AND WEAKNESSES

The possibility of ranking activities of daily living at their best and at their worst is a very nice introduction to the study of disabilities of off periods, as well as of quality of on periods. The lack of separation between on/off and wearing-off, treatment of the condition as a single phenomenon, and inconsistency in scale range with 0–4 and 1–4 points available for different items, as well as the impossibility of a 0 score for wearing-off and on-off phenomena, are all serious shortcomings of this scale with respect to generating a total score. Furthermore, the scale requires open comments from the evaluator. Although the scale can be used through all disease stages, item confusion might be affected by comorbidities.

FINAL ASSESSMENT

In conclusion, this scale was a very important first step toward the development of a tool for evaluating motor complications. However, important limitations have now been overcome by its successors. Therefore, this scale is ranked as "Listed," because it has not been used by substantially by investigators outside the developers, and the clinimetric profile is ill-defined.

Intermediate Scale for Assessment of PD (ISAPD)

STRUCTURE

The ISAPD was designed in 1987[6] applying a statistical procedure to the selection of items, based on the Northwestern University Disability Scale,[14] the UCLA-Cornell Scale,[15] and the Webster Scale.[16] In a modification of the methods section as proposed by Lieberman et al.[17] and Larsen et al.,[5] a subscale for the evaluation of complications of therapy (dyskinesias and fluctuations) was included. The research objective was "to develop a relatively short, functional and valid scale to form a standard nucleus for future clinical trials or to be applied in daily practice."[18] It was designed to be used only in PD patients. The ISAPD is a rapid scale for use in daily practice and research.[19] It comprises 11 items, scored from 0 (*normal*) to 3 (*severe*) by interview, and two items requiring examination (total, 13 items), and is geared mainly to the evaluation of functional aspects. In addition, it includes a four-item subscale for the assessment of motor complications (dyskinesias and fluctuations).

KEY EVALUATION ISSUES

The psychometric properties of the ISAPD as a global scale have been found to be satisfactory,[20-23] displaying adequate reliability and validity for the assessment of disability.[20] However, "complications of therapy" items were only used for evaluating construct validity, and were excluded from the evaluation of the other parameters. Furthermore, no analyses have focused specifically on motor fluctuations. The motor fluctuation component of the scale has not been used by multiple authors.

STRENGTHS AND WEAKNESSES

The psychometric properties of the ISAPD as a global scale have been found to be satisfactory; therefore the scale appears to be a valid instrument to assess functional state in PD patients in simple and rapid fashion. Nevertheless, for motor fluctuations, with only four questions that combine motor fluctuations with dyskinesia, it cannot be considered a substantive scale for motor fluctuations.

FINAL ASSESSMENT

For motor fluctuations, the ISAPD is ranked as "Listed," because it has not been substantially used by investigators other than its developers, and because the clinimetric properties of the motor fluctuation component are not established.

Unified Parkinson's Disease Rating Scale (UPDRS)

STRUCTURE

The Unified Parkinson's Disease Rating Scale (UPDRS) was developed by a Development Committee in 1984[7] and since then has become the most widely used rating scale for PD for many authors in different languages. UPDRS assessments have been used as primary outcome measures in studies of clinical correlates of PD, during use of novel therapeutics in PD, and for diagnostic classification systems. Section IV is constructed differently than the rest of the UPDRS, with a mixture of five-point options and dichotomous (yes/no) ratings that are difficult to analyze together. For motor fluctuation evaluation, UPDRS Part IV has questions that estimate the amount of time spent with poor medication response and the types of off-function, whether predictable, unpredictable, gradual in onset, or sudden.

KEY EVALUATION ISSUES

The average time required to apply the complete version is 17 minutes. Clinimetric properties of activities of daily living as well as of motor sections of the UPDRS have been studied extensively, but very little work has focused on Part IV (complications of therapy) where motor fluctuations are assessed. The scale has been widely used by the movement disorder community.

STRENGTHS AND WEAKNESSES

MDS Task Force members who evaluated the scale considered these items insufficient to assess severity of impairment or disability related to non-motor domains of PD, to the point that most studies of patients with motor fluctuations have used self-scoring on-off diaries, and not this part of the scale.[24]

FINAL ASSESSMENT

In conclusion, UPDRS is a multidimensional, reliable, and valid scale, with some drawbacks derived from its internal consistency, discriminant validity, and pragmatic application. The UPDRS ADL and motor sections are widely used, so much so that it is considered today the gold standard. Nevertheless, Complication of Therapy Section IV presents structural drawbacks and lacks proper validation. Because it has been widely used by investigators and clinicians, it receives the classification of "Suggested,"

though it qualifies weakly as a recommendation for in-depth study of motor fluctuations.

SCOPA-MOTOR SCALE (S-MS)

Structure

The Short Parkinson's Evaluation Scale (SPES) was developed as an attempt to construct a simple, relatively quick, and valid scale for use in clinical practice and as a basic measure in clinical research.[25] This scale was short, conceptually clear, and displayed good reliability and validity.[9] The instrument was considered easy to use by evaluators, but was only used in a few studies.[24-29] It was later refined under strict clinimetric criteria under the new name of SCOPA–Motor Scale, or S-MS, and is part of the Scales for Outcomes in the Parkinson's Disease (SCOPA) research project,[9] with improvements to the conceptual structure of the sections, the rules governing examination, and the definition of ranks of response. S-MS's length (21 items, 25 scores in three sections) is shorter than corresponding sections in the UPDRS (35 items, 48 scores). S-MS allows a proportionate saving in terms of time spent on patient assessment and furnishes high-quality data from a clinimetric point of view. The S-MS–Complications section contains two items for evaluation of dyskinesias and two for appraisal of fluctuations (presence and severity in both sections). Scores for each item range from 0 (*normal*) to 3 (*severe*). Hence, possible scores range from 0 to 12 for the motor complications sections and 0 to 6 for motor fluctuations. To establish presence, the item asks what proportion of the waking day the patient is "off" on average, 0 = *none* 1 = *some of the time*, 2 = *a considerable part of the time*, and 3 = *most or all of the time*; and for severity of off-periods, 0 = *absent*, 1 = *mild end-of-dose fluctuations*, 2 = *moderate end-of-dose fluctuations* (unpredictable fluctuations may occur occasionally) and 3 = *severe end-of-dose fluctuations* (unpredictable on-off oscillations occur frequently).

Key evaluation issues

The S-MS has been designed for use only in PD and has been used by several authors, but not by groups outside of the SCOPA developers. It is a consistent, precise, and potentially responsive measuring tool. It possesses high construct (convergent) validity, as well as satisfactory discriminative validity. The mean time required to complete the scales is 8.1 minutes (SD 1.9).[30] *Construct validity* of the complications section of SCOPA–Motor Scale presents a Spearman's r of 0.91, and *internal consistency* presents a Cronbach's alpha of 0.91.[31] S-MS floor and ceiling effects have proven satisfactory across all sections except for "Complications," a finding shared with the equivalent UPDRS subscale, probably due to the fact that motor complications are usually absent in early, mild disease stages, tending to occur only several years after date of onset. Minimal clinical relevant difference and minimal clinical relevant incremental difference for the motor complications section of S-MS have not been established, nor is there any information on the clinimetric behavior of the scale in unselected PD populations.

Strengths and weaknesses

S-MS is unable to discriminate different types of motor fluctuations, but it has been properly validated. It has not been widely adopted by investigators outside the developers.

Final assessment

The scale is reviewed as "Suggested," because it has been clinimetrically evaluated and applied to PD populations, though not widely adopted.

Movement Disorders Society version of the Unified Parkinson's Disease Scale (MDS-UPDRS)

STRUCTURE

In 2001, the Movement Disorder Society sponsored a critique of the UPDRS, underlining the strengths of the scale but also identifying a series of ambiguities and weaknesses,[32] concluding with the recommendation that the development of a new version was needed, retaining the strengths of the original scale, but resolving problems identified and incorporating a number of clinically pertinent PD-related problems poorly captured in the original version. The MDS therefore commissioned a revision of the scale, and a new version, the MDS-sponsored UPDRS revision, was written (MDS-UPDRS).[8]

An important addition to the MDS-UPDRS is a set of detailed instructions. Although measurement of the OFF time, (time spent in the OFF state in the MDS-UPDRS, formerly Off duration) is still ranked in the UPDRS in five categories according the percentage of the waking day that the patient remains in that state. Differences between the MDS-UPDRS and the original scale include the addition of "functional impact of fluctuations," through a new item written to run parallel with "functional impact of dyskinesias." Complexity of motor fluctuations previously covered in the UPDRS by three yes/no answers to questions of predictability, unpredictability, and sudden occurrence, is now more consolidated through a series of questions to fit the 0 to 4 rating format of the rest of MDS-UPDRS, so that partial parallelism between both scales can be mapped. ON and OFF definitions are provided to ensure rater uniformity. The scale uses historical and objective information to assess motor fluctuations that include OFF-state dystonia, obtaining information from patient and/or caregiver, as well as from a physical examination, to answer three questions summarizing function over the past week, including the day of the visit. As in other sections, rates are scored using full numbers only (no half points allowed), and all items must be completed. Some answers are based on percentages and therefore require calculating how many hours the patient is awake in general. MDS-UPDRS evaluates time spent in OFF state, estimated calculating the number of hours that patient/caregiver reports as off, divided by the hours of the waking day. Items rank from zero (no off time) to 4 (over 75% of the day off). The second question evaluates functional impact of motor fluctuations on activities of daily living and social interactions. This question concentrates on the difference between the ON and the OFF state. If a patient has no OFF time, the rating will be 0, but if patients have very mild fluctuations, it is still possible to be rated 0 on this item if no impact on personal activities occurs. At the opposite end of the spectrum, the maximum score is 4, meaning fluctuations affect daily living to the point that, during OFF periods, the patient can barely perform activities or participate in social interactions performed during ON ones. The third item determines the usual predictability of OFF function whether due to dose, time of day, food intake, or other factors. Patient is asked if he can count on them *always* coming at a special time, *mostly* coming at a special time, *only sometimes* occurring at a special time, or whether they are totally unpredictable.

KEY EVALUATION ISSUES

The time needed by the rater to administer MDS-UPDRS Part IV is five minutes.[8] MDS-UPDRS Part IV shows an internal consistency of alpha 0.79, and strong concurrent validity based on its high correlations with UPDRS sum of items 32 through 39,(all items covering dyskinesias) and motor fluctuations on the UDPRS versus total Part IV from the MDS-UPDRS (r 0.89). As a measure of internal validity, correlations among the MDS-UPDRS parts have been examined. These analyses confirm that each Part assesses a different aspect of PD, with most parts, except I and II, showing relatively low correlation. Part IV of MDS-UPDRS presents an expected floor effect, but no ceiling effect.[8] MDS-UPDRS has excellent factor validity, and factor analysis confirms that items cluster in clinically pertinent domains. Because data are collected using three different methods, namely: patient questionnaire, investigator assessments, and a combination of both, as in the case of the "motor complications" section, authors do not anticipate that the total score (combined parts I–IV) will be the recommended outcome, and advise that each Part (I–IV) be reported separately, and not collapsed into a single "Total MDS-UPDRS" summary score. Minimal clinical relevant difference and minimal clinical relevant incremental difference, as well as item responsiveness for the MDS-UPDRS motor complications section,

have not been established yet. Moreover, there is no information on clinimetric behavior of this scale in unselected PD populations. The MDS-UPDRS, including Part IV and the items focusing on motor complications, is being used by several research teams involved in the study of new interventions and the monitoring of disease progression and biomarker research.

STRENGTHS AND WEAKNESSES

MDS-UPDRS is a scale that retains the strengths of the original UPDRS scale, resolves problems identified in the previous version, and incorporates a number of clinically pertinent motor complications problems toward their identification. Nevertheless, it is an extremely new scale and needs to tested by different authors in unselected PD populations.

FINAL ASSESSMENT

The MDS-UPDRS component of the scale focusing on motor fluctuations is reviewed as "Suggested" at the time of this publication. Although used in PD and having strong support, it is still a new scale and insufficient wide usage has been published. The authors are aware of several programs utilizing the scale, and believe it is likely to be recommended eventually.

The Treatment Response Scale (TRS)

TRS was developed based on previous scales.[33-34] This scale has been used to grade motor status throughout the day, from *normal function* to *severe OFF* (score 0–3/0–5) as well as dyskinesias from *none* to *severe*. The TRS has, to date, only been used in studies with L-dopa/carbidopa gel infusion.[33-34] The scale was used by other authors in just one small study to assess efficacy of continuous daily levodopa duodenal infusion.

CLINIMETRIC TESTING

A validation study has not been published, but a validation process in ongoing.

STRENGTHS AND WEAKNESSES

With respect to characterization of duration and severity of OFF-time, it is relatively simple to apply. The scale was not designed to assess wearing-off specifically, but rather to grade changes in motor conditions (both occurrence of OFF periods and dyskinesia) in patients undergoing infusion therapies. An additional weakness is that there is no general agreement on which parts of the symptomatology should be included in the TRS score.

FINAL ASSESSMENT

The TRS is a "Listed" scale that was not intended primarily as a scale for wearing-off but rather as a tool for research.

QUESTIONNAIRES FOR MOTOR FLUCTUATIONS DETECTION (TABLES 9-2 AND 9-5)

A second strategy for measuring motor fluctuations is the use of patient-based questionnaires that provide a series of questions that the patient answers to assess various elements of dyskinesia timing, severity, and disruption. Clinical researchers have developed three versions of this type of patient survey.

The initial efforts to inventory motor and non-motor symptoms of wearing-off consisted of a panel of ten movement-disorder specialists who developed a prototype patient questionnaire based on a review of the literature and a consensus view of the most common motor and non-motor symptoms associated with wearing-off.[15] These 32 motor and non-motor symptoms were incorporated into a four-page survey (the WOQ-32) that included a brief set of instructions and definitions and a graph illustrating motor fluctuations. For the purposes of evaluating this tool, the group defined "wearing-off" as any (>1) of the 32 symptoms that patients currently experienced during their normal day and that improved or resolved following a dose of anti-Parkinsonian medication.

Nineteen of the 32 symptoms were subsequently found to be statistically relevant

TABLE 9-5. Strengths and Weaknesses of Motor Fluctuation Questionnaires and Diaries.

	STRENGTH	WEAKNESS
WOQ-32	Better identification of WO than UPDRS.	Length of the questionnaire requires considerable time on the patient's part. Open questions.
QQ-WOQ	Global accuracy for WO detection greater than 85%.	Not in generalized use.
WOQ-9	Short and quick.	Low specificity for WO detection (influence of comorbidities). Not in generalized use.
Hauser Parkinson's Disease Diary	Provides information on daily function throughout a full 24 hour cycle.	Patients require special training. Compliance is a known problem with diary date.
CAPSIT-PD ON-OFF Diary	Provides information on daily function throughout a full 24-hour cycle.	Patients require special training. Compliance is a known problem with diary date.

WOQ-32: Wearing-off Questionnaire. WOQ-19 or QQ-WOQ: QUICK questionnaire for wearing off detection. WOQ-9: Wearing-Off Questionnaire 9 questions. Hauser Diary is the Parkinson's Disease Diary. CAPSIT-PD diary is the Core Assessment Program for Surgical Interventional Therapies in Parkinson's Disease ON-OFF Diary.

for inclusion into the WOQ-19 (also called "QUICK"), which has been translated into Flemish[21] and Spanish[18,22] using a back-translation procedure to ensure cultural and linguistic equivalence. The WOQ-19 consists of 19 symptoms related to PD: tremor, difficulty in speech, anxiety, sweating, mood changes, weakness, problems with balance, slowness, reduced dexterity, numbness, general stiffness, panic attacks, cloudy mind/dullness of thinking, abdominal discomfort, muscle cramping, difficulty getting out of the chair, experience hot and cold, pain, and aching. Patients are asked to mark which of these symptoms they are experiencing currently, "during a normal day," and whether they usually improve after the next dose of medication. A "positive response" is registered when any of these symptoms is reported to improve after a dose of medication. In addition, the WOQ-19 explores whether the improvement after treatment doses occurs only with the first daily dose, other doses, or all daily doses.

As some of the items in the 19-item questionnaire did not appear to have high specificity for wearing-off, the original survey data were further reassessed to focus on the nine symptoms (WOQ-9) believed to be the most "important" or significant out of the original 32 symptoms in terms of wearing-off.[17] Motor symptoms associated with wearing-off included tremor, reduced dexterity, muscle cramping, slowness, and stiffness. Non-motor symptoms consisted of cloudy mind/slowness of thinking, mood change, pain/aching, and anxiety/panic. In this chapter, the four are reviewed together, because they are all versions of the original scale and each is related to the others.

Wearing-Off Questionnaire (WOQ): version WOQ-32, version WOQ-19 (QUICK Questionnaire or QQ), and version WOQ-9

STRUCTURE

The prototype WOQ-32 was evaluated in 289 male and female patients with idiopathic PD at least 30 years of age and showing symptoms for less than five years. Overall, 165 patients (57.1%) were identified as experiencing wearing-off by the WOQ-32. Thirty-seven percent of subjects indicated that the symptoms were very troublesome, and 55.2% indicated they were slightly troublesome. By comparison, 85 (29.4%) subjects with wearing-off fluctuations were identified by the Clinical Assessment Question and 127 (43.9%) subjects by question 36 of the UPDRS.[15]

Two published studies have evaluated translated versions of the WOQ-19. The first study was an observational study, undertaken to report its usefulness in detecting both motor and non-motor wearing-off in 160 Belgian PD patients.[21] Most neurologists considered the questionnaire "useful" or "very useful" in detecting wearing-off, more so for non-motor phenomena (61%) than for motor symptoms (56%). The second study was an observational, cross-sectional, multi-center study to evaluate the feasibility and performance of the WOQ-19 in a Spanish population (n = 94).[22] Overall, 75 (79.8%) patients were identified as having wearing-off with the WOQ-19, compared with 51 patients (55.4%) with a follow-up questionnaire, and 33 (35.1%) patients using the UPDRS. The validity results are given below.

The sensitivity and specificity of the WOQ-9 has been studied in the United States in PD patients receiving treatment with anti-Parkinsonian medication.[23] In this study, patients reported having wearing-off more frequently than had been identified by their physician. Patients agreed with physician assessment in 76 of 79 cases. Physicians disagreed with patient assessment in 81 of 157 cases. Thus the WOQ-9 was shown to be a highly sensitive (96.2%) tool, which may be useful for the identification of end-of-dose wearing-off. However, the specificity was observed to be low (40.9%).

KEY EVALUATION ISSUES

The WOQ-19 has been used in a number of studies as a screening tool to identify patients in the early stages of wearing-off. In these studies, patients were required to experience at least one or two of the 19 items to be diagnosed as having wearing-off.

Similarly, the WOQ-9 has recently been used as a screening tool in an open-label, six-week study, which evaluated the efficacy of switching from either levodopa/carbidopa or levodopa/benserazide to levodopa/carbidopa/entacapone.[24] The identification of at least one symptom of wearing-off, via the WOQ-9, was used as an inclusion criterion, and it was reported that use of this questionnaire improved the identification of the target patient population for this study as well as aiding in the evaluation of the benefits of switching regarding both motor and non-motor symptoms. It has also been reported that the recruitment rate for this study was rapid, leading to the suggestion that use of such tools aids in the more rapid identification of PD patients currently experiencing wearing-off.[24-25]

WOQ-9 and the WOQ-19 have undergone clinimetric testing focusing on the validation of the scales. The sensitivity and specificity of the WOQ-9 as a screening tool for the recognition of wearing-off was compared with a standard neurologist's assessment in 216 patients, with diagnosis of PD for five years.[23] In this study, patients completed the WOQ-9 and a patient demographics form prior to being evaluated during a regularly scheduled visit. Overall, 157 (72.7%) patients reported wearing-off using the WOQ-9. In contrast, physicians reported that only 79 (36.6%) of patients in this study had wearing-off. The WOQ-9 was shown to be a highly sensitive screening tool, with its sensitivity calculated to be 96.2%. However, as a large number of positive results obtained from the questionnaire did not correlate with the physician's assessment, the specificity of the WOQ-9 was very low (40.9%). The WOQ-19 was evaluated in 222 patients (36.0% without wearing-off; 64.0% with mild or moderate/severe wearing-off). The diagnosis of wearing-off by the participant neurologist was considered the "gold standard." Patients independently completed the WOQ-19 just before the clinical assessment. A cutoff with two positive symptoms showed sensitivity of 88%, specificity of 80%, positive predictive value of 88.7%, negative predictive value of 79%, diagnostic accuracy of 85%, positive and negative likelihood ratios of 4.4 and 0.15, with an area under the ROC curve of 0.90 (CI95%: 0.86–0.94%).[35-36]

STRENGTHS AND WEAKNESSES

The WOQ-32, WOQ-19, and WOQ-9 forms are in public domain and have been specifically designed to screen for the presence or absence of motor and non-motor symptoms related to wearing-off in PD. The WOQ-19 and WOQ-9 have been found to possess adequate screening properties for detection of wearing-off, but specificity of the WOQ-9 has been reported to be low. Whether this reflects poor specificity or under-recognition of wearing-off needs further clarification. These questionnaires were designed to be easily completed by patients and then to be used by the treating physician in patient–physician discussions.

All three versions are patient-rated scales and depend on the patient's understanding wearing-off. The scales were designed to be screening tools for the presence or absence of wearing-off and therefore cannot be used as rating instruments of the severity of wearing-off. Because there are questions that focus on non-motor aspects of wearing-off (dysautonomia and sleep disorders), the questionnaires in any of the three formats cannot be used specifically for examining the presence or absence of motor wearing-off. The specificity of these scales for wearing-off requires further study.

FINAL ASSESSMENT

The WOQ-32 is a "Suggested" diagnostic screening tool for wearing-off, because it has been used in PD and has been used by authors other than the developers, but there are insufficient clinimetric data on it. The WOQ-19 and WOQ-9 can be considered "Recommended" diagnostic screening tools for screening for the presence or absence of wearing-off in PD, because they also have undergone at least some clinimetric testing. The task force members suggest that further clinimetric studies, including further tests of specificity and sensitivity in a larger cohort, be assessed with the WOQ-19 and WOQ-9.

SELF EVALUATION DIARIES (TABLES 9-2 AND 9-5)

The final category of motor fluctuation assessments involves a prospectively gathered inventory of the time spent, usually in 30-minute increments, as ON (medications working with good Parkinson's control) versus OFF (medications not working and poor Parkinson's control). These data sets are often gathered for three days before an office visit and then the total number of hours OFF and total hours ON allow analysis of motor fluctuations. Diaries can also capture dyskinesia and distinguish between dyskinesia that is troublesome or not troublesome (see Chapter 8). The number of changes between ON and OFF can also be calculated as an index of motor fluctuations. These assessments require that patients complete their data entry frequently throughout the assessment period, and the instructions specify that data must be entered at the times indicated, not summarized at the end of the day based on recollection. Timely compliance is mandatory and full education on the difference between ON and OFF is essential to the accurate interpretation of these home-based data sets that have no input from physicians or other health care officials.

Structure

The prototype of this methodology is the Parkinson's Disease Diary developed by Hauser and colleagues.[12] Home-based diaries used by patients to document motor states have been developed for both research and practice settings. In most instances, patients choose between four categories: sleep, off, on without troublesome dyskinesias, and on with troublesome dyskinesias.[12] A three-part breakdown into Sleep, Good Time (on without troublesome dyskinesia), and Bad Time (combined off and on with troublesome dyskinesia) has also been utilized[37]; although the disadvantage of this latter version is the inability to discriminate OFF periods.

Written instructions and descriptions for each category are included, and in clinical practice, a training day running through the test with a patient observer is necessary. In a research setting, this training is generally incorporated into the study protocol with requirements of equivalent ratings between rater and patient as a prerequisite for study participation. In such instances,

pre-study training involves several 30-minute observations and a specified agreement between rater and subject. In trained subjects, diary sets are generally considered reliable if there are no more than four absent or multiple responses (more than one check mark, per half-hour time period, per diary). Training tapes for on and off definitions are available, but clinical situations and definitions vary widely among patients.[38] In addition to the Hauser Parkinson's Disease Diary, the CAPSIT-PD (Core Assessment Program for Surgical Intervention Therapies in Parkinson's Disease) ON-OFF diary is also available and differentiates between OFF, Partial OFF, ON, and ON with dyskinesias.[39]

Key evaluation issues

Both the Hauser and CAPSIT-PD diaries are tools specifically developed for Parkinson's disease and has been the source of multiple clinical trials reported by others outside the original developmental teams. Without specific training for diary use, however, patients can disagree with examiners on up to 80% of entries made every half hour.[38] After one month's training using an experimental teaching tape, patients can increment rater-matching score levels from 57.4% (baseline) to 93.1% (after training), underlining the need for proper patient education prior to use of this tool. The Parkinson's Disease Home Diary has been assessed for reliability using test-retest calculations.[12] Overall, 83% of 302 patients completed six days of the diaries with no missing or duplicate entries, suggesting that the diary is simple and feasible.[37] The percent of the awake day ON without dyskinesia or with non-troublesome dyskinesia was found to be reliable (Intraclass Correlation coefficient > 0.70). Diary results were not influenced by age, gender, or country. Predictive validity as assessed by estimating the strength of association between results from patient diaries and responses to five VAS items was moderate (R = 0.36–0.57).

There is no comparison with clinician ratings or objective scores during diary category times, or data on the predictive validity of diary entries.

Overall patient–clinician agreement in CAPSIT-PD diary entries during a four-hour observation period was good ($\kappa = 0.62$; weighted $\kappa = 0.84$). Agreement for individual diary categories was good for OFF and ON with dyskinesias ($\kappa \geq 0.72$), but moderate for partial OFF and ON ($\kappa = 0.49$). The overall validity of patient-kept diaries was also supported by expected differences between motor assessment scores between diary categories during the four-hour observation period.[36] One day's home diary data failed to predict outcomes from the full four weeks for all diary categories, and data from three days failed to yield good predictions for the time spent in "off" and "partial off." Data from one week yielded good predictions in all instances except "partial off," which could not be well predicted even when two weeks' home diary data were considered.[39]

Strengths and weaknesses

Diaries are presently the most practical means of following a patient throughout several days of motor fluctuations, and the clinimetric studies support that carefully trained subjects can provide accurate data. Patient education, however, is time-consuming, and may require regular reeducation. It is labor-intensive for patients to keep the diaries with them and complete them every half-hour, especially if diaries are to be completed several days in a row. The compliance rate appears to fall when patients are requested to complete a greater number of consecutive days of diaries. Electronic diaries that sound an alarm when an entry has been missed have been shown to increase entry compliance, but such diaries are costly.[40]

Final assessment

Home diaries, both the Hauser Parkinson's Disease Diary and the CAPSIT-PD ON-OFF Diary are considered "Recommended," but with the caveat that they should be used with subject training and verification that they are completed at the designated times that patients are required to report on their motor fluctuation state.

CONCLUSION AND FUTURE PERSPECTIVES

Wearing-off is a common manifestation in treated PD patients with a significant impact on global disability. Its identification is now facilitated by the use in the clinic of dedicated questionnaires. However, the precise assessment of wearing-off in PD is more complex and in theory would require a continuous evaluation of a patient's motor function throughout the day. Because this is not possible outside of very laborious research techniques that require patients to be in a hospital or outpatient unit with continual monitoring, all current methods utilize shortcuts that make an assessment feasible, but do so at the cost of losing potentially important information.

Even if continuous motor function monitoring through the day were developed, such data would best be described mathematically, perhaps as an area-under-the-curve function, and would probably have little obvious meaning to the non-expert. Today, we commonly describe an amount (hours) or a percentage (of the waking day) for OFF time, ON time, and ON time without troublesome dyskinesia. These terms are readily understood, their general meaning is clear but by their very nature are imprecise. Many patients experience a transition over some time from their best to their worst motor state, and there is no uniform definition that captures all the nuances of ON and OFF. Does a patient go from ON to OFF when his function deteriorates 1%, 25%, 50%, 75%, or 99%? We define ON time as time when medication is providing (clear) benefit for motor signs of PD, and we define OFF time as time when medication has worn off and is no longer providing (substantial) benefit for motor signs. But there is an ambiguous zone covering the transition between these two states, thereby making any evaluation of ON and OFF time imprecise. A further problem is the current lack of a clear definition for "wearing-off." In particular, we found that the scales currently used to assess the severity of wearing-off do not generally distinguish between types of motor fluctuations (e.g., wearing-off, sudden ON-OFF fluctuations, or delayed-ON). In order to better capture wearing-off, we suggest that the predictability of OFF periods be built detailed into the instrument. Additionally, severity of OFF varies between patients. Some patients may experience more OFF time but may have better overall function than another patient with a much smaller amount of OFF time, but more dramatic worsening in mobility in the OFF state. In addition, the presence of disabling non-motor features during off-time like pain, bladder dysfunction, or mood changes may worsen patients' perception of severity of their motor condition.

Finally, explaining to patients and caregivers the terminology and significance of the assessment can be complex. This could be partially overcome if one uses available videotapes and dedicated sessions that may help patients and caregivers become familiarized with the scales or diaries used.

Technology is likely to help improve assessments of motor fluctuations in the future. Clinical trials have begun to use electronic patient-completed PD diaries. There are advantages to this approach. An electronic device can potentially be carried on a belt holster or in a pocket (like a cell phone) to provide greater convenience for the patient in having access to the recording device. The device can be set to provide a signal at appropriate time points to remind the patient to provide input. Perhaps most important, the time of the data input can be recorded, and potentially, data that are too delayed when entered can be excluded. In addition, electronic devices may query both motor state and severity in a presentation that is less complicated than paper diaries. The main drawbacks of electronic diaries are that they may require good dexterity to manipulate and many elderly individuals are not comfortable with electronic devices.

Farther in the future, there may be electronic methods to monitor patient motor function at home throughout a normal day. One concept is that a patient could install prepackaged software and a special sensing device on their home computer. They may then wear special devices, perhaps on the wrists and ankles, to communicate positions in space and movement to the computer sensors. Software would then capture and analyze this data, ultimately putting it in a useful and digestible format and relaying it over the Internet to a central source or physician's office. However, there are many obstacles to overcome for this to become reality. Right now, sensors should be able to detect and analyze patient movement within the same room, but this geographic area of motion capture may need to be expanded. Perhaps the greatest difficulty is in creating algorithms and methods to truly understand patient motor function based on the input received. It will be important to consistently and accurately distinguish tremor and dyskinesia. Moreover, it is not yet clear how to judge patient motor function when they are sitting still, for example. Despite these potential hurdles, technology can be expected to improve assessment of motor function and fluctuations in the future.

In conclusion, current scales to assess severity of wearing-off are primarily focused on the extent of off-time and do not gather extensive information on the severity of associated motor and non-motor features as a critical factor in the assessment. It would be desirable for such a scale to capture severity of wearing-off to allow a comprehensive evaluation of clinical benefit of specific therapeutic strategies. The MDS-UPDRS gathers the complexity, predictability, and severity of motor fluctuations as well as the time, but has not yet been sufficiently used in published studies to attain the "Recommended" designation,. In the authors' views, this tool will become the standard, however, along with the WOQ-19 or WOQ-9 and one of the diaries already developed, especially if electronic data-capturing methods can be incorporated into diary methodology on a regular basis. Based on the availability of these scales, the MDS Task Force on PD Rating Scales felt there was no need to recommend the development of a new scale for motor fluctuations.

RECOMMENDED SCALES
WO-19, QQ-WO
WO-9
HAUSER DIARY
CAPSIT-PD DIARY

References

1. Marsden CD, Parkes JD. Success and problems of long-term levodopa therapy in Parkinson's disease. *Lancet.* 1977;1:345–349.

2. Quinn NP. Classification of fluctuations in patients with Parkinson's disease. *Neurology.* 1998;51(suppl 2):S25–S29.

3. Nutt JG, Holford NH. The response to levodopa in Parkinson's disease: imposing pharmacological law and order. *Ann Neurol.* 1996;39:561–567.

4. Lloret SP, Rossi M, Cardinali DP, Merello M. Actigraphic evaluation of motor fluctuations in patients with Parkinson's disease. *Int J Neurosci.* 2010;120(2):137–143.

5. Larsen TA, Calne S, Calne DB. Assessment of Parkinson's disease. *Clin Neuropharmacol.* 1984;7:165–169.

6. Martinez-Martin P. *Parametros evolutivos en la enfermedad de Parkinson* (thesis). Madrid: Universidad Complutense; 1987:132.

7. Fahn S, Elton RL, Members of the UPDRS Development Committee. Unified Parkinson's Disease Rating Scale. In: Fahn S, Marsden CD, Calne DB, Goldstein M, eds. *Recent Developments in Parkinson's Disease.* vol. 2. Florham Park, NJ: Macmillan Health Care Information; 1987:153–164.

8. Goetz CG, Tilley B, Shaftman S, et al. Movement Disorder Society-sponsored revision of the Unified Parkinson's Disease Rating Scale (MDS-UPDRS): scale presentation and clinimetric testing results. *Mov Disord.* 2008;23:2129–2170.

9. Marinus J, Visser M, Stiggelbout AM, et al. A short scale for the assessment of motor impairments and disabilities in Parkinson's disease: the SPES/SCOPA. *J Neurol Neurosurg Psychiatry.* 2004;75:388–395.

10. Stacy M, Bowron A, Guttman M, et al. Identification of motor and non-motor wearing-off in Parkinson's disease: comparison of a patient questionnaire versus a clinician assessment. *Mov Disord.* 2005;20:726–733.

11. Stacy MA, Murphy JM, Greeley DR, Stewart RM, Murcke H, Menge X; on behalf of the COMPASS-I Study Investigators. The sensitivity and specificity of the 9-item Wearing-off Questionnaire. *Parkinsonism Relat Disord.* 2008;14:205–212.

12. Hauser RA, Zesiewicz TA, Adler CH, et al. A home diary to assess functional status in patients with Parkinson's disease with motor fluctuations and dyskinesia. *Clin Neuropharmacol.* 2000;23:75–81.

13. Antonini A, Martinez-Martin P, Chaudhuri RK, et al. Wearing-off scales in Parkinson's disease: critique and recommendations. *Mov Disord.* 2011;26:2169–2175.

14. Canter CJ, de la Torre R, Mier M. A method of evaluating disability in patients with Parkinson's disease. *J Nerv Ment Dis.* 1961;133:143–147.

15. Markham CH, Diamond SG. Evidence to support early levodopa therapy in Parkinson's disease. *Neurology.* 1981;31:125–131.

16. Webster DD. Critical analysis of the disability in Parkinson's disease. *Mod Treat.* 1968;5:257–282.

17. Lieberman A, Dziatolowsky M, Gopinathan G, et al. Evaluation of Parkinson's disease. In: Goldstein M, Calne DB, Lieberman A, Thorner MD, eds. *Ergot Compounds and Brain Function: Neuroendocrine and Neuropsychiatric Aspects.* New York, NY: Raven Press; 1980:277–286.

18. Martinez-Martin P. Rating scales in Parkinson's disease. In: Jankovic J, Tolosa E, eds. *Parkinson's Disease and Movement Disorders.* 2nd ed. Baltimore, MD: Williams and Wilkins; 1993:281–292.

19. Jankovic J, McDermott M, Carter J, et al. Variance expression of Parkinson's disease: a base-line analysis of the DATATOP cohort. *Neurology.* 1990;40:1529–1534.

20. Martinez-Martin P, Gil-Nagel A, Morlán Gracia L, et al. Intermediate scale for assessment of Parkinson's disease. Characteristics and structure. *Parkinsonism Relat Disord.* 1995;1:97–99.

21. Ramaker C, Marinus J, Stiggelbout AM, et al. Systematic evaluation of rating scales for impairment and disability in Parkinson's disease. *Mov Disord.* 2002;17:867–876.

22. Longstreth WT, Koepsell TD, van Belle G. Clinical neuroepidemiology. Diagnosis. *Arch Neurol.* 1987;44:1091–1099.

23. Martinez-Martin P, Prieto L, Forjaz MJ. Longitudinal metric properties of disability rating scales for Parkinson's disease. *Value Health.* 2006;9:386–393.

24. Martinez-Martin P, Gil-Nagel A, Morlfin Gracia L, Balseiro Gimez J, Martinez-Sarris J; and Cooperative Multicentric Group. Unified Parkinson's Disease Rating Scale characteristics and structure. *Mov Disord.* 1994;9:76–83.

25. Rabey JM, Bass H, Bonuccelli U, et al. Evaluation scale: a new friendly scale for the evaluation of Parkinson's disease in clinical

drug trials. *Clin Neuropharmacol.* 1997;20: 323–337.

26. Werber EA, Rabey JM. The beneficial effect of cholinesterase inhibitors on patients suffering from Parkinson's disease and dementia. *J Neural Transm.* 2001;108:1319–1325.

27. Reichmann H, Brecht HM, Kraus PH, et al. [Pramipexole in Parkinson disease. Results of a treatment observation]. *Nervenarzt.* 2002;73:745–750.

28. Klein C, Zoldan J, Korczyn AD, et al. Pergolide as an adjunct therapy in Parkinson's disease evaluated using the SPES. *Rev Med Hosp Gen* (Mex). 2000;63:155–164.

29. Rabey JM, Klein C, Molochnikov A, et al. Comparison of the Unified Parkinson's Disease Rating Scale and the Short Parkinson's Evaluation Scale in patients with Parkinson's disease after levodopa loading. *Clin Neuropharmacol.* 2002;25:83–88.

30. Verbrugge LM, Jette AM. The disablement process. *Soc Sci Med.* 1994;38:1–14.

31. Martínez-Martín P, Benito-León J, Burguera JA, et al. The SCOPA–motor scale for assessment of Parkinson's disease is a consistent and valid measure. *J Clin Epidemiol.* 2005;58:674–679.

32. Goetz CG, Fahn S, Martinez-Martin P, et al. Movement Disorder Society-sponsored revision of the Unified Parkinson's Disease Rating Scale (MDS-UPDRS): process, format, and clinimetric testing plan. *Mov Disord.* 2007;22:41–47.

33. Nyholm D, Nilsson Remahl AI, Dizdar N, et al. Duodenal levodopa infusion monotherapy vs oral polypharmacy in advanced Parkinson disease. *Neurology.* 2005;64(2):216–223.

34. Nyholm D, Constantinescu R, Holmberg B, Dizdar N, Askmark H. Comparison of apomorphine and levodopa infusions in four patients with Parkinson's disease with symptom fluctuations. *Acta Neurol Scand.* 2009;119(5):345–348.

35. Stacy M. An abbreviated wearing-off patient questionnaire (WOPQ): sensitivity analysis. In: Poster presented at: the 9th International Congress of Parkinson's Disease and Movement Disorders; March 5–8, 2005; New Orleans, LA.

36. Stacy M; and EODWO Group. Wearing-off in Parkinson's disease: a patient survey vs programmed clinical evaluation. *Mov Disord.* 2003;18:1094.

37. Hauser RA, Deckers F, Lehert P. Parkinson's disease home diary: further validation and implications for clinical trials. *Mov Disord.* 2004;19:1409–1413.

38. Goetz CG, Stebbins GT, Blasucci LM, et al. Efficacy of a patient-training videotape on motor fluctuations for on-off diaries in Parkinson's disease. *Mov Disord.* 1997;12:1039–1041.

39. Reimer J, Grabowski M, Lindvall O, Hagell P. Use and interpretation of on/off diaries in Parkinson's disease. *J Neurol Neurosurg Psychiatry.* 2004;75:396–400.

40. Lyons KE, Pahwa R. Electronic motor function diary for patients with Parkinson's disease: a feasibility study. *Parkinsonism Relat Disord.* 2007;13:304–307.

10

GLOBAL SCALES TO STAGE DISABILITY IN PD: THE HOEHN AND YAHR SCALE

Werner Poewe

Summary

The Hoehn and Yahr (HY) scale is the most widely used and universally accepted staging system for overall functional disability in Parkinson's disease. It meets criteria for (1) specific use in PD, (2) usage by multiple authors in many types of studies covering the full range of durations and severities of PD, and (3) has acceptable clinimetric properties in terms of reliability and convergent validity. Therefore, it is a **Recommended** scale by the Movement Disorder Society Task Force on Parkinson's Disease Scales criteria.

Its main conceptual problems, making full clinimetric assessment difficult, relate to its categorical structure and the mixing of objective impairment and functional disability. Another limitation lies in the fact that the five stages of the original scale are probably too broad, resulting in insufficient responsivity to change. A modified version introducing intermediate stages (Stage 1.5 and Stage 2.5) has not been formally evaluated clinimetrically. Nevertheless, the Hoehn and Yahr scale has gained universal acceptance, is simple and easy to use by specialists as well as non-specialists, and has convincing convergent validity with a wide range of scales used to rate impairment and health-related quality of life in PD.

INTRODUCTION

Despite all the advances made in the symptomatic treatment of the motor and, more recently, also some of the non-motor, symptoms of Parkinson's disease, the disorder is relentlessly progressive and eventually leads to significant disability requiring institutional care in up to 50% of patients surviving for more than 15 years.[1] As comprehensively reviewed in this volume, a considerable number of scales have been developed over time to screen for PD or rate the severity of its cardinal motor features,

the motor complications developing with sustained dopaminergic therapies, as well as the many non-motor aspects of the disease. In addition, several generic and disease-specific scales are have been extensively tested for their utility and clinimetric performance in relation to assessing health related quality of life in PD.[2] On the other hand, a more global framework that will allow clinicians and researchers to classify patients to overall severity stages as their disease progresses can offer important additional benefits for studies of the natural history of PD. Such scales characterize different patient cohorts for clinical trials and naturalistic studies, capturing progression rates to key disability milestones, as well as assessing potential interventions to delay or reduce global disability.

The Hoehn and Yahr (HY) scale was originally introduced more than 40 years ago in a seminal paper describing the natural history and progression of a large cohort of patients with Parkinson's disease in the pre-levodopa era.[3] Ever since, the HY scale has been used widely and has gained global acceptance as a gold-standard reference system describing severity stages of PD-related functional disability and impairment. In 2004, the Movement Disorders Society (MDS) Task Force on Parkinson's Disease Rating Scales reviewed the HY scale and, despite some shortcomings regarding scale concept and clinimetric testing, the panel designated it as "Recommended" in its original form for demographic presentation of patient groups, including the use in clinical research.[4] This chapter is largely based on the 2004 report by the MDS-sponsored Task Force report.

Scale description

STRUCTURE

The HY scale was originally designed as a simple descriptive staging system to provide a global clinical estimate of PD severity, based on key aspects of disability, as well as features of objective impairment. The original scale defined five stages of progressive impairment and disability, while in the 1990s, intermediate stages between stages 1 and 2 (1.5) as well as 2 and 3 (2.5) of the original scale began to be used in some clinical trials (Table 10-1).

The anchors of the original and modified HY scale combine two principle concepts to describe progression of overall PD-related dysfunction: first, the topographical extent of motor impairment (unilateral versus bilateral); and, second, the degree of impairment of balance and gait. Increasing PD severity is thus described as a progression from unilateral (Stage 1) to bilateral motor symptoms (Stage 2)—both without balance difficulties—to the emergence of postural instability (Stage 3). Stage 3 patients remain independent, but loss of physical independence with maintained ability to stand or walk defines Stage 4, while Stage 5 designates patients who are wheelchair- or bed-bound. As noted in the MDS Task Force 2004 report, the original description by the authors of the HY scale did not imply that all PD patients uniformly start with levels of dysfunction defined as Stage 1 nor sequentially decline to Stage 5.

HANDLING COMORBIDITIES

PD prevalence increases with age, accompanied by an increase in age-related comorbidities,

Table 10-1. Comparison Between the Original and Modified Hoehn and Yahr Scales

HOEHN AND YAHR SCALE	MODIFIED HOEHN AND YAHR SCALE
1: Unilateral involvement only, usually with minimal or no functional disability	1.0: Unilateral involvement only
	1.5: Unilateral and axial involvement
2: Bilateral or midline involvement without impairment of balance	2.0: Bilateral involvement without impairment of balance
	2.5: Mild bilateral disease with recovery on pull test
3: Bilateral disease: mild to moderate disability with impaired postural reflexes; physically independent*	3.0: Mild to moderate bilateral disease; some postural instability; physically independent
4: Severely disabling disease; still able to walk or stand unassisted	4.0: Severe disability; still able to walk or stand unassisted
5: Confinement to bed or wheelchair unless aided	5.0: Wheelchair-bound or bedridden unless aided

*Stage 3 is a summary of the author's original, more narrative description.

including cerebrovascular or osteoarthritic disease. Impairments and functional disabilities resulting from stroke, peripheral neuropathy, vestibular or visual impairment, myelopathy, or hip arthrosis can confound the staging of PD-related impairment and disability in the HY staging system. The question of how issues of comorbidity should be handled has not been specifically addressed in the original description of the HY scale or later work. The MDS Task Force review highlighted the two principal approaches that could be applied for patients with confounding comorbidity. The "purist" approach would try to assign patients to different HY stages only on the basis of PD-related dysfunction, trying to disregard all additional impairment or disability components due to non-PD-related conditions. The disadvantage of this approach is the high degree of subjectivity entering decisions about the different contributions of PD itself versus comorbidity on a given impairment or disability status. In addition, the basic concept underlying the HY scale is to provide a picture of the overall functioning of an individual patient, which would be invalidated by separation by source of disability or impairment. Given that standardized instructions for rating PD in the context of comorbidities do not exist for the HY system, the Task Force recommendation was to use the HY system in a "rate-as-you-see" approach—describing a PD patient's stage based on the overall clinical level of functioning, regardless of potential impacts of comorbidity.

Key evaluation issues

USE IN PD AND APPLICATIONS ACROSS THE DISEASE SPECTRUM

Ever since its introduction, the HY scale has remained the most commonly and most widely used scale to describe severity of PD worldwide.[5] It is the standard staging system used to describe patient populations enrolled in clinical trials of anti-Parkinsonian interventions and the second most frequently used outcome measure after the UPDRS in all randomized, controlled drug trials for PD published between 1966 and 1998.[5] It

provides an overall assessment of severity based on clinical features and functional disability.[6]

The HY scale has been used extensively in natural history studies of PD and for the description of large populations of PD patients. Studies from both the pre-L-dopa and L-dopa eras involving large cohorts of PD patients have found similar percentages of cases assigned to the different stages of the HY scale.[3,7–11] In these studies, Stage 1 and Stage 5 account for the smallest number of subjects, followed by Stage 4, while the majority of patients, ranging from 52% to 77%, fall into Stages 2 or 3.

Prospective studies using the HY scale longitudinally over the long-term course of PD would be able to generate valuable data on the time course of PD progression as reflected by latencies to reach successive stages of this scale. Most of the available data, however, come from retrospective cohorts suggesting latencies of six to seven years to Stage 3 in the pre-levodopa era.[3,7] Some studies have suggested that the advent of L-dopa treatment has resulted in prolonged latencies to successive stages, compared to the pre-L-dopa era,[8] although this does not seem to be supported by prospective data of the Sydney Multicentre Study cohort where combined median latencies from Stage 1 or 2 to HY Stage 3 were only about 3.5 years, despite combined therapies with dopamine agonists and L-dopa.[12] Other studies have suggested that latencies to progress by one HY stage may be dependent on the patient's age at disease onset, where patients with onset at 50 years had latencies of around nine years, versus five years for patients at 70 years.[13]

A recent retrospective analysis of 695 carefully documented PD cases with sufficiently frequent and regular assessments on the modified HY scale found that transition times were about two years for moving from HY Stages 1 to 2, 3 to 4, and 4 to 5, and only progression from HY Stage 2 to 2.5 was significantly longer—around five years.[14] Similar to the study by Alves and colleagues,[13] transition times were shorter in older patients, possibly reflecting effects of comorbidity, as well as longer disease duration and higher UPDRS scores at entry.

The emergence of balance problems and thus transition into Stage 3 of the HY scale seems to carry unfavorable prognostic implications, since, the medium time to loss of full physical independence from Stage 3 is only around two years. In line with such observations, Goetz and colleagues[15] found that Stage 2 patients could be maintained on stable UPDRS scores with an increasing medication dose, whereas Stage 3 patients experienced progression of UPDRS scores despite medication adjustments.[15] Reaching Hoehn and Yahr Stage 3 has also been associated with higher risks of subsequently progressing to dementia, and reduced survival.[16]

USE BY MULTIPLE AUTHORS

The HY scale is the standard staging system used to describe patient populations enrolled in clinical trials of anti-Parkinsonian interventions, and the second most frequently used outcome measure after the UPDRS in all drug trials for PD.[4] It is easy to apply and quick to administer, and lends itself both to research and patient-care settings, where the HY scale has been used by raters without special expertise in movement disorders as well as by specialists.[17] The HY staging system is commonly used to categorize patients into early versus advanced disease, not only for purposes of clinical trials but also in studies of surrogate markers of PD progression.[18] In addition, the HY scale has been utilized in studies in other types of degenerative Parkinsonism, including progressive supranuclear palsy or multiple-system atrophy, where transitions to HY Stage 3, anchored on balance and gait problems, occur much faster than in PD.[19]

CLINIMETRIC ISSUES

Despite its widespread use and acceptance, few formal clinimetric examinations of reliability and validity for the HY scale have been conducted. Reliability testing assesses the scale's measurement error, whereas validity testing assesses the scale's ability to measure its designated domains. The available clinimetric data on the HY scale have been recently reviewed by the MDS Task Force[4] and are summarized below with some limited additions from more recent papers.

RELIABILITY

Scale reliability reflects the consistency of ratings by different raters (inter-rater reliability) or different ratings over time performed by the same rater (inter-rater reliability). Published reports of the HY scale's reliability have focused on this latter type of assessment. Overall, available studies document a moderate to significant level of inter-rater reliability, with nonweighted and weighted kappa scores ranging between 0.44 and 0.71.[17,20,21] The stability of inter-rater reliability has been shown across experienced movement disorder specialists and inexperienced neurology residents.[21] No formal assessments of test-retest reliability (intra-rater reliability) have been conducted, and because the scale is effectively a single question with five answer options, internal consistency cannot be calculated.

VALIDITY

Clinimetric examinations of validity of the HY scale have been limited, partly due to its ordinal level of measurement. Face validity (*Does the scale measure what it is designed to measure?*) is difficult to establish for the HY scale because of its combination of disability and impairment criteria. Likewise, no direct tests of the HY scale criteria validity (*Does the scale provide results comparable to a gold standard?*) have been conducted. Rather, most studies used the Hoehn and Yahr scale as a reference standard against which the validity of other scales is assessed.[22] Such studies do, however, generally find significant correlations between HY stages and other measures.[10,23–26] There are significant correlations between the HY stages of PD and measures of quality of life, both with respect to general health-based scales[2,22] as well as with disease-specific instruments like the PD Questionnaire-39 (PDQ-39)[27] and the PD Quality of Life scale (PDQUALIF).[28] Studies with both types of scales have found worse quality of life with more advanced HY stages.[28] Studies of objective and quantitative motor impairment tests and objective assessments of tasks involved in daily living have identified significant correlations between objective motor performance and early versus late HY stages.[9,29]

The HY scale has an inconsistent relationship with self-care measures, some disability ratings, and the Webster score,[30] but has high Spearman's correlations with standard PD rating scales like the UPDRS, the Columbia University Rating Scale, the Northwestern University Disability scale, and the Extensive Disability Scale.[23,24] In addition, there have been significant correlations between HY stages and imaging measures of PD progression in studies using dopamine-transporter SPECT scanning[18,31] and [18F]fluorodopa PET scanning.[32,33] Overall, these studies suggest at least convergent validity of the HY scale.

RESPONSIVENESS

Despite studies showing prolonged latencies to higher HY stages with L-dopa treatment,[7] the scale seems relatively insensitive to treatment-induced change, particularly in the lower categories.[6] The MDS-sponsored "Management of Parkinson's Disease: An Evidence-Based Review"[34] summarized treatment results from a large series of clinical trials, with an emphasis on randomized controlled trials. Several agents found efficacious in this report due to statistically significant effects on primary outcomes did not significantly alter the HY score: among six randomized, controlled double-blind studies on the efficacy of an agonist for PD, despite statistically significant changes in the UPDRS, only one reported significant improvements in HY stages.[35] The others showed no change in the HY scores,[36,37] did not report the HY findings despite collecting the data,[38,39] or did not report using the HY scale as an efficacy outcome.[40,41] Furthermore, even with drug treatment of PD that otherwise leads to clinically pertinent improvements, Stage 2 patients do not revert regularly to Stage 1. Some studies of modern dopaminergic therapies find the percentages of patients reaching the higher stage of the HY scale over 10 years to be similar to figures from the pre-L-dopa era.[12]

On the other hand, a recent study comparing the responsiveness of various outcome measures to assess progression of PD over one or four years found the HY scale to be more sensitive to change over time compared to health-related quality of life measures, and—in a sub-sample of patients followed by a specialized clinic for one year—the HY scale appeared even more responsive to progression than the UPDRS motor score.[22]

MINIMAL CLINICALLY RELEVANT DIFFERENCE AND MINIMAL CLINICALLY RELEVANT INCREMENTAL DIFFERENCE

As reviewed by the MDS Task Force report on the HY scale, the necessary assumptions needed to establish a minimal clinically relevant difference (MCRD) are not met by the HY scale, because the different categorical ratings are too broad, and an MCRD is very likely smaller than one categorical increment in the original scale—the latter being very probably clinically significant. The same limitation also applies to the definition of minimal clinically relevant incremental difference (MCRID), and the lack of difference in HY stages after treatment in trials assessing interventions in both early and advanced PD with clear effects on primary outcomes like the UPDRS or ON-/OFF-diaries illustrates this problem.

Strengths and weaknesses: additional considerations

The main strengths of the HY scale are its focus on a global clinical impression of overall PD severity, global acceptance and use, and simplicity combined with acceptable data to support reliability and conversion validity. Several limitations, however, exist. First, there is conceptual inconsistency in that the scale merges aspects of motor impairment as assessed by neurological examination (unilaterality, postural reflex data) with functional disability. As has been pointed out, these two concepts are not necessarily equivalent. Unilaterality would define Stage I, but affected patients, depending on the severity and type of their motor symptoms, might still be more significantly disabled by severe tremor or bradykinesia of the dominant hand and thereby have more overall functional disability than some Stage 2 patients with mild bilateral disease or even some Stage 3 patients with postural reflex abnormality but otherwise relatively mild motor symptoms.

Another weakness is the reduction of the entire spectrum of PD severity into only five categories, making each stage too broad to be sensitive to changes in response to treatment. Furthermore, this reductionist approach forces a wide heterogeneity of motor-symptom severities into one stage.

Finally, the main anchor to capture advancing disability in the HY scale is focused on gait and balance problems, while other significant factors important to overall disability in PD like drug-related motor complications or non-motor symptoms are not captured or incorporated into the staging system.

Final assessment

The HY scale is the most widely used scale to globally stage PD patients by level of functional disability and impairment. The scale meets criteria for specific use in PD, wide usage by multiple authors in multiple settings covering the entire spectrum of PD severities, and, although still limited, clinimetric studies supporting its reliability and convergent validity. The HY scale therefore meets criteria for a "Recommended" scale for the assessment of global disability stages in PD as defined by the MDS Task Force.

FUTURE PERSPECTIVES

Although the HY scale has been the most extensively used instrument to assess global disability in PD in a wide spectrum of research settings over several decades, there are still very limited data on the long-term progression of PD as reflected by the HY system from large and well-defined patient cohorts. Such studies would be needed to better define latencies of progression to the different stages and their correlation with clinical features like age at onset, comorbidity, and treatment parameters, and would eventually improve our understanding of the heterogeneity of progression in PD.

In its current form, the five-stage HY scale may be too broad to adequately capture the clinical evolution of PD progression. Furthermore, it does not incorporate key drivers of global disability in PD like levodopa-induced motor complications and, probably even more important, the non-motor features of this illness. Non-motor symptoms like cognitive decline, dementia, hallucinosis, orthostatic hypotension, urinary incontinence insomnia, fatigue, and daytime sleepiness become increasingly prevalent as the disease progresses and contribute in a major fashion to the global disability of advanced PD. The development of a modified version of the HY scale taking into account these aspects may be the focus of future studies—not only to better reflect PD progression in the modern treatment era, but also to enhance the clinimetric validity and responsiveness of the scale.

REFERENCES

1. Hely MA, Reid WG, Adena MA, et al. The Sydney multicenter study of Parkinson's disease: the inevitability of dementia at 20 years. *Mov Disord.* 2008;23:837–844.
2. Schrag A, Selai C, Jahanshahi M, et al. The EQ-5D—a generic quality of life measure is a useful instrument to measure quality of life in patients with Parkinson's disease. *J Neurol Neurosurg Psychiatry.* 2000;69:67–73.
3. Hoehn MM, Yahr MD. Parkinsonism: onset, progression and mortality. *Neurology.* 1967;17:427–442.
4. Goetz CG, Poewe W, Rascol O, et al. Movement Disorder Society Task Force report on the Hoehn and Yahr staging scale: status and recommendations. *Mov Disord.* 2004;19: 1020–1028.
5. Mitchell SL, Harper DW, Lau A, et al. Patterns of outcome measurement in Parkinson's disease clinical trials. *Neuroepidemiology.* 2000;19: 100–108.
6. Diamond SG, Markham CH. Evaluating the evaluations: or how to weigh the scales of parkinsonian disability. *Neurology.* 1983;33:1098–1099.
7. Marttila RJ, Rinne UK. Disability and progression in Parkinson's disease. *Acta Neurol Scand.* 1977;56:159–169.
8. Maier Hoehn MM. Parkinsonism treated with levodopa: progression and mortality. *J Neural Transm Suppl.* 1983;19:253–264.

9. Pinter MM, Pogarell O, Oertel WH. Efficacy, safety, and tolerance of the non-ergoline dopamine agonist pramipexole in the treatment of advanced Parkinson's disease: a double-blind, placebo-controlled, randomised, multicentre study. *J Neurol Neurosurg Psychiatry.* 1999;66:436–441.

10. van Hilten JJ, van der Zwan AD, Zwinderman AH, et al. Rating impairment and disability in Parkinson's disease: evaluation of the Unified Parkinson's Disease Rating Scale. *Mov Disord.* 1994;9:84–88.

11. Sato K, Hatano T, Yamashiro K, et al. Prognosis of Parkinson's disease: time to stage III, IV, V, and to motor fluctuations. *Mov Disord.* 2006;21:1384–1395.

12. Hely MA, Morris JGL, Traficante R, et al. The Sydney multicentre study of Parkinson's disease: progression and mortality at 10 years. *J Neurol Neurosurg Psychiatry.* 1999;67:300–307.

13. Alves G, Wentzel-Larsen T, Aarsland D, et al. Progression of motor impairment and disability in Parkinson disease: a population-based study. *Neurology.* 2005;65:1436–1441.

14. Zhao YJ, Wee HL, Chan YH, et al. Progression of Parkinson's disease as evaluated by Hoehn and Yahr stage transition times. *Mov Disord.* 2010;25:702–708.

15. Goetz CG, Stebbins GT, Blasucci LM. Differential progression of motor impairment in levodopa-treated Parkinson's disease. *Mov Disord.* 2000;15:479–484.

16. Roos RA, Jongen JC, Van der Velde EA. Clinical course of patients with idiopathic Parkinson's disease. *Mov Disord.* 1996;11:236–242.

17. Geminiani G, Cesana BM, Tamma F, et al. Interobserver reliability between neurologists in training of Parkinson's disease rating scales. A multicenter study. *Mov Disord.* 1991;6:330–335.

18. Wang J, Zuo CT, Jiang YP, et al. 18F-FP-CIT PET imaging and SPM analysis of dopamine transporters in Parkinson's disease in various Hoehn and Yahr stages. *J Neurol.* 2007;254:185–190.

19. Muller J, Wenning GK, Jellinger K, et al. Progression of Hoehn and Yahr stages in Parkinsonian disorders: a clinicopathologic study. *Neurology.* 2000;55:888–891.

20. Ginanneschi A, Degl'Innocenti F, Magnolfi S, et al. Evaluation of Parkinson's disease: reliability of three rating scales. *Neuroepidemiology.* 1988;7:38–41.

21. Ginanneschi A, Degl'Innocenti F, Maurello MT, et al. Evaluation of Parkinson's disease: a new approach to disability. *Neuroepidemiology.* 1991;10:282–287.

22. Schrag A, Spottke A, Quinn NP, et al. Comparative responsiveness of Parkinson's disease scales to change over time. *Mov Disord.* 2009;24:813–818.

23. Hely MA, Chey T, Wilson A, et al. Reliability of the Columbia scale for assessing signs of Parkinson's disease. *Mov Disord.* 1993;8:466–472.

24. Martinez-Martin P, Gil-Nagel A, Gracia LM, et al. Unified Parkinson's Disease Rating Scale characteristics and structure. The Cooperative Multicentric Group. *Mov Disord.* 1994;9:76–83.

25. Rabey JM, Bass H, Bonuccelli U, et al. Evaluation of the Short Parkinson's Evaluation Scale: a new friendly scale for the evaluation of Parkinson's disease in clinical drug trials. *Clin Neuropharmacol.* 1997;20:322–337.

26. Stebbins GT, Goetz CG. Factor structure of the Unified Parkinson's Disease Rating Scale: motor examination section. *Mov Disord.* 1998;13:633–636.

27. Jenkinson C, Fitzpatrick R, Peto V, et al. The Parkinson's Disease Questionnaire (PDQ-39): development and validation of a Parkinson's disease summary index score. *Age Ageing.* 1997;26:353–357.

28. Welsh M, McDermott MP, Holloway RG, et al. Development and testing of the Parkinson's disease quality of life scale. *Mov Disord.* 2003;18:637–645.

29. Reynolds NC Jr, Montgomery GK. Factor analysis of Parkinson's impairment. An evaluation of the final common pathway. *Arch Neurol.* 1987;44:1013–1016.

30. Henderson L, Kennard C, Crawford TJ, et al. Scales for rating motor impairment in Parkinson's disease: studies of reliability and convergent validity. *J Neurol Neurosurg Psychiatry.* 1991;54:18–24.

31. Staffen W, Mair A, Unterrainer J, et al. Measuring the progression of idiopathic Parkinson's disease with [123I] beta-CIT SPECT. *J Neural Transm.* 2000;107:543–552.

32. Eidelberg D, Moeller JR, Ishikawa T, et al. Assessment of disease severity in parkinsonism with fluorine-18-fluorodeoxyglucose and PET. *J Nucl Med.* 1995;36:378–383.

33. Vingerhoets FJ, Snow BJ, Lee CS, et al. Longitudinal fluorodopa positron emission tomographic studies of the evolution of idiopathic parkinsonism. *Ann Neurol.* 1994;36:759–764.

34. Goetz CG, Koller WC, Poewe W, et al. Management of Parkinson's disease: an

evidence-based review. *Mov Disord.* 2001;12: 1–166.

35. Lieberman A, Ranhosky A, Korts D. Clinical evaluation of pramipexole in advanced Parkinson's disease: results of a double-blind, placebo-controlled, parallel-group study. *Neurology.* 1997;49:162–168.

36. Guttman M. Double-blind comparison of pramipexole and bromocriptine treatment with placebo in advanced Parkinson's disease. International Pramipexole-Bromocriptine Study Group. *Neurology.* 1997;49:1060–1065.

37. Pinter MM, Helscher RJ, Nasel CO, et al. Quantification of motor deficit in Parkinson's disease with a motor performance test series. *J Neural Transm Park Dis Dement Sect.* 1992;4:131–141.

38. Parkinson Study Group. Safety and efficacy of pramipexole in early Parkinson disease. A randomized dose-ranging study. *JAMA.* 1997;278:125–130.

39. Shannon KM, Bennett JP Jr, Friedman JH. Efficacy of pramipexole, a novel dopamine agonist, as monotherapy in mild to moderate Parkinson's disease. The Pramipexole Study Group. *Neurology.* 1997;49:724–728.

40. Hubble JP, Koller WC, Cutler NR, et al. Pramipexole in patients with early Parkinson's disease. *Clin Neuropharmacol.* 1995;18: 338–347.

41. Parkinson Study Group. Pramipexole vs levodopa as initial treatment for Parkinson disease: a randomized controlled trial. *JAMA.* 2000;284:1931–1938.

11

QUALITY OF LIFE SCALES

Pablo Martinez-Martin, Carmen Rodriguez-Blazquez, and Kelly E. Lyons

Summary

Parkinson's disease is a complex disorder manifested by a wide variety of symptoms, progressive disability, and complications that strongly affect patients' quality of life. Health-related quality of life (HRQOL) is considered an important patient-reported outcome for trials of interventions and monitoring the consequences of disease in physical, mental, and social domains. A long debate about the definition of HRQOL remains, but it is generally accepted that it refers to the impact of the disease and its treatment on patients, assessed from their perspective.

Following the methodology imposed by previous work of the Movement Disorder Society Task Force, a review of the psychometric attributes of those generic and specific HRQOL scales applied in studies on PD was completed. Considering the scales from three perspectives, including use in PD, use by multiple research groups, and clinimetric properties, a final classification as **Recommended**, **Suggested**, or **Listed** was applied to each reviewed instrument. Four generic scales (EQ-5D, NHP, SF-36, and SIP) and five specific (PDQ-39, PDQ-8, PDQL, PIMS, and SCOPA-PS) reached the level of "Recommended." The PDQ-39 is the most thoroughly tested and applied questionnaire. Three other generic measures (15-D, SEIQOL-DW, and WHOQOL-BREF) and the specific PDQUALIF are "Suggested." With additional effort in completing the stipulated requirements, they could reach the Recommended level in the future.

At present, a wide variety of HRQOL measures for application in PD are available and the task force does not recommend the development of a new scale. Selection of the most appropriate instrument for a particular objective requires consideration of the characteristics of each scale and the goals of the assessment.

INTRODUCTION

Parkinson's disease is a complex disorder with motor impairment and a wide variety of non-motor symptoms that result in progressive disability and severe complications, factors that have a significant impact on physical, mental, and social well-being and, subsequently, on quality of life.

In recent years and in agreement with the biopsychosocial model of medicine, clinical data have been increasingly supplemented with patient-reported outcomes (PROs), which refer to a patient's report of a health condition and its treatment.[1] These include patient reports regarding symptoms, functional status, psychological well-being, health-related quality of life (HRQOL), satisfaction with care, global impression of health, and others.

In medical settings, "quality of life" is used as an umbrella term referring to a wide range of PROs. A lack of clearly delimited conceptual framework and consistent terminology in this area has led to both misunderstanding and sometimes misuse of PRO measures. Confusion arises because there are no universally accepted definitions for many of the concepts, and the boundaries between them are often unclear.

Global quality of life has been approached across such disciplines as sociology and economy, but in the clinical context, emphasis should be placed on addressing HRQOL, a more restricted concept combining experiences and expectations related to health status, health care, and social support.[2,3] In summary, HRQOL refers to the dimensions of global quality of life that are affected by health status and by health care. The theoretical framework of HRQOL is largely based on a multidimensional perspective derived from the World Health Organization's (WHO) definition of *health* as a "state of complete physical, mental and social well-being, and not merely the absence of disease or infirmity."[4] Therefore, although there is a variety of domains that could be considered in the concept of HRQOL, the three major dimensions of physical status and functioning, psychological status and well-being, and social interactions and well-being are the starting points of most approaches to HRQOL assessment.[5–8]

HRQOL focuses on the impact of disease and treatment on patients, assessed from their perspective.[9–11] Nonetheless, the term "HRQOL" frequently involves a combination of objective functioning and subjective perceptions of health[11,12] For some authors, HRQOL focuses on health status, level of impairment, disability, and, to a lesser extent, handicap.[13]

Health status (HS) refers to perceived health in descriptive terms of physical and mental symptoms, disability, and social dysfunction related to the health condition, but is different from HRQOL in that it lacks judgements and reactions. Therefore, HS may influence and predict HRQOL, but should not be considered equivalent to HRQOL.[11] In fact, studies have shown that, from the perspective of patients, health status and quality of life are distinct constructs, with different predictors.[14] Therefore, HS could be considered a relevant factor influencing HRQOL, which—in turn—is an aspect of global quality of life.

In practice, instruments measuring HRQOL assess the physical, emotional and social well-being and satisfaction related to health and care, combining objective functioning and subjective perceptions and judgements; whereas instruments aimed at measuring HS focus mainly on the impact of disease on physical, mental, and social functioning, but do not include judgements and reflections about well-being and satisfaction with health.

Because of the impact of PD on patients' HRQOL, the profusion of studies including HRQOL measures, and the existence of a wide variety of HRQOL scales, the Movement Disorder Society (MDS) organized a systematic review of the psychometric properties of the scales used to measure HRQOL in PD. MDS-sponsored reviews of scales for assessing other aspects of PD have already been published.[15–21] Taking into account the lack of agreement on the concepts inherent to HRQOL and the loose use of this term in some settings, the task force performed a comprehensive review, including all instruments typically recognized by clinicians as HRQOL scales that have been applied in studies on PD.

METHODS

Administrative organization and critique process

This review followed the same working methods as those applied by the MDS Task Force on Rating Scales for PD for other constructs (for example, apathy, anxiety, depression, dyskinesias) in PD.[15–21]

This chapter is an adaptation of a peer-reviewed manuscript published previously (Martinez-Martin et al.) and uses the same methodology as described in Chapter 6.

Literature search strategy

All specific instruments recognized by clinicians as "QoL scales" for PD and the generic ones that have been applied in studies on PD more than anecdotally (i.e., with published data about the instrument design, validation, and application in PD) were included in the review. These scales were identified by a systematic literature search. Medline on PubMed (online) was searched for relevant papers with the terms *Parkinson's disease, parkinsonism* or *Parkinson disease,* and "quality of life," "QoL," "health-related quality of life," and "HRQOL," published before January 2010. For each scale, a search was conducted for the terms *Parkinson's disease, parkinsonism* or *Parkinson disease,* and the name of the scale. Additionally, published papers known to the task force members were included in this review.

The reviewed scales are categorized as generic or specific for PD and, within each of these groups, following the temporal order of their first publication. The description of each scale in terms of its administrative characteristics is provided in Table 11-1 and the results of the evaluation strategy for each scale are summarized in Table 11-2.

REVIEW OF HRQOL GENERIC SCALES

Sickness Impact Profile (SIP)

Scale description—*Structure.* The SIP is a generic health status questionnaire consisting of 136 items grouped in 12 categories and two dimensions: physical and psychosocial. It may be used as patient self-report or by an interviewer, and it takes approximately 30 minutes to administer. Higher scores, from 0 (*no dysfunction*) to 100 (*maximal dysfunction*), indicate worse health status.[23] Time frame is "today."

Table 11-1. Descriptive Characteristics of the Health-Related Quality of Life Scales

ACRONYM*	TYPE	NUMBER OF ITEMS	NUMBER OF DOMAINS	TIME FRAME
SIP	*Generic*	136	12	Today
NHP	*Generic*	38	6	At present time
EQ-5D	*Generic*	5	5	Today
SF-36	*Generic*	36	8	Last 4 weeks
SEIQOL-DW	*Generic*	–	5	At present time
15-D	*Generic*	15	15	At present time
WHOQOL-BREF	*Generic*	26	4	Last 4 weeks
QLS -MD	*Generic*	12	1	Last 4 weeks
QLS-DBS		5	1	
BELA-p-k	Specific	19	4	At present time
PDQ-39	Specific	39	8	Last month
PDQ-8	Specific	8	8	Last month
PIMS	Specific	10	4	At present time
PDQL	Specific	37	4	Last 3 months
PDQUALIF	Specific	32	7	Flexible
Fragebogens PLQ	Specific	44	9	Past week
PPS	Specific	39	3	?
SCOPA-PS	Specific	11	1	Last month

*For acronym interpretation, see the text.

General population norms are available for the SIP (Table 11-1).

Additional points. The instrument is available in multiple languages [24,25] and may be obtained from Medical Outcomes Trust at www.outcomes-trust.org. A shortened version, the SIP 68, has been developed.[26]

Key evaluation issues—It has been applied in studies on PD and has been used by multiple authors other than the developers.[27,28] The SIP covers areas of importance to PD patients in both physical and psychosocial domains. In terms of clinimetric issues, internal consistency and test-retest analysis showed the satisfactory reliability of the scale.[23,26] Convergent and discriminant validity were appropriate as evaluated by the multitrait-multimethod technique. SIP category scores explained 30% to 60% of the variance in the criterion measures used. Studies have reported associations of the SIP with constructs important in PD such as the UPDRS, Hoehn and Yahr, and SF-36.[24,27] Responsiveness has been reported in some studies.[27–29] The minimally important difference (MID) has not been determined for the SIP in PD.

Strengths and weaknesses—The SIP is a widely used measure, it has general population norms, and its validity has been supported in PD samples. Criticisms of the scale are related to the length of the instrument, the scoring method (relative contribution of each category to the overall score has little justification), the presence of ceiling effects in older adults, and the better sensitivity to worsened health state over improved health state.

Final assessment—The SIP is "Recommended" for use in PD.

NOTTINGHAM HEALTH PROFILE (NHP)

Scale description—*Structure.* The NHP is a measure of perceived health status.[30] The instrument contains 38 items, in a yes/no format, covering emotional reactions, energy, pain, physical mobility, sleep, and social isolation. Affirmative responses in each domain are multiplied by a domain-specific weight, with domain scores ranging from 0 (good health) to 100 (poor health). The time frame is "at the moment" (Table 11-1). The NHP index of distress (NHPD) is a measure of illness-related distress containing 24 items of the NHP, omitting those related to physical disability.[31]

Additional points. The NHP and scoring is in the public domain and has been translated into 23 languages. It takes around to 10 minutes to complete, and there are norms available for the general population. The NHP can be obtained at www.cebp.nl/media/m83.pdf. It has been validated in many patient populations.[32,33]

Key evaluation issues—The NHP has been applied by multiple authors in studies on PD.[34–37] With regard to the clinimetric issues, the NHP has shown adequate internal consistency, except for sleep, energy, and social isolation domains. NHP content is considered relevant for PD patients,[38] and it has satisfactory known-groups and convergent validity.[35]

NHP sensitivity to change over time or in response to treatment has been demonstrated in several studies,[33,34,36,37,39,40] although it showed a substantial floor effect in mild PD patients relative to the PDQ-39.[35]

Strengths and weaknesses—The NHP strengths include rapid application, availability of general population norms, and assessment of change over time and response to interventions. The main weakness of the NPH is that it has significant floor effects when used in PD patients.

Final assessment—The NHP is "Recommended" for use in PD.

EUROQOL 5-DIMENSIONS (EQ-5D)

Scale description—*Structure.* The EQ-5D is a standardized generic measure of health status.[41] It provides a descriptive profile and a single index value for health status that can be used in the clinical and economic evaluation of health care. The time frame is "today." The EQ-5D has five domains (mobility, self-care, usual activities, pain/discomfort and anxiety/depression). Each domain is represented by one item with three possible response levels, from 1 (no problems or symptoms) to 3 (serious problems or symptoms) (Table 11-1). It also contains a question about change in health state in the preceding 12 months and a visual analogue scale (VAS) to assess current health status, scored from 0 (worst imaginable) to 100 (best imaginable). Higher scores represent better health. The descriptive responses can be combined into a single profile (EQ-Index) representing one of 245 possible health states. The index ranges from 0 (death) to 1 (perfect health). Negative values, for health states considered worse than death, are possible.[42] Norms are available for the general population.

Additional points. The EQ-5D is useful for economic evaluations and allows for comparisons among different populations and health conditions. It is owned by the EuroQol Group, and licensing fees may be determined by the EuroQol Executive Office. It has been widely translated (EuroQol website: www.euroqol.org).

Key evaluation issues—The EQ-5D has been applied by multiple authors in studies on PD.[43–46] Concerning the clinimetric issues, studies on the psychometric properties of the EQ-5D in PD are insufficient. In this population, the EQ-5D has some ceiling effect and does not discriminate between patients in Hoehn and Yahr 1 to 2.5.[44] The face and content validity is adequate in PD, and it shows satisfactory convergent validity with the SF-36 and PDQ-39.[43] The EQ index is significantly correlated with the UPDRS and other clinical scales.[43,46] The EQ-5D has been responsive to medical and surgical interventions in PD patients.[47–52]

Strengths and weaknesses—The EQ-5D is unique in that it provides a summary score unique features of the that can be used to calculate quality adjusted life years (QALYs) for economic analysis. It is a brief and widely used measure, with general population norms, that is available in many languages and has been used in many disease states.

Reliability in PD has not been tested, but has been established in a variety of other populations. The EQ-5D should be used with caution in mild PD populations as it may not be responsive in this group.

Final Assessment—The EQ-5D is "Recommended" for use in PD.

MEDICAL OUTCOMES STUDY 36-ITEM SHORT-FORM HEALTH SURVEY (SF-36)

Scale description—*Structure.* The SF-36 is a measure of health status.[53] It consists of 36 questions in eight domains: physical function, role-physical, bodily pain, general health, vitality, social function, role-emotional, and mental health. A score between 0 and 100 is calculated for each domain, as well as for the summary scales for physical and mental function, which are weighted averages of the individual domain scales. Higher scores represent better health status. The time frame of the SF-36 is four weeks (Table 11-1).

Additional points. There are several versions (e.g. SF-36v2, SF-12, SF-8), all in the public domain. The SF-36 has been translated into numerous languages, and may be obtained at www.sf-36.org/tools/sf36.shtml. Normative data are available for different populations and health conditions, but not for PD.

Key evaluation issues—The SF-36 has been used by multiple authors in studies to assess patients with PD.[54–60]

Clinimetric issues. Studies have reported missing responses, particularly for older patients with PD, ranging from 3% to 20%,[55,57,58] and floor and ceiling effects have been reported for some SF-36 subscales.[57,58,61] The internal consistency of the SF-36 was good, except for the social subscale, and stability was good for most subscales.[54,56,58,59] There is evidence of convergent and discriminant validity.[54,56,62] Evidence to support the two subscales measuring physical and mental health in PD was not found.[58,63] The SF-36 was responsive to change over time in several subscales but not the physical and mental summary indices.[64] Responsiveness to change over time was superior to the PDQ-39 and PDQUALIF, but accounted for less PD-specific content.[60] When used to measure change due to treatment, the SF-36 was less sensitive than the PDQ-39.[49] The minimal detectable change estimated per domain has been determined.[59]

Strengths and weaknesses

In PD, there is partial evidence of reliability, validity, and responsiveness. It can be used for

PD when the eight subscales are applied and reported, but the two physical and mental composite scores do not appear to be valid in this population.

Final assessment—SF-36 is "Recommended" for use in PD.

SCHEDULE FOR THE EVALUATION OF INDIVIDUAL QUALITY OF LIFE—DIRECT WEIGHTING (SEIQOL-DW)

Scale description—*Structure.* The SEIQOL is a non-standardized tool designed to assess an individual's QoL,[65] defined by the authors as "what the individual determines it to be or what the patient tells himself it is."[66] For use in the clinical setting, a simpler assessment, the SEIQOL-Direct Weighting (SEIQOL-DW), was developed.[67,68] The assessment has three stages: (1) a semi-structured interview, where the respondent identifies the five areas of life considered most important to his or her overall QoL; (2) respondent rating of the current state for each domain on a 0 to 100 vertical visual analogue scale; and (3) respondent quantification of the relative importance (weight) of each domain in colored laminated circular disks, on a scale from 0 to 100. This scale assesses current QoL (Table 11-1) and has been validated in several countries.

Additional points. Also available are the SEIQOL-DR (Disease-related)[69] and a computer-administered version of SEIQOL-DW.[70] SEIQOL-DW requires minimal training, is copyrighted, and may be obtained at http://www.proqolid.org.

Key evaluation issues—The SEIQOL-DW has been used by multiple authors,[71-73] but seldom in PD.[74] Regarding the SEIQOL-DW clinimetric issues: in non-PD conditions, the measure has shown satisfactory acceptability,[72] moderate to acceptable reproducibility,[68,70,72] and moderate/weak convergent validity.[73] Acceptability, stability, and known-groups validity have not been formally tested in PD. Content validity is adequate, although limited to five domains. It has shown a moderate correlation with the PDQ-39.[74] Due to the complexity

of PD, changes over time are difficult to evaluate with the SEIQOL-DW due to potential changes in many domains. The management of disks may limit its use in PD.[74]

Strengths and weaknesses

The main advantage of this scale is the individualized assessment. It has been rarely applied in PD, and most of SEIQOL-DW psychometric properties have not been tested in this condition.

Final assessment—The SEIQOL-DW is "Suggested" for use in PD.

QUALITY OF LIFE QUESTIONNAIRE 15D (15D)

Scale description—*Structure.* The 15D was designed to measure HRQOL defined as a multidimensional concept including mobility, vision, hearing, breathing, sleeping, eating, speech, elimination, usual activities, mental function, discomfort/symptoms, depression, distress, vitality, and sexual activity.[75] Each question has five response options, from *normal* to *complete disability/dysfunction*. Higher scores reflect greater impact on HRQOL. Either an individual or a population profile based on the 15 dimensions and an index score ranging from 0 to 1 based on preference weightings can be calculated.[75-77] The time frame is "present health state" (Table 11-1).

Additional points. The 15D takes about 10 to 15 minutes to complete. The instrument is available in 25 languages. It is copyrighted and can be obtained free of charge for academic purposes at www.15d-instrument.net/15d.

Key evaluation issues—The 15D has been used by multiple authors, and occasionally in PD.[78-80] In terms of clinimetric issues, the instrument has shown satisfactory psychometric properties in non-PD populations,[75] and has been validated in PD patients across a wide range of ages and disability.[78] Acceptability, internal consistency, and stability of the 15D have not been reported in the PD population. Content and discriminative validity appear acceptable in PD patients. PD patients with depression or dementia were shown to have worse HRQOL than those without these symptoms. The 15D was strongly correlated with the PDQ-39 and with some parts of the UPDRS. Responsiveness and MID have not been tested in PD. The validation of the 15D in PD patients was completed only in Finland.[78]

Strengths and weaknesses

The 15D has been used in healthy individuals and in those with a variety of disease states. It is available in multiple languages and can be completed quickly and easily, producing a profile and also an index score usable in studies of health economics. Psychometric properties have been extensively tested in multiple health states, but not in PD.

Final assessment—The 15D is "Suggested" for use in PD.

WHO QUALITY OF LIFE ASSESSMENT SHORT VERSION (WHOQOL-BREF)

Scale description—*Structure.* The WHOQOL-BREF[81,82] is a short form of the WHOQOL-100.[83] The scale has 26 questions in the four domains of physical health, psychological, social relationships, and environment, as well as two general questions about quality of life and health that are not included in the summary score. Items are rated in an ordinal scale with five options of response, with the lowest value being the worst score. Items in each domain are added to obtain raw scores, which are transformed to scores ranging from 0 to 100 for each domain. Higher scores indicate better quality of life. The time frame is "the past four weeks" (Table 11-1).

Additional points. The WHOQOL-BREF can be completed in 5 to 10 minutes. It is multidimensional, multicultural, and available in multiple languages. It is copyrighted by WHO and can be obtained by contacting permissions@who.int.

Key evaluation issues—The WHOQOL-BREF has been used by multiple authors and occasionally in PD.[84,85] With regard to the clinimetric issues, in the general population, the scale showed no ceiling or floor effects; internal consistency and stability were good; and content and construct validity were demonstrated.[81,82] The WHOQOL-BREF has not been validated in the PD population.

In one study, the scale was shown to be correlated with disease severity.[85] In another study, the scale was shown to differentiate between PD patients and caregivers based on the physical and psychological domains.[84]

Strengths and weaknesses

This is a brief, easily administered, widely available, and validated scale. However, it has been rarely used in PD patients and has not been validated in this population.

Final assessment—WHOQOL-BREF is "Suggested" for use in PD.

QUESTIONS ON LIFE SATISFACTION—MOVEMENT DISORDERS (QLS-MD) MODULE AND QUESTIONS ON LIFE SATISFACTION—DEEP BRAIN STIMULATION (QLS-DBS) MODULE

Scale description—*Structure.* The QLS-MD and QLS-DBS[86] are two modules of an existing life-satisfaction questionnaire that includes modules of general life satisfaction (QLS-A) and satisfaction with health (QLS-G).[87] The QLS-MD has 12 questions on various aspects of health in PD, essential tremor, and dystonia, and the QLS-DBS has five items on HRQOL of patients under DBS treatment for the same disease states. Items are scored on a five-point scale for both importance to the patient and satisfaction with its current state, with higher scores meaning greater importance and higher level of satisfaction. Time frame is "the past four weeks" (Table 11-1).

Additional points. The modules take approximately 10 minutes to complete. They were developed in German and translated to English. The scale is available in the literature, and copyright is not mentioned.[86]

Key evaluation issues—The QLS-MD and QLS-DBS were developed and validated primarily in PD, but have been used only by the developers, and seldom applied in PD.[86]

Clinimetric issues: Floor and ceiling effects are overall adequate; internal consistency and content validity are satisfactory for both modules; and convergent validity was moderate to high with the SF-36 and EQ-5D for both modules.[86] No other psychometric properties were explored.

Strengths and weaknesses

These modules are short and easily completed, although they provide little information about psychological or social issues. Some relevant attributes of the scale have not been tested.

Final assessment—The QLS-MD and QLS-DBS are "Listed" for use in PD.

SPECIFIC INSTRUMENTS FOR PD

Belastungsfragebogen Parkinson Kurzversion (BELA-P-k)

Scale description—*Structure.* The BELA-P-k contains 19 items grouped into four dimensions of achievement capability/physical symptoms, fear/emotional symptoms, social functioning, and partner-bonding/family.[88,89] (Table 11-1). Each item explores both the extent to which the patient is bothered by the psychosocial problem (0 = *not at all* to 4 = *a great deal*) and the need for help (0 = *not important* to 4 = *very important*). Two subscale scores "Bothered by" (Bb) and "Need for Help" (NfH) are obtained by summing up the item scores. A higher score indicates the patient is more bothered by and has a greater need for help with the specific psychosocial problem. It is really a psychosocial assessment administered by a rater through a semistructured interview. It may be completed with the help of a partner.

The time frame is "the present," but answers are based on a comparison to past ability/experiences.

Additional points. It is available in German (original), Dutch, and English,[89] and is available for use with permission of the authors.

Key evaluation issues—The BELA-P-k was developed for use in PD, but seldom used by authors other than the developers.[89,90] Concerning its clinimetric issues, the validation study included patients with a wide range of duration and staging.[89] Acceptability and

reproducibility have not been tested. The internal-consistency coefficients for the total Bb and NfH scales were excellent. Content validity was satisfactory, and convergent validity with other HRQOL measures were generally moderate or high. Discriminative validity for PD severity levels was poor.[90] The correlation between total Bb and NfH subscales (internal validity) was high.

Strengths and weaknesses

The BELA-P-k is a relatively short instrument, informative for psychosocial problems, with satisfactory psychometric properties. There is only one validation study available, and important psychometric properties are not tested.

Final assessment—The BELA-P-k is "Suggested" for use in PD.

PARKINSON'S DISEASE QUESTIONNAIRE (PDQ-39)

Scale description—*Structure.* The PDQ-39 is composed of 39 items grouped in eight subscales including mobility, activities of daily living, emotional well-being, stigma, social support, cognitions, communication, and bodily discomfort.[91] The time frame is "over the last month" and responses are scored from 0 (*never*) to 4 (*always*) (Table 11-1). Subscales scores range from 0 to100 and are obtained by summing the items and transforming to a percentage based on the maximum possible subscale score. A Summary Index (PDQ-39 SI), the arithmetic mean of the sub-scales, can also be calculated.[92] Higher scores represent worse QoL.

Additional points. PDQ-39 does not include sexuality and sleep problems. It has been translated and validated in many languages and different cultural settings. The scale, manual, and license may be obtained from the University of Oxford at www.publichealth.ox.ac.uk/research/hsru/PDQ/Intropdq.

Key evaluation issues—The PDQ-39, developed and validated for use in PD,[54,91,92] has been used in various studies by multiple authors.[46,50,93–104] It is applicable across all severity levels of PD, although patients in more advanced disease stages may find some items not relevant and the questionnaire too long.[96] Regarding the clinimetric issues: the PDQ-39 SI is a multidimensional measure lacking relevant floor and ceiling effects; however, a floor effect for the social support domain has been reported in some studies.[95,97,100] Studies have found adequate score distribution.[98,100] It has satisfactory internal consistency parameters globally, although some domains have not reached predefined thresholds, and some items have scaling problems.[92,94,97,98,100,101] Stability was adequate for the PDQ-39 SI and most domains,[91,95,97,100,102] but some items demonstrated a weak or moderate level of agreement.[100,102] Content validity was generally good, with some shortcomings and problems related to missing areas and interpretation.[94,95] Convergent validity of the PDQ-39 SI with summary indexes of other HRQOL instruments has been satisfactory.[46,97,98,100,102]

Correlations between PDQ-39 domains and corresponding domains of other QoL measures and clinical rating scales are, as a whole, moderate or high.[91,93,95,100,102,104] Discriminative validity for Hoehn and Yahr stages and perceived PD severity levels has been established.[54,91,98,100,102] The PDQ-39 has been widely applied in different ethnic/cultural settings[105] and used as an outcome measure in clinical trials. It has been shown to be responsive.[50,51,99,103] A MID and other interpretability parameters have been calculated for the PDQ-39 SI.[102,106,107]

Strengths and weaknesses

The PDQ-39 is widely available, allowing cross-cultural comparisons. It has been extensively analyzed, showing adequate psychometric properties. Familiarity and wide use are also relevant advantages. However, it lacks items on some relevant HRQOL aspects and has reliability limitations in some domains.

Final Assessment—PDQ-39 is "Recommended" for use in PD.

PARKINSON'S DISEASE QUESTIONNAIRE SHORT FORM (PDQ-8)

Scale description—*Structure*. The PDQ-8 is a shorter version of the PDQ-39.[108] It includes one item from each PDQ-39 domain (Table 11-1). For each item, the response options range from 0 (*never*) to 4 (*always*). The total score is obtained by summing the eight items and standardizing on a scale of 0 to 100 (PDQ-8 SI). Higher scores reflect worse HRQOL, and the time frame is "the past four weeks."[108,109]

Additional points. Conditions of usage are the same as for the PDQ-39. It has been cross-culturally adapted and validated in many languages and countries.

Key evaluation issues—The PDQ-8 has been used in diverse studies by multiple authors.[110–116] With regard to its clinimetric attributes, there has been no evidence of floor or ceiling effects for the PDQ-8 SI[109,112,113,115]; internal consistency is satisfactory and test-retest has been found to be adequate.[109–113,115] A high level of agreement between patient and caregiver was demonstrated, albeit the agreement showed a trend to decrease at advanced stages of PD and in the presence of depression.[111] As expected, correlation between the PDQ-8 and PDQ-39 (criterion validity) was very high (r ≥ 0.90).[108–110,112] Convergent validity with other HRQOL measures [94,110,112] and the correlation with other clinical scales was moderate or high.[110,114] It is considered unidimensional,[109] but more research is necessary to confirm this property.[115] The PDQ-8 has been used as an outcome measure for some interventions and was sensitive to changes in health status.[117,118] MID has been calculated in one study.[116]

Strengths and weaknesses

The PDQ-8 is applicable across all PD stages, although patients with severer impairment could have difficulties with the response options, similar to the PDQ-39. The PDQ-8's brevity significantly decreases respondent burden and completion time. Nonetheless, a simplified three-category scale has been proposed.[115]

Final Assessment—The PDQ-8 is "Recommended" for use in PD.

PARKINSON'S IMPACT SCALE (PIMS)

Scale description—*Structure*. The PIMS is a 10-item scale with four domains: physical aspects of disease, psychological aspects, social aspects, and sexuality (Table 11-1). Scores range from 0 to 40, and lower scores indicate better HRQOL. Patients rate the degree of impact of each item as 0 = *no change*, 1 = *slight*, 2 = *moderate*, 3 = *moderately severe*, or 4 = *severe*.[119] Ratings are based on "the present time."

Additional points. The scale is in the public domain.[119] It can be completed by the patient or by an interviewer and has also been validated in caregivers.[120]

Key evaluation issues—The PIMS has been validated in some studies[119–121] but has been rarely used by authors other than developers.[122] In terms of clinimetric issues, internal consistency was satisfactory,[119] and a four-factor structure of the PIMS has been reported.[120] The scale showed an ability to discriminate between fluctuating and non-fluctuating patients.[120,121] A close convergent validity with other specific HRQOL questionnaires has been demonstrated.[122] The PIMS showed high sensitivity and moderate specificity to capture changes in HRQOL.[121]

Strengths and weaknesses

The PIMS is brief, concise, and has also been validated for use in caregivers. There is no evidence of its use in large or long-term prospective studies; hence there are limited sensitivity data available. In addition, some tested attributes need to be explored with a more robust methodology.

Final Assessment—The PIMS is "Recommended" for use in PD.

PARKINSON'S DISEASE QUALITY OF LIFE QUESTIONNAIRE (PDQL)

Scale description—*Structure.* The PDQL has 37 items covering four subscales including Parkinsonian symptoms, systemic symptoms, social function, and emotional function. Responses for each item range from 1 (*all of the time*) to 5 (*never*).[123] The PDQL-Summary Index (SI) is obtained from the sum of all items and ranges from 37 to 185, with higher scores representing better HRQOL. The time frame is "over the last three months" (Table 11-1).

Additional points. Most of the items address the impact of the physical manifestations of PD. Permission from the authors is required and can be obtained at www.mapi-trust.org. The scale has been translated into several languages.

Key evaluation issues—The PDQL has been validated in some studies[123–125] and has been used by multiple authors.[102,122,126–129] Score distributions, including floor and ceiling effects, are adequate for the PDQL-SI. Internal consistency has also been found satisfactory, as a whole.[102,123,125] Test-retest reliability has been satisfactory, both for items and the summary index.[102] The PDQL showed high convergent validity with other HRQOL scales. Also, the internal validity and the validity for known groups (HY stages, disability levels) were satisfactory.[102,122–125] Data about responsiveness and MID are available from clinical trials,[126–128] observation over time,[129] and formal studies on change.[64]

Strengths and weaknesses

The PDQL is available in several languages. It has adequate psychometric properties and is applicable across all stages of the disease, but it may be difficult for patients in advanced stages to complete. As a disadvantage, the PDQL does not cover relevant HRQOL areas in depth (physical function, mental health, social function, cognitive function, and sleep and rest). The long time frame can make the assessment difficult and imprecise.

Final Assessment—The PDQL is "Recommended" for use in PD.

PARKINSON'S DISEASE QUALITY OF LIFE SCALE (PDQUALIF)

Scale description—*Structure.* The PDQUALIF is a 33-item measure that includes seven dimensions with 32 domain specific items and one item of global HRQOL.[130,131] The seven subscales measure social/role function, self image/sexuality, sleep, outlook, physical function, independence, and urinary function. The total score ranges from 0 to 128, with the higher scores indicating worse HRQOL. The user may define the time frame ("today," "in the past week," etc.) (Table 11-1).

Additional points. The scale is available in several languages and can be obtained at www.mapi-trust.org.

Key evaluation issues—The PDQUALIF has been validated in some studies[60,131] and used in a variety of studies, but only by the developers.[132–134] In relation to the clinimetric issues, some ceiling and floor effects were noted in the first validation study. Internal consistency indexes for the subscales ranged from moderate to satisfactory values. Test-retest reliability estimates for the total score and seven subscale scores were globally satisfactory. The PDQUALIF items showed moderate to substantial stability. Convergent and discriminant validity of the PDQUALIF were satisfactory, as a whole. Factor analysis supported a seven-factor solution.[131] In one study, the SF-36 was found to have better responsiveness; however, the PDQUALIF had content that more significantly explained PD patients' HRQOL.[60]

Strengths and weaknesses

The instrument's emphasis is on non-motor symptoms. The PDQUALIF includes a global item of overall HRQOL not found in other specific instruments. It has been used by the Parkinson Study Group in randomized clinical trials of PD.[132–134] Further refinements of the instrument to enhance scaling and instrument properties and eliminating ceiling and floor effects are needed.

Final Assessment—The PDQUALIF is "Suggested" for use in PD.

FRAGEBOGEN PARKINSON LEBENSQUALITÄT (PLQ)

Scale description—*Structure.* This questionnaire consists of 44 items in nine domains, including depression, physical achievement, concentration, leisure, restlessness, activity limitation, insecurity, social integration, and anxiety (Table 11-1). Each item is scored from 1 to 5 based on either intensity, applicability, or quality, depending on the question. Higher scores

reflect worse HRQOL and the time frame is "the past week."[135]

Additional points. The scale is in the public domain but is only available in German. It can be obtained from the developer at Helgoland@paracelsus-kliniken.de.

Key evaluation issues—The PLQ has been used only by the developers of the scale.[135]

The internal consistency of the PLQ was satisfactory. The test-retest reliability was not appropriately evaluated, and the construct validity is uncertain. The content validity of the PLQ is adequate as it covers many domains. Responsiveness has been tested in a small sample ($n = 16$) with poor evidence.[135]

Strengths and weaknesses

The PLQ is relatively short and covers many domains. It includes relevant items for PD patients. Nonetheless, the PLQ is only available in German, and some relevant psychometric properties have not been evaluated.

Final Assessment—The PLQ is "Listed" for use in PD.

PARKINSON'S PROBLEM SCHEDULE (PPS)

Scale description—*Structure.* The PPS is a questionnaire administered by a health care professional that contains 39 items, reflecting activities, behaviors and emotions that are potential problems for PD patients (Table 11-1). The presence of the problems is rated "yes" or "no." Then, severity and stress are both rated on a 5-point Likert scale ranging from 0 = *not at all*, to 4 = *extremely*.[136] Higher scores reflect more problems.

Additional points. The PPS measures the total experience of PD as an illness. There are no validated versions in other languages available.

Key evaluation issues—The PPS has been used only by the developers of the scale.[136]

With regard to its clinimetric properties, score distributions were not evaluated. Internal consistency for subscales was satisfactory. Test-retest reliability was not tested. Face validity is adequate and construct validity was moderate. Responsiveness was not evaluated.

Strengths and weaknesses

The PPS is difficult to obtain, has no translations available, and many relevant psychometric properties were not explored. There are three ratings per item, but only the severity rating is evaluated. A health care professional is needed to administer the questionnaire. In the development of the scale, very few patients with advanced PD were included.

Final Assessment—The PPS is "Listed" for use in PD.

SCALES FOR OUTCOMES IN PARKINSON'S DISEASE–PSYCHOSOCIAL (SCOPA-PS)

Scale description—*Structure.* The SCOPA-PS is a questionnaire that consists of 11 items. Each item is scored on a 4-point Likert scale ranging from 0 to 3. Higher scores reflect worse psychosocial functioning. The time frame is "the past month"[137] (Table 11-1). This questionnaire was developed to quantify the psychosocial impact in PD. Physical and mental domains are not included in the scale.

Additional points. The scale is in the public domain and can be obtained at www.scopa-propark.eu. It was validated in several cultural settings and has been translated into a variety of languages.[100,138,139]

Key evaluation issues—The SCOPA-PS has been independently tested by multiple authors.[138–140]

The scale has no floor or ceiling effects. The item related to sexual problems frequently has missing values. Internal consistency of the scale is satisfactory.[137,140] Test-retest reliability of the SCOPA-PS is good and known-groups analysis revealed adequate discriminative validity.[137,140] Convergent validity is satisfactory with other generic and specific HRQOL scales. Factor analysis showed one single dimension accounting for 48.58% of the variance.[137] However, other studies have identified two factors embedded in the SCOPA-PS.[139,140] Responsiveness of the SCOPA-PS was examined by different methods in a study of change over time.[138]

Strengths and weaknesses

The SCOPA-PS is a short questionnaire with independent validation studies. It is easy to obtain and free to use. However, it evaluates only psychosocial functioning.

Final Assessment—The SCOPA-PS is "Recommended" for use in PD.

CONCLUSIONS AND RECOMMENDATIONS

This review was focused on the HRQOL scales applied to PD patients. For pragmatic reasons, the concept of HRQOL was broad, and the review was inclusive. As a result, the reviewed scales are multidimensional PROs that provide a subjective approach and judgement of physical, mental, and social aspects related to health, but also to functioning and perceptions. More specifically, the reviewed instruments can be classified as measures of health status, psychosocial adjustment, or genuine HRQOL, but in the clinical setting they are often collectively referred to as "QoL or HRQOL questionnaires." The condition for inclusion of an instrument in the review was the availability of enough data to allow a description of the scale and information on the key evaluation issues.

Several instruments are available to measure HRQOL in PD patients. Some of these PROs were specifically developed and validated for use in PD (specific scales), whereas others are used to assess HRQOL in multiple disorders and healthy populations (generic scales). Four of the eight reviewed generic measures (SIP, NHP, EQ-5D, and SF-36),[23,30,41,53] and five of the nine specific scales (PDQ-39, PDQ-8, PIMS, PDQL, and SCOPA-PS)[91,108,119,123,137] were classified as "Recommended" (Table 11-2), according to the MDS-Task Force criteria.

An advantage of the generic instruments is that they cover aspects of general health not included in the specific instruments. For example, the impact of some adverse effects caused by the treatment could be captured by the generic measure but not by the specific one. In addition, they allow for comparison between different disorders and with healthy populations. The

Table 11-2. Key Evaluation Points of the Health-Related Quality of Life Scales

ACRONYM*	TYPE	CRITERIA 1	CRITERIA 2	CRITERIA 3	MSD-TF CLASSIFICATION
SIP	Generic	X	X	X	Recommended
NHP	Generic	X	X	X	Recommended
EQ-5D	Generic	X	X	X	Recommended
SF-36	Generic	X	X	X	Recommended
SEIQOL-DW	Generic	X	X	–	Suggested
15-D	Generic	X	X	–	Suggested
WHOQOL-BREF	Generic	X	X	–	Suggested
QLS-MD QLS-DBS	Generic	X	–	–	Listed
BELA-p-k	Specific	X	–	–	Listed
PDQ-39	Specific	X	X	X	Recommended
PDQ-8	Specific	X	X	X	Recommended
PIMS	Specific	X	X	X	Recommended
PDQL	Specific	X	X	X	Recommended
PDQUALIF	Specific	X	–	X	Suggested
Fragebogens PLQ	Specific	X	–	–	Listed
PPS	Specific	X	–	–	Listed
SCOPA-PS	Specific	X	X	X	Recommended

*For acronym interpretation, see the text.

domains included in these scales may be perceived as unrelated to their condition by patients with specific disorders, sometimes giving rise to high proportion of missing data and low acceptability. Lacking specific dimensions, the generic scales may show a low responsiveness.

Importantly, normative values for the general population exist for the "Recommended" SIP, NHP, SF-36, and EQ-5D, providing a benchmark for comparison of results in the PD population. These four measures are quite different with respect to the number of items, dimensions, and content, covering a wide spectrum of aspects that may be affected by health problems. In addition, the EQ-5D provides utility values for econometric issues. These generic questionnaires have an impressive background of data, are widely available, and are frequently applied in PD studies. Therefore, there is no need to develop new generic scales from the perspective of PD.

In general, the following factors should be considered in making a selection of the most appropriate scale: relevance of the content for patients; objective of the study; characteristics and availability of the instruments (including cross-cultural validation and legal issues, if required); the balance between required information and burden of respondent; and capacity of the researchers for analyzing data that is more complex than the simple summing of items. In the near future, such initiatives as the COSMIN study (COnsensus-based Standards for the selection of health Measurement INstruments) will help us choose the most appropriate scale on the basis of their measurement properties.[14,142]

Concerning the specific measures, they consider aspects closely related to PD and subsequently they are well accepted by patients, who appreciate how their main problems are reflected in the scale. These instruments are more responsive than the generic ones, but they cannot be used for assessing other conditions and may ignore important aspects of general health.

The PDQ-39 is the most thoroughly tested and used HRQOL questionnaire for PD. It possesses, as a whole, adequate psychometric properties and adequately covers physical, mental, and social domains, though nocturnal sleep and sexuality are not included in this scale.[94,143] PDQ-39 and its short form, PDQ-8,[108] are widely available and have been used in diverse epidemiological studies and clinical trials.

The PDQL is the second most frequently used HRQOL instrument specific for PD. It has satisfactory psychometric attributes but does not adequately cover self-care, sleep, cognition, close relationships, or role functioning.[94,143] It is available in different languages and has been applied to various studies.

The PIMS has very few independent and cross-cultural validation studies[122] and has been used only occasionally in applied research. It has limitations in content, with no items on walking, transfers, self care, motor features, cognition and other mental aspects, or social stigma.[94]

Finally, the SCOPA-PS is really an instrument focused on psychosocial adjustment more than on HRQOL.[137] Consequently, it lacks the physical and mental health domains. However, it has been tested psychometrically in several studies and showed satisfactory attributes. It is available and validated in several languages; it has been applied in epidemiological studies only.

In conclusion, none of the "Recommended" specific measures is completely free of limitations, but after consideration of their advantages, disadvantages, and characteristics, they cover the needs for studies on HRQOL in PD. Furthermore, some of the "Suggested" scales may obtain the status of "Recommended" in the future if psychometric testing is completed and satisfactory. Refinement of the existent instruments, such as the addition of items about sleep and sexuality to the PDQ-39/PDQ-8, may improve the characteristics of these specific questionnaires, but there is no need for development of a new specific scale.

The above-mentioned recommendations for selection of the most appropriate generic scale should also be considered for the specific instruments. With regard to limitations of use, some comorbidities can impede the patients' self-assessment. For example, blindness or illiteracy may prevent reading of questions, requiring help by another person who may influence the patient's response. Mental deterioration, particularly in the case of moderate and severe dementia, may make the assessment unreliable or impossible,[144–146] and evaluations by proxy may not be valid.[111,147,148]

In addition to the consequences of the motor impairment, HRQOL questionnaires reflect the impact of non-motor symptoms (NMS) on PD patients. Generic measures include assessment for nocturnal sleep, mental functioning, pain, depression, anxiety, sexual functioning, and fatigue. In addition, PD specific HRQOL measures also address NMS in PD patients such as cognitive functioning, perceptual problems, paresthesias, and daytime somnolence.[149,150] Recently, a close association has been demonstrated between NMS, as a whole, and HRQOL measures,[46,104] a finding that is not surprising when it is considered that some NMS are recognized determinant factors for HRQOL.[143,151]

Taking into account the complexity of manifestations and complications of PD, and the variety of therapies and treatments available and investigated, HRQOL measurement represents at present an indispensable resource in clinical research. It provides information about effects of treatment from the unique perspective of the patient in a more reliable way than the informal interview.[152] Therefore, performing clinical trials that include HRQOL endpoints (even as main outcome of the study) and providing information on the HRQOL outcomes is needed.[50,51,99,103,153,154] Concerning clinical practice, HRQOL evaluation helps investigators prioritize interventions and understand important aspects of the condition and treatment that are impossible to assess through any other method. For obtaining the most appropriate information, it is strongly recommended to combine the generic and specific measures most relevant for patients.[38]

Finally, it is convenient to highlight that the reviewed scales were developed and for the most part validated following the classical test theory principles and methodology, which have important weaknesses. As an alternative, the item response theory methodology (Rasch analysis, for example) has scientific superiority, but there are some impediments limiting its use.[155] In the future, new developments in design of measures and data capture systems (e.g., computer adaptive testing based on item response theory) will facilitate the use of HRQOL measures and the efficiency in their application and interpretation.

Acknowledgments

This chapter is based on the systematic review carried out in 2010 by the Movement Disorder Society–sponsored Task Force on Health-Related Quality of Life Scales for Parkinson's Disease: Pablo Martinez-Martin, Martine Jeukens-Visser, Kelly E. Lyons, C. Rodriguez-Blazquez, Caroline Selai, Andrew Siderowf, Mickie Welsh, Werner Poewe, Oliver Rascol, Cristina Sampaio, Glenn T. Stebbins, Christopher G. Goetz, and Anette Schrag (*Mov Disord* 2011:26: 2371–2380)

RECOMMENDED SCALES
SIP
NHP
EQ-5D
SF-36
PDQ-39
PDQ-8
PIMS
PDQL
SCOPA-PS

REFERENCES

1. Acquadro C, Berzon R, Dubois D, et al. Incorporating the patient's perspective into drug development and communication: an ad hoc task force report of the Patient-Reported Outcomes (PRO) Harmonization Group Meeting at the Food and Drug Administration, February 16, 2001. *Value Health*. 2003;6:522–531.
2. Bowling A. *Measuring Health: A Review of Disease-Specific Quality of Life Measurement Scales*. 3rd ed. Maidenhead, Berkshire: Open University Press; 2005:1–9.
3. Fayers PM, Machin D. *Quality of Life*. 2nd ed. Chichester, England: John Wiley & Sons Ltd; 2007:3–30.
4. World Health Organization. *Handbook of Basic Documents*. 5th ed. Geneva: WHO, Palais des Nations; 1952:3–20.
5. Berzon R, Hays RD, Shumaker SA. International use, application and performance of health-related quality of life instruments. *Qual Life Res*. 1993;2:367–368.
6. Spilker B. Introduction. In: Spilker B. *Quality of Life and Pharmacoeconomics in Clinical Trials*. 2nd ed. Philadelphia, PA: Lippincott-Raven; 1996:1–10.
7. Fitzpatrick R, Davey C, Buxton MJ, Jones DR. Evaluating patient-based outcome measures for use in clinical trials. *Health Technol Assess*. 1998;2:26.
8. Fitzpatrick R, Alonso J. Quality of life in health care: concepts and components. In: Martinez-Martin P, Koller WC, eds. *Quality of Life in Parkinson's Disease*. Barcelona: Masson, SA; 1999:1–15.
9. Schipper H, Clinch JJ, Olweny CLM. Quality of life studies: definitions and conceptual issues. In: Spilker B, ed. *Quality of Life and Pharmacoeconomics in Clinical Trials*. 2nd ed. Philadelphia, PA: Lippincott-Raven Publishers; 1996:11–23.
10. Martínez-Martín P. An introduction to the concept of quality of life in Parkinson's disease. *J Neurol*. 1998;245(suppl 1):2–5.
11. Den Oudsten BL, Van Heck GL, De Vries J. Quality of life and related concepts in Parkinson's disease: a systematic review. *Mov Disord*. 2007;22:1528–1537.
12. Hunt SM. The problem of quality of life. *Qual Life Res*. 1997;6:205–212.
13. Doward LC, McKenna SP. Defining patient-reported outcomes. *Value Health*. 2004;7 (suppl 1):4–8.
14. Smith KW, Avis NE, Assmann SF. Distinguishing between quality of life and health status in quality of life research: a meta-analysis. *Qual Life Res*. 1999;8:447–459.
15. Movement Disorder Society Task Force on Rating Scales for Parkinson's Disease. The Unified Parkinson's Disease Rating Scale (UPDRS): status and recommendations. *Mov Disord*. 2003;18:738–750.

16. Schrag A, Barone P, Brown RG, et al. Depression rating scales in Parkinson's disease: critique and recommendations. *Mov Disord.* 2007;22:1077–1092.

17. Fernandez HH, Aarsland D, Fenelon G, et al. Scales to assess psychosis in Parkinson's disease: critique and recommendations. *Mov Disord.* 2008;23:484–500.

18. Leentjens AFG, Dujardin K, Marsh L, et al. Apathy and anhedonia rating scales in Parkinson's disease: critique and recommendations. *Mov Disord.* 2008;23: 2004–2014.

19. Leentjens AFG, Dujardin K, Marsh L, et al. Anxiety rating scales in Parkinson's disease: critique and recommendations. *Mov Disord.* 2008;23:2015–2023.

20. Friedman JH, Alves G, Hagell P, et al. Fatigue rating scales critique and recommendations by the Movement Disorders Society Task Force on Rating Scales for Parkinson's Disease. *Mov Disord.* 2010;25:805–822.

21. Colosimo C, Martinez-Martin P, Fabbrini G, et al. Task force report on scales to assess dyskinesia in Parkinson's disease: critique and recommendations. *Mov Disord.* 2010;25: 1131–1142.

22. Goetz CG, Tilley BC, Shaftman SR, et al. Movement Disorder Society-sponsored revision of the Unified Parkinson's Disease Rating Scale (MDS-UPDRS): scale presentation and clinimetric testing results. *Mov Disord.* 2008;23:2129–2170.

23. Bergner B, Bobbitt R, Carter W, Gilson B. The Sickness Impact Profile: development and final revision of a health status measure. *Med Care.* 1981;19:787–805.

24. Welsh MD, Dorflinger E, Chernik D, Waters C. Illness impact and adjustment to Parkinson's disease: before and after treatment with tolcapone. *Mov Disord.* 2000;15:497–502.

25. Deyo RA. Pitfalls in measuring the health status of Mexican Americans: comparative validity of the English and Spanish Sickness Impact Profile. *Am J Public Health.* 1984;74:569–573.

26. Pollard WE, Bobbitt RA, Bergner M, Martin DP, Gilson BS. The Sickness Impact Profile: reliability of a health status measure. *Med Care.* 1976;14:146–155.

27. Longstreth WT, Nelson L, Linde M, Munoz D. Utility of the Sickness Impact Profile in Parkinson's disease. *J Geriatr Psychiatry Neurol.* 1992;5:142–148.

28. Welsh M, Dorflinger E, Chernik D, Waters C. Illness impact and adjustment to Parkinson's

disease: before and after treatment with tolcapone. *Mov Disord.* 2000;15:497–502.

29. Volkmann J, Albanese A, Kulisevsky J, et al. Long-term effects of pallidal or subthalamic deep brain stimulation on quality of life in Parkinson's disease. *Mov Disord.* 2009;24:1154–1161.

30. Hunt SM, McEwen J, McKenna SP. Measuring health status: a new tool for clinicians and epidemiologists. *J R Coll Gen Pract.* 1985;35:185–188.

31. Wann-Hansson C, Klevsgard R, Hagell P. Cross-diagnostic validity of the Nottingham Health Profile index of distress (NHPD). *Health Qual Life Outcomes.* 2008;6:47–60.

32. Hunt SM, McKenna SP, McEwen J, Williams J, Papp E. The Nottingham Health Profile: subjective health status and medical consultations. *Soc Sci Med—Part A Med Soc.* 1981;15:221–229.

33. Hunt SM, McKenna SP, McEwen J, Backett EM, Williams J, Papp E. A quantitative approach to perceived health status: a validation study. *J Epidemiol Community Health.* 1980;34:281–286.

34. Karlsen KH, Tandberg E, Aarsland D, Larsen JP. Health related quality of life in Parkinson's disease: a prospective longitudinal study. *J Neurol Neurosurg Psychiatry.* 2000;69:584–589.

35. Hagell P, Whalley RE, McKenna SP, Lindvall O. Health status measurement in Parkinson's disease: validity of the PDQ-39 and Nottingham Health Profile. *Mov Disord.* 2003;18:773–783.

36. Hariz GM, Lindberg M, Hariz MI, Bergenheim AT. Gender differences in disability and health-related quality of life in patients with Parkinson's disease treated with stereotactic surgery. *Acta Neurol Scand.* 2003;108:28–37.

37. Erola T, Karinen P, Heikkinen E, et al. Bilateral subthalamic nucleus stimulation improves health-related quality of life in parkinsonian patients. *Parkinsonism Relat Disord.* 2005;11:89–94.

38. Hagell P, Reimer J, Nyberg P. Whose quality of life? Ethical implications in patient-reported health outcome measurement. *Value Health.* 2009;12:613–617.

39. Forsaa EB, Larsen JP, Wentzel-Larsen T, Herlofson K, Alves G. Predictors and course of health-related quality of life in Parkinson's disease. *Mov Disord.* 2008;23:1420–1427.

40. Dereli EE, Yaliman A. Comparison of the effects of a physiotherapist-supervised exercise programme and a self-supervised exercise programme on quality of life in patients with

Parkinson's disease. *Clin Rehabil.* 2010;24: 352–362.

41. The EuroQol Group. EuroQol—a new facility for the measurement of health-related quality of life. *Health Policy.* 1990;16:199–208.

42. Badia X, Herdman M, Kind P. The influence of ill-health experience on the valuation of health. *Pharmacoeconomics.* 1998;13:687–696.

43. Schrag A, Selai C, Jahanshahi M, Quinn NP. The EQ-5D—a generic quality of life measure is a useful instrument to measure quality of life in patients with Parkinson's disease. *J Neurol Neurosurg Psychiatry.* 2000;69:67–73.

44. Siderowf A, Ravina B, Glick HA. Preference-based quality-of-life in patients with Parkinson's disease. *Neurology.* 2002;59:103–108.

45. Reuther M, Spottke EA, Klotsche J, et al. Assessing health-related quality of life in patients with Parkinson's disease in a prospective longitudinal study. *Parkinsonism Relat Disord.* 2007;13:108–114.

46. Martinez-Martin P, Rodriguez-Blazquez C, Abe K, et al. International study on the psychometric attributes of the non-motor symptoms scale in Parkinson disease. *Neurology.* 2009;73:1584–1591.

47. Noyes K, Dick AW, Holloway RG. Pramipexole v. levodopa as initial treatment for Parkinson's disease: a randomized clinical-economic trial. *Med Decis Making.* 2004;24:472–485.

48. Noyes K, Dick AW, Holloway RG. Pramipexole versus levodopa in patients with early Parkinson's disease: effect on generic and disease-specific quality of life. *Value Health.* 2006;9:28–38.

49. Siderowf A, Jaggi JL, Xie SX, et al. Long-term effects of bilateral subthalamic nucleus stimulation on health-related quality of life in advanced Parkinson's disease. *Mov Disord.* 2006;21:746–753.

50. Martinez-Martin P, Deuschl G. Effect of medical and surgical interventions on health-related quality of life in Parkinson's disease. *Mov Disord.* 2007;22:757–765.

51. Martinez-Martin P, Kurtis MM. Systematic review of the effect of dopamine receptor agonists on patient health-related quality of life. *Parkinsonism Relat Disord.* 2009;15 (suppl 4):S58–S64.

52. Ebersbach G, Hahn K, Lorrain M, Storch A. Tolcapone improves sleep in patients with advanced Parkinson's disease (PD). *Arch Gerontol Geriatr.* 2010;51:e125–e128.

53. Ware JE, Sherbourne CD. The MOS 36-item short-form health survey (SF-36): I. Conceptual framework and item selection. *Med Care.* 1992;30:473–483.

54. Jenkinson C, Peto V, Fitzpatrick R, Greenhall R, Hyman N. Self-reported functioning and well-being in patients with Parkinson's disease: comparison of the short-form health survey (SF-36) and the Parkinson's disease questionnaire (PDQ-39). *Age Ageing.* 1995;24:505–509.

55. Hobson P, Meara J. Self-reported functioning and well-being in patients with Parkinson's disease: comparison of the short-form 36 and the Parkinson's disease questionnaire. *Age Ageing.* 1996;25:334–335.

56. Rubenstein LM, Voelker MD, Chrischilles EA, Glenn DC, Wallace RB, Rodnitzky RL. The usefulness of the functional status questionnaire and medical outcomes study short form in Parkinson's disease research. *Qual Life Res.* 1998;7:279–290.

57. Kuopio AM, Martilla RJ, Helenius H, Toivonen M, Rinne UK. The quality of life in Parkinson's disease. *Mov Disord.* 2000;15:216–223.

58. Hagell P, Tornqvist AL, Hobart J. Testing the SF-36 in Parkinson's disease. Implications for reporting rating scale data. *J Neurol.* 2008;255:246–254.

59. Steffen T, Seney M. Test-retest reliability and minimal detectable change on balance and ambulation tests, the 36-item short-form health survey, and the Unified Parkinson Disease Rating Scale in people with parkinsonism. *Phys Ther.* 2008;88:733–746.

60. Brown CA, Cheng EM, Hays RD, Vassar SD, Vickrey BG. SF-36 includes less Parkinson's disease (PD)-targeted content but is more responsive to change than two PD-related health-related quality of life measures. *Qual Life Res.* 2009;18:1219–1237.

61. Den Oudsten BL, Van Heck GL, de Vries J. The suitability of patient-based measures in the field of Parkinson's disease: a systematic review. *Mov Disord.* 2007;22:1390–1401.

62. Chrischilles EA, Rubenstein LM, Voelker MD, Wallace RB, Rodnitsky RL. The health burdens of Parkinson's disease. *Mov Disord.* 1998;13:406–413.

63. Banks P, Martin C. The factor structure of the SF-36 in Parkinson's disease. *J Eval Clin Pract.* 2009;15:460–463.

64. Schrag A, Spottke A, Quinn NP, Dodel R. Comparative responsiveness of Parkinson's disease scales to change over time. *Mov Disord.* 2009;24:813–818.

65. O'Boyle CA, McGee H, Hickey A, O'Malley K, Joyce CR. Individual quality of life in

patients undergoing hip replacement. *Lancet.* 1992;339:1088–1091.

66. Joyce CR, Hickey A, McGee HM, O'Boyle CA. A theory-based method for the evaluation of individual quality of life: the SEIQoL. *Qual Life Res.* 2003;12:275–280.

67. Hickey AM, Bury G, O'Boyle CA, Bradley F, O'Kelly FD, Shannon W. A new short form individual quality of life measure (SEIQoL-DW): application in a cohort of individuals with HIV/AIDS. *BMJ.* 1996;313:29–33.

68. Browne JP, O'Boyle CA, McGee HM, McDonald NJ, Joyce CR. Development of a direct weighting procedure for quality of life domains. *Qual Life Res.* 1997;6:301–309.

69. Wettergren L, Bjorkholm M, Langius-Eklof A. Validation of an extended version of the SEIQoL-DW in a cohort of Hodgkin's lymphoma survivors. *Qual Life Res.* 2005;14:2329–2333.

70. Ring L, Lindblad AK, Bendtsen P, Viklund E, Jansson R, Glimelius B. Feasibility and validity of a computer administered version of SEIQoL-DW. *Qual Life Res.* 2006;15: 1173–1177.

71. Hickey AM, Bury G, O'Boyle CA, Bradley F, O'Kelly FD, Shannon W. A new short form individual quality of life measure (SEIQoL-DW): application in a cohort of individuals with HIV/AIDS. *BMJ.* 1996;313:29–33.

72. Moons P, Marquet K, Budts W, De Geest S. Validity, reliability and responsiveness of the Schedule for the Evaluation of Individual Quality of Life-Direct Weighting (SEIQoL-DW) in congenital heart disease. *Health Qual Life Outcomes.* 2004;2:27.

73. Neudert C, Wasner M, Borasio GD. Patients' assessment of quality of life instruments: a randomised study of SIP, SF-36 and SEIQoL-DW in patients with amyotrophic lateral sclerosis. *J Neurol Sci.* 2001;191: 103–109.

74. Lee MA, Walker RW, Hildreth AJ, Prentice WM. Individualized assessment of quality of life in idiopathic Parkinson's disease. *Mov Disord.* 2006;21:1929–1934.

75. Sintonen H. The 15D-measure of health-related quality of life. I. Reliability, validity, and sensitivity of its health state descriptive system. Working paper 41. Melbourne: National Centre for Health Program Evaluation, 1994.

76. Sintonen H. The 15D-measure of health-related quality of life. II. Feasibility, reliability and

validity of its valuation system. Working paper 42. Melbourne: National Centre for Health Program Evaluation, 1995.

77. Sintonen H. The 15D instrument of health-related quality of life: properties and applications. *Ann Med.* 2001;33:328–336.

78. Haapaniemi TH, Sotaniemi DA, Sintonen H, Taimela E. The generic 15D instrument is valid and feasible for measuring health-related quality of life in Parkinson's disease. *J Neurol Neurosurg Psychiatry.* 2004;75:976–983.

79. Nyholm D, Nilsson Remahl AI, Dizdar N, et al. Duodenal levodopa infusion monotherapy vs oral polypharmacy in advanced Parkinson disease. *Neurology.* 2005;64:216–223.

80. Kristiansen IS, Bingefors K, Nyholm D, Isacson D. Short-term cost and health consequences of duodenal levodopa infusion in advanced Parkinson's disease in Sweden: an exploratory study. *Appl Health Econ Health Policy.* 2009;7:167–180.

81. Saxena S, Carlson D, Billington R. The WHO quality of life assessment instrument (WHOQOL-Bref): the importance of its items for cross-cultural research. *Qual Life Res.* 2001;10:711–721.

82. Skevington SM, Lotfy M, O'Connell KA. The World Health Organization's WHOQOL-BREF quality of life assessment: psychometric properties and results of the international field trial: a report from the WHOQOL Group. *Qual Life Res.* 2004;13:299–310.

83. WHOQOL Group. The World Health Organization Quality of Life Assessment (WHOQOL): development and general psychometric properties. *Soc Sci Med.* 1998;46:1569–1585.

84. Schestatsky P, Zanatto VC, Margis R, et al. Quality of life in a Brazilian sample of patients with Parkinson's disease and their caregivers. *Rev Bras Psiquiatr.* 2006;28:209–211.

85. Hirayama MS, Gobbi S, Gobbi LT, Stella F. Quality of life (QoL) in relation to disease severity in Brazilian Parkinson's patients as measured using the WHOQOL-BREF. *Arch Gerontol Geriatr.* 2008;46:147–160.

86. Kuehler A, Henrich G, Schroeder U, Conrad B, Herschbach P, Ceballos-Baumann A. A novel quality of life instrument for deep brain stimulation in movement disorders. *J Neurol Neurosurg Psychiatry.* 2003;74:1023–1030.

87. Henrich G, Herschbach P. Questions on life satisfaction (FLZM)—a short questionnaire for assessing subjective quality of life. *Eur J Psychol Assess.* 2000;16:150–159.

88. Ellgring H, Seiler S, Perleth B, Frings W, Gasser T, Oertel W. Psychosocial aspects of Parkinson's disease. *Neurology.* 1993;43(suppl):41–44.

89. Spliethoff-Kamminga NG, Zwinderman AH, Springer MP, Roos RA. Psychosocial problems in Parkinson's disease: evaluation of a disease-specific questionnaire. *Mov Disord.* 2003;18:503–509.

90. Spliethoff-Kamminga NGA, Zwinderman AH, Springer MP, Roos RAC. Difference in quality of life and psychosocial well-being between Parkinson disease patient members and non-members of the Dutch Parkinson Disease Association. In: Spliethoff-Kamminga NGA. *Psychosocial Problems in Parkinson's Disease* [doctoral thesis]. The Netherlands: Leiden University; 2004:79–89.

91. Peto V, Jenkinson C, Fitzpatrick R, Greenhall R. The development and validation of a short measure of functioning and well-being for individuals with Parkinson's disease. *Qual Life Res.* 1995;4:241–248.

92. Jenkinson C, Fitzpatrick R, Peto V, Greenhall R, Hyman N. The Parkinson's disease questionnaire (PDQ-39): development and validation of a Parkinson's disease summary index score. *Age Ageing.* 1997;26:353–357.

93. Katsarou Z, Bostantjopoulou S, Peto V, Alevriadou A, Kiosseoglou G. Quality of life in Parkinson's disease: Greek translation and validation of the Parkinson's disease questionnaire (PDQ-39). *Qual Life Res.* 2001;10:159–163.

94. Marinus J, Ramaker C, van Hilten JJ, Stiggelbout AM. Health-related quality of life in Parkinson's disease: a systematic review of disease specific instruments. *J Neurol Neurosurg Psychiatry.* 2002;72:241–248.

95. Hagell P, McKenna SP. International use of health status questionnaires in Parkinson's disease: translation is not enough. *Parkinsonism Relat Disord.* 2003;10:89–92.

96. Hagell P. Feasibility and linguistic validity of the Swedish version of the PDQ-39. *Expert Rev Pharmacoecon Outcomes Res.* 2005;5:131–136.

97. Luo N, Tan LC, Li SC, Soh LK, Thumboo J. Validity and reliability of the Chinese (Singapore) version of the Parkinson's disease questionnaire (PDQ-39). *Qual Life Res.* 2005;14:273–279.

98. Martinez-Martin P, Serrano-Duenas M, Vaca-Baquero V. Psychometric characteristics of the Parkinson's disease questionnaire (PDQ-39)-Ecuadorian version. *Parkinsonism Relat Disord.* 2005;11:297–304.

99. Deuschl G, Schade-Brittinger C, Krack P, et al. A randomized trial of deep-brain stimulation for Parkinson's disease. *N Engl J Med.* 2006;355:896–908.

100. Carod-Artal FJ, Martinez-Martin P, Vargas AP. Independent validation of SCOPA-psychosocial and metric properties of the PDQ-39 Brazilian version. *Mov Disord.* 2007;22:91–98.

101. Hagell P, Nygren C. The 39-item Parkinson's disease questionnaire (PDQ-39) revisited: implications for evidence based medicine. *J Neurol Neurosurg Psychiatry.* 2007;78:1191–1198.

102. Martinez-Martin P, Serrano-Duenas M, Forjaz MJ, Serrano MS. Two questionnaires for Parkinson's disease: are the PDQ-39 and PDQL equivalent? *Qual Life Res.* 2007;16:1221–1230.

103. Gallagher DA, Schrag A. Impact of newer pharmacological treatments on quality of life in patients with Parkinson's disease. *CNS Drugs.* 2008;22:563–586.

104. Martinez-Martin P, Rodriguez-Blazquez C, Kurtis MM, Ray Chaudhuri K; on behalf of the NMSS Validation Group. The impact of non-motor symptoms on health-related quality of life of patients with Parkinson's disease. *Mov Disord.* 2011, Jan 24. doi:10.1002/mds.23462.

105. Jenkinson C, Fitzpatrick R, Norquist J, Findley L, Hughes K. Cross-cultural evaluation of the Parkinson's disease questionnaire: tests of data quality, score reliability, response rate, and scaling assumptions in the United States, Canada, Japan, Italy, and Spain. *J Clin Epidemiol.* 2003;56:843–847.

106. Peto V, Jenkinson C, Fitzpatrick R. Determining minimally important differences for the PDQ-39 Parkinson's disease questionnaire. *Age Ageing.* 2001;30:299–302.

107. Fitzpatrick R, Norquist JM, Jenkinson C. Distribution-based criteria for change in health-related quality of life in Parkinson's disease. *J Clin Epidemiol.* 2004;57:40–44.

108. Jenkinson C, Fitzpatrick R, Peto V, Greenhall R, Hyman N. The PDQ-8: development and validation of a short-form Parkinson's disease questionnaire. *Psychol Health.* 1997;12:805–814.

109. Jenkinson C, Fitzpatrick R. Cross-cultural evaluation of the short-form 8-item Parkinson's disease questionnaire (PDQ-8): results from America, Canada, Japan, Italy and Spain. *Parkinsonism Relat Disord.* 2007;13:22–28.

110. Katsarou Z, Bostantjopoulou S, Peto V, Kafantari A, Apostolidou E, Peitsidou E. Assessing quality of life in Parkinson's disease: can a short-form questionnaire be useful? *Mov Disord.* 2004;19:308–312.

111. Martinez-Martin P, Benito-Leon J, Alonso F, Catalan MJ, Pondal M, Zamarbide I. Health-related quality of life evaluation by proxy in Parkinson's disease: approach using PDQ-8 and EuroQoL-5D. *Mov Disord.* 2004;19:312–318.

112. Tan LC, Luo N, Nazri M, Li SC, Thumboo J. Validity and reliability of the PDQ-39 and the PDQ-8 in English-speaking Parkinson's disease patients in Singapore. *Parkinsonism Relat Disord.* 2004;10:493–499.

113. Tan LC, Lau PN, Au WL, Luo N. Validation of PDQ-8 as an independent instrument in English and Chinese. *J Neurol Sci.* 2007;255:77–80.

114. Chaudhuri KR, Martinez-Martin P, Brown RG, et al. The metric properties of a novel non-motor symptoms scale for Parkinson's disease: results from an international pilot study. *Mov Disord.* 2007;22:1901–1911.

115. Franchignoni F, Giordano A, Ferriero G. Rasch analysis of the short-form 8-item Parkinson's disease questionnaire (PDQ-8). *Qual Life Res.* 2008;17:541–548.

116. Luo N, Tan LC, Zhao Y, Lau PN, Au WL, Li SC. Determination of the longitudinal validity and minimally important difference of the 8-item Parkinson's disease questionnaire (PDQ-8). *Mov Disord.* 2009;24:183–187.

117. Onofrj M, Thomas A, Vingerhoets F, et al. Combining entacapone with levodopa/DDCI improves clinical status and quality of life in Parkinson's disease (PD) patients experiencing wearing-off, regardless of the dosing frequency: results of a large multicentre open-label study. *J Neural Transm.* 2004;111:1053–1063.

118. Linazasoro G; and Spanish Dopamine Agonists Study Group. Conversion from dopamine agonists to cabergoline: an open-label trial in 128 patients with advanced Parkinson disease. *Clin Neuropharmacol.* 2008;31:19–24.

119. Calne S, Schulzer M, Mak E, et al. Validating a quality of life rating scale for idiopathic parkinsonism: Parkinson's Impact Scale (PIMS). *Parkinsonism Relat Disord.* 1996;2:55–61.

120. Calne SM, Mak E, Hall J, et al. Validating a quality-of-life scale in caregivers of patients with Parkinson's disease: Parkinson's Impact Scale (PIMS). *Adv Neurol.* 2003;91:115–122.

121. Schulzer M, Mak E, Calne SM. The psychometric properties of the Parkinson's Impact Scale (PIMS) as a measure of quality of life in Parkinson's disease. *Parkinsonism Relat Disord.* 2003;9:291–294.

122. Serrano-Duenas M, Serrano S. Psychometric characteristics of PIMS compared to PDQ-39 and PDQL to evaluate quality of life in Parkinson's disease patients: validation in Spanish (Ecuadorian style). *Parkinsonism Relat Disord.* 2008;14:126–132.

123. de Boer AG, Wijker W, Speelman JD, de Haes JC. Quality of life in patients with Parkinson's disease: development of a questionnaire. *J Neurol Neurosurg Psychiatry.* 1996;61:70–74.

124. Hobson P, Holden A, Meara J. Measuring the impact of Parkinson's disease with the Parkinson's disease quality of life questionnaire. *Age Ageing.* 1999;28:341–346.

125. Serrano-Duenas M, Martinez-Martin P, Vaca-Baquero V. Validation and cross-cultural adjustment of PDQL-questionnaire, Spanish version (Ecuador) (PDQL-EV). *Parkinsonism Relat Disord.* 2004;10:433–437.

126. de Bie MA, de Haan RJ, Nijssen PCG, et al. Unilateral pallidotomy in Parkinson's disease: a randomised, single-blind, multicentre trial. *Lancet.* 1999;354:1665–1669.

127. Esselink RA, de Bie RM, de Haan RJ, et al. Unilateral pallidotomy versus bilateral subthalamic nucleus stimulation in PD: a randomized trial. *Neurology.* 2004;62:201–207.

128. Yousefi B, Tadibi V, Khoei AF, Montazeri A. Exercise therapy, quality of life, and activities of daily living in patients with Parkinson disease: a small scale quasi-randomised trial. *Trials.* 2009;10:67.

129. Reuther M, Spottke EA, Klotsche J, et al. Assessing health-related quality of life in patients with Parkinson's disease in a prospective longitudinal study. *Parkinsonism Relat Disord.* 2007;13:108–114.

130. Welsh M, McDermott M, Holloway R, et al. Development and testing of the Parkinson's disease quality of life scale: the PDQUALIF [abstract]. *Mov Disord.* 1997;12:836.

131. Welsh M, McDermott MP, Holloway RG, et al. Development and testing of the Parkinson's disease quality of life scale (PDQUALIF). *Mov Disord.* 2003;18:637–645.

132. Parkinson Study Group. A controlled trial of rasagiline in early Parkinson disease. The TEMPO Study. *Arch Neurol.* 2002;59: 1937–1943.

133. Parkinson Study Group. Pramipexole vs Levodopa as initial treatment for Parkinson's disease. *Arch Neurol.* 2004;61:1044–1053.

134. Parkinson Study Group. A randomized placebo-controlled trial of rasagiline in levodopa-treated patients with Parkinson disease and motor fluctuations. The PRESTO Study. *Arch Neurol.* 2005;62:241–248.

135. Van den Berg M. Leben mit Parkinson: Entwicklung und psychometrische Testung des Fragenbogens PLQ. *NeuroRehabilitation.* 1998;4:221–226.

136. Brod M, Mendelsohn GA, Roberts B. Patients' experiences of Parkinson's disease. *J Gerontol Psychol Sci.* 1998;53B:213–222.

137. Marinus J, Visser M, Martinez-Martin P, van Hilten JJ, Stiggelbout AM. A short psychosocial questionnaire for patients with Parkinson's disease: the SCOPA-PS. *J Clin Epidemiol.* 2003;56:61–67.

138. Martinez-Martin P, Carod-Artal FJ, da Silveira Ribeiro L, et al. Longitudinal psychometric attributes, responsiveness, and importance of change: an approach using the SCOPA-Psychosocial Questionnaire. *Mov Disord.* 2008;23:1516–1523.

139. Virues-Ortega J, Carod-Artal FJ, Serrano-Duenas M, et al. Cross-cultural validation of the scales for outcomes in Parkinson's disease—psychosocial questionnaire (SCOPA-PS) in four Latin American countries. *Value Health.* 2009;12:385–391.

140. Martinez-Martin P, Carroza-García E, Frades-Payo B, et al. [Psychometric attributes of the scales for outcomes in Parkinson's disease-psychosocial (SCOPA-PS): validation in Spain and review]. *Rev Neurol.* 2009;49:1–7.

141. Mokkink LB, Terwee CB, Knol DL, et al. Protocol of the COSMIN study: COnsensus-based Standards for the selection of health Measurement INstruments. *BMC Med Res Methodol.* 2006;6:2.

142. Mokkink LB, Terwee CB, Patrick DL, et al. The COSMIN checklist for assessing the methodological quality of studies on measurement properties of health status measurement instruments: an international Delphi study. *Qual Life Res.* 2010;19: 539–549.

143. Damiano AM, Snyder C, Strausser B, et al. A review of health-related quality-of-life concepts and measures for Parkinson's disease. *Qual Life Res.* 1999;8:235–243.

144. Selai C, Trimble MR. Assessing quality of life in dementia. *Aging Mental Health.* 1999;3:101–111.

145. Mack JL, Whitehouse PJ. Quality of life in dementia: state of the art–report of the International Working Group for Harmonization of Dementia Drug Guidelines and the Alzheimer's Society Satellite Meeting. *Alzheimer Dis Assoc Disord.* 2001;15:69–71.

146. Banerjee S, Samsi K, Petrie CD, et al. What do we know about quality of life in dementia? A review of the emerging evidence on the predictive and explanatory value of disease specific measures of health-related quality of life in people with dementia. *Int J Geriatr Psychiatry.* 2009;24:15–24.

147. Vogel A, Mortensen EL, Hasselbalch SG, et al. Patient versus informant reported quality of life in the earliest phases of Alzheimer's disease. *Int J Geriatr Psychiatry.* 2006;21: 1132–1138.

148. Conde-Sala JL, Garre-Olmo J, Turro-Garriga O, Lopez-Pousa S, Vilalta-Franch J. Factors related to perceived quality of life in patients with Alzheimer's disease: the patient's perception compared with that of caregivers. *Int J Geriatr Psychiatry.* 2009;24:585–594.

149. Schrag A, Jahansahi M, Quinn NP. What contributes to quality of life in patients with Parkinson's disease? *J Neurol Neurosurg Psychiatry.* 2000;69:308–312.

150. Visser M, van Rooden SM, Verbaan D, Marinus J, Stiggelbout AM, van Hilten JJ. A comprehensive model of health-related quality of life in Parkinson's disease. *J Neurol.* 2008;255:1580–1587.

151. Martinez-Martin P, Carod Artal FJ, de Pedro J. Non-motor symptoms and health-related quality of life. In: Chaudhuri KR, Tolosa E, Schapira A, Poewe W, eds. *Non-Motor Symptoms of Parkinson's Disease.* Oxford: Oxford University Press; 2009:309–320.

152. Food and Drug Administration, US Department of Health and Human Services. *Guidance for Industry. Patient-Reported Outcome Measures: Use in Medical Product Development to Support Labeling Claims.* Rockville, MD: FDA; 2009.

153. Rodrigues J, Walters SE, Watson P, Stell R, Mastaglia FL. Globus pallidus stimulation improves both motor and nonmotor aspects of quality of life in advanced Parkinson's disease. *Mov Disord*. 2007;22:1866–1870.

154. Zahodne LB, Okun MS, Foote KD, et al. Greater improvement in quality of life following unilateral deep brain stimulation surgery in the globus pallidus as compared to the subthalamic nucleus. *J Neurol*. 2009;56:1321–1329.

155. Martinez-Martin P, Rodriguez Blazquez C, Frades Payo B. Specific patient-reported outcomes measures for Parkinson's disease: analysis and applications. *Expert Rev Pharmacoeconomics Outcomes Res*. 2008;8:401–418.

12

MEASUREMENTS OF COSTS AND SCALES FOR OUTCOMES IN HEALTH ECONOMIC STUDIES OF PARKINSON'S DISEASE

Richard Dodel

Summary

In health economic evaluations, operational techniques are applied in quantifying the economic burden to a society and its various participants (patient, healthcare provider, society). Health economic evaluations can be divided into non-comparative cost of illness (COI) studies, which quantify the economic burden of a disease from a specified perspective, and comparative studies, which evaluate cost-effectiveness of different treatment options (CE).

In this review, approaches to evaluate cost of illness and cost-effectiveness studies were assessed as well as direct (standard gamble, time trade-off, and visual analogue scales) and indirect models/instruments to evaluate health status and utilities (AQol, EQ-5D, HUI, Index of Health Related Quality of Life Quality of Well-being scale, Rossor scale, SF-6D, 15D).

No validated models/instruments have been identified to evaluate CE or COI in PD patients. Among the scales used for cost-utility (CU) analyses, only a few of the outcome instruments have been used in the PD population. Only limited clinimetric data were available for those instruments with respect to PD, although clinimetric data for these scales have been acquired for conditions other than PD. The Standard Gamble, Time Trade-OFF, EQ-5D, 15D, SF-6D, and HUI met the criteria for "Recommended (with limitations)," but only the EQ-5D has been assessed in detail in patients with PD. The task force recommends further study of these instruments in the PD population to establish core clinimetric properties. For assessment of COI, the development of a COI instrument specifically for PD is recommended.

INTRODUCTION

Recent projections have estimated that the number of Parkinson's disease (PD) patients will approximately double until the year 2030.[1,2] Therefore, evaluative research including economic evaluations contributing to the decision-making processes associated with resource allocation is needed to ensure that health resources are allocated in ways that best benefit the society. In recent years health economic analyses have also been initiated in patients with Parkinson's disease. There are different approaches in health economics, which are outlined in Table 12-1: **Noncomparative studies:** *Cost of illness* (COI) studies evaluate the economic burden of a certain disease within a healthcare setting and a number of those studies

Table 12-1 Basic Forms of Health Economic Evaluations (Adapted from Schöffski[125])

Health Economic Analysis					
Not Comparative		**Comparative**			
Cost analysis	Cost-of-illness analysis	Cost-minimization analysis	Cost benefit analysis	Cost-effectiveness analysis	Cost-utility analysis

have been performed in respect to PD in various countries (Table 12-2). **Comparative studies**: *Cost-effectiveness* (CE) studies investigate the value of different treatment options and provide a method to help decision-makers determine the value of new therapeutical approaches.[3,4] In CE analyses, two or more competing interventions are compared with regard to both their costs and their health effects and are subdivided depending on their outcome. A *cost-minimization* analysis is when the analysis focuses solely on the costs of competing interventions (i.e., finding the minimal-cost strategy). If benefits are measured in terms of willingness to pay, the analysis is termed a "cost-benefit" analysis. Cost-minimization studies as well as cost-benefit studies are rarely performed in health economics. Health effects can be expressed also in disease-specific terms (e.g., progression, change in functional scales, change in symptoms (CE study), or by using one of several methods to calculate quality-adjusted life years or QALYs (*cost-utility* [CU] analyses). Particularly, the evaluation of utilities has become a major topic in outcome research.

Currently, 19 comparative analyses have been performed for interventions in PD.[5–7] Among the different approaches, outcome measurements included clinical constructs such as years of beneficial treatment, adequate treatment months, motor complications, UPDRS, and time to levodopa initiation, among others. Comprehensive reviews with thorough discussions and recommendations for future modeling in PD have recently been published.[5–7] As cost-effectiveness evaluation is a strategy that may incorporate scale-based information/data, but instead of single outcome scale measures uses statistical models incorporating several measurements of importance, no recommendation according to the MDS Task Force criteria (see Chapter 6) is feasible. The aim of this chapter is to review the literature on measures and scales to estimate cost and to evaluate outcomes in health economic studies of patients with Parkinson's disease.

METHODS

Following the definitions described in Chapter 6, classification was made according to the following definitions: (1) "Recommended": a scale that has been applied to PD populations; there are data on its use in clinical studies beyond the group who developed the scale; and, it has been clinimetrically studied and considered valid, reliable, and sensitive in the PD population; (2) "Suggested": a scale that has been applied to PD populations, but only one of the other criteria was fulfilled; (3) "Listed": only one criterion (it has been applied to PD population) was fulfilled. Whereas several chapters in this book are based on a final, peer-reviewed publication in the journal *Movement Disorders*, the contents of this essay are still in review at the time of publication.

Evaluation of clinimetric properties

A systematic literature search was performed involving the databases NHS CRD (National Health Service Centre for Reviews and Dissemination) and PubMed until december 15, 2011. "Parkinson" [Mesh] and "cost" were used as search terms in PubMed and only "Parkinson" in the CRD database. To be included, publications had to be health economic analyses. In order to extract the data, a standardized assessment form was used for multiattribute utility assessments, which was based on guidelines and recommendations for assessing health status and quality-of-life instruments,[8,9] and another standardized assessment form was used for COI studies.[10]

None of the scales addressed the potential variability, which is due to variations in relation to medication ("on" versus "off" states; DBS on/off), or other PD-related factors. As these topics

Table 12-2. Cost of Illness Studies in PD

AUTHOR[#]	COUNTRY	YEAR OF COSTING	TIME-SPAN	SETTING	INCIDENCE OR PREVALENCE BASED STUDIES	PERSPECTIVE ON COSTING	TOP-DOWN/ BOTTOM-UP APPROACH	INDIRECT COSTS EVALUATED (HCA: HUMAN CAPITAL APPROACH; FCM: FRICTION COST METHOD)	NUMBER OF PATIENTS INCLUDED	CURRENCY
von Campenhausen[96]	Austria	2008	6 months	Outpatient monocenter cohort	prevalence-based	societal, patients	bottom-up	HCA	81	EUR
Guttman[97]	Canada	1993	1 year	Outpatient community-based	prevalence-based	payer's	bottom-up	N.E.	15,306	USD
Wang[98]	China	2004	1 year	Hospital-based monocenter cohort	prevalence-based	societal	bottom-up	HCA	190	RMB, EUR, USD
Winter[99]	Czech Republic	2008	6 months	Outpatient monocenter cohort	prevalence-based	societal, patients	bottom-up	HCA	100	EUR
Keränen[100]	Finland	1998	1 year	Outpatient multicenter cohort	prevalence-based	societal	bottom-up	HCA	258	EUR, USD
Le Pen[101]	France	1996	6 months	Outpatient multicenter cohort	prevalence-based	payer**	bottom-up	N.M.	294	EUR, USD
Barth[102]	Germany	2003	5 months	Outpatient monocenter cohort	prevalence-based	societal	bottom-up	HCA	75	EUR
Dengler[103]	Germany	2002	3 years	Outpatient monocenter cohort	prevalence-based	societal	bottom-up	HCA	117	EUR
Dodel[104]	Germany	1995	3 months	Outpatient multicenter cohort	prevalence-based	payer, patients	bottom-up	N.E.	40	DM, USD, GBP
Ehret[105]	Germany	2006	3 months	Outpatient multicenter cohort	prevalence-based	payer	bottom-up	N.E.	425	EUR
Reese[106]	Germany	2006	6 months	Outpatient monocenter cohort	prevalence-based	societal	bottom-up	HCA	86	EUR
Spottke[107]	Germany	2000–02	6 months	Outpatient multicenter cohort	prevalence-based	societal	bottom-up	HCA	145	EUR
Winter[108]	Germany	2009	1 year	Outpatient multicenter cohort	prevalence-based	societal	bottom-up	HCA	145	EUR

(continued)

Table 12-2. (continued)

AUTHOR#	COUNTRY	YEAR OF COSTING	TIME-SPAN	SETTING	INCIDENCE OR PREVALENCE BASED	PERSPECTIVE ON COSTING	TOP-DOWN/ BOTTOM-UP APPROACH	INDIRECT COSTS EVALUATED	NUMBER OF PATIENTS INCLUDED	CURRENCY
Winter[109]	Germany	2004	1 year	Outpatient multicenter cohort	prevalence-based	societal	bottom-up	HCA	278	EUR
Ragothaman[110]	India	2004	6 months	Outpatient monocenter cohort	prevalence-based	payer, patients	bottom-up	N.E.	175	INR, USD
Winter[111]	Italy	2009	6 months	Outpatient monocenter cohort	prevalence-based	societal, patients	bottom-up	HCA	70	EUR
Winter[112]	Russia	2008	6 months	Outpatient monocenter cohort	prevalence-based	societal, patients	bottom-up	HCA	100	EUR
Cubo[113]	Spain	2004	3 months	Outpatient multicenter cohort	prevalence-based	payer	bottom-up	N.E.	78	EUR
Hagell[114]	Sweden	2000	1 year	Monocenter hospital-based cohort	prevalence-based	societal	bottom-up	HCA	127	SEK, USD, EUR
Findley[115]	UK	1998	1 year	Outpatient multicenter cohort	prevalence-based	payer, patients	bottom-up	N.E.	423	GBP
McCrone[116]	UK	2003	1 year	Community-based cohort	prevalence-based	payer, patients	bottom-up	N.E.	155	GBP
Huse[117]	USA	2002	approx. 2.5 years	Retrospective health insurance database	prevalence-based	payer, patients	bottom-up	N.E.	20,016	USD
Leibson[118]	USA	N.S.*	18 years	Retrospective population-based medical database	prevalence-based	payer	bottom-up	N.E.	92	USD
Noyes[119]	USA	2002	9 years	Retrospective database	prevalence-based	payer	bottom-up	N.E.	717	USD

*Year of cost adjustment was not stated. Apparently, costs were calculated as a mean of costs during the period of data collection (1987–2004). Abbreviations: N.S., not stated; RMB, Chinese yuan = renminbi.

†None of available studies has published questionnaires used for data collection. However, questionnaires can be usually received from authors on request. Abbreviations: N.E., not estimated; N.M. non-monetary assessment. HCA: Human capital approach; FCM: Friction cost method.

**Indirect costs were evaluated using non-monetary terms (e.g., loss of working days).

were not specifically addressed in the validation studies, these were not assessed below, but investigators would be expected to consider such factors in further study designs.

RESULTS

Cost-of-illness assessment in patients with Parkinson's disease

Results from COI studies in PD patients are available in a large number of countries as outlined in Table 12-2. The methods applied in those studies, however, differ in several respects (e.g., type of cost included, perspective on costing, such as social perspective vs. specific-payer perspective), incidence vs. prevalence approach, top-down vs. bottom-up study; prices and costs; representativeness of the sample), therefore the results cannot easily be compared across the different countries (Table 12-2). Only a few transnational studies applying the same methodology have been performed in patients with PD.[11,12] Most studies used data on individual patients. This approach, also known as a "bottom-up" approach, allows more precise data than the "top-down" approach, which calculates costs by breaking down highly aggregated statistical data, such as reports of national statistics. The disadvantage of the bottom-up approach, however, among others, is that small samples of patients have to be "inflated" to national estimates, and often the patient sample is not representative.[13]

In the available studies on PD patients, all the questionnaires were developed by the respective groups and evaluated various factors with quite different methodologies (Table 12-2). None of the questionnaires used was tested appropriately, and most of the questionnaires are not publicly available. As shown, there is a large number of methodological differences in the selected studies, both from a clinical point of view (e.g., the cohort investigated), as well as from an economical point of view (including cost, and how cost, charges, prices have been derived, etc.) (Table 12-3). Furthermore, most of the studies adhere only loosely to the national or international guidelines for health-economic evaluations, which provide a framework for an appropriate evaluation.[14–17] All these limitations make a comparison within and particularly among countries and healthcare systems difficult. Therefore, a recommendation of the most appropriate questionnaire to apply for the cost of illness in patients with PD is currently not feasible. Instead, we propose to use a set of minimal data that should be obtained in a study evaluating the costs of PD; this should adhere to the respective national and international guidelines to perform health-economic evaluations, and we recommend that future researchers consult them before starting a study for the evaluation of costs in PD.[17] Furthermore, current recommendations for sample selection and sample size should be implemented to ensure that results are valid and applicable to the general PD population. None of the measurement tools used was evaluated with respect to basic clinimetric issues, and the questionnaires used in the PD populations have not been published. Only one task force criterion was fulfilled ("applied in PD population"), and thus all applied instruments have been categorized as "Listed."

Cost-effectiveness assessments

As CE analysis uses statistical models incorporating several measurements of importance, no evaluation according to the MDS Task Force criteria is feasible.

Utility analysis: direct and indirect measurements of preference-based outcomes

In health economics health-related quality of life rather than global quality of life is an important outcome (the term "quality of life" will be used here as an umbrella, loose term particularly referred to quality of life aspects related to the health status). Traditional measures of QOL are most important as descriptions of patients' outcomes, but are of limited value for evaluating consequences of different interventions or to demonstrate cost-effectiveness. Since it is the individual who experiences and evaluates this state, the challenge is to find ways of measuring this individual perspective that are sensitive, valid, and reliable, and yield respondent information that can be considered alongside clinical data.

Table 12-3. Resource Components Included

COMPONENT	DODEL[104]	FINDLEY[115]	BARTH[102]	CUBO[113]	DENGLER[103]	EHRET[105]	GUTTMAN[97]	HAGELL[114]	HUSE[117]	KERÄNEN[100]	LEIBSON[118]	LE PEN[101]	MCCRONE[116]
Direct medical costs													
Inpatient care	×	×	×	×	×	×	×	×	×	×	×	×	×
Outpatient visits	×	×	×	×	×	×	×	×	×	×	×	×	×
Rehabilitation	×		×	×	×		×		×	×	×	×	×
PD drugs	×	×	×	×	×	×	×	×	×	×		×	×
Other drugs	×	×	×	×	×	×	×	×	×			×	×
Adaptations	×	×*	×	×	×				×		×		×
Direct non-medical costs													
Community services	×		×	×	×	×		×				×	×
Travel costs			×	×	×			×				×	×
Special accommodation			×	×	×	×		×				×	×
Informal care costs			×	×	×					×			×
*Indirect costs***													
Sick leave			×	×	×			×				×	
Early retirement			×	×	×			×		×		×	

COMPONENT	NOYES[119]	RAGOTHAMAN[110]	REESE[106]	SPOTTKE[107]	VON CAMPENHAUSEN[96]	WANG[98]	WINTER[112]	WINTER[111]	WINTER[108]	WINTER[99]	WINTER[112]
Direct medical costs											
Inpatient care	×	×	×	×	×	×	×	×	×	×	×
Outpatient visits	×	×	×	×	×	×	×	×	×	×	×
Rehabilitation	×		×	×	×	×	×	×	×	×	×
PD drugs	×	×	×	×	×	×	×	×	×	×	×
Other drugs	×	×				×					
Adaptations			×	×	×	×	×	×	×	×	×
Direct non-medical costs											
Community services		×	×	×	×	×	×	×	×	×	×
Travel costs		×		×		×		×		×	
Special accommodation			×	×	×	×	×	×	×	×	×
Informal care costs			×	×	×	×	×	×	×	×	×
Indirect costs											
Sick leave			×	×	×	×	×	×	×	×	×
Early retirement			×	×	×	×	×	×	×	×	×

*The study reported an estimate of all patient expenditures.

**Indirect costs were included in the data collection, but the sample is too small for analysis.

To evaluate a certain health status, different instruments and methods have been established. In contrast to profile-health-status approaches, such as the generic SF-36 or the disease-specific PDQ-39, where functional performance or capacity in a large set of dimensions is evaluated, preference-based health outcome measurements ("utilities") characterize how health outcomes are valued by a certain individual.[18,19] It is important to recognize that two individuals with identical self-assessed health status as measured by a generic health assessment instrument may evaluate their health quite differently. A straightforward definition of *utility* is that it is a cardinal measure of the strength of one's preference. The basic idea of *health state utilities* and *quality-adjusted life-years* (QALYs) is simple. Utilities are cardinal values that are assigned to each health state on a scale that is established by assigning a value of 1.0 to being healthy and 0.0 to being dead. The utility values reflect the value of the health states depending on the respondent's preferences and in contrast to multi-dimensional profile measures (e.g., SF-36) can be combined into a weighted index, where 1.00 represents best possible HRQOL states, 0.00 death-equivalent states, and negative values states worse than death. Where a utility state exists over time, the value of the state and the time spent in it can be used to calculate the QALY-value of the state (i.e., QALYs reflect both the quality and quantity of life). The calculation of QALYs allows for direct comparison between different programs.

The most common approaches to **direct utility assessment** include standard gamble (SG), time trade-off (TTO), or the use of a visual analogue scale (VAS). Alternative approaches are the person trade-off[20] and the willingness to pay.[21] We will describe the different methods briefly—for more comprehensive discussions of measurement and scaling issues, we refer the reader to a series of review articles.[22–28]

In addition, **indirect methods** are available. Multi-attribute utility (MAUs) instruments break down HRQOL states into their constituent parts, described as the "instrument descriptive system" (i.e., the questions or items that are asked of study participants). Each item is then valued by respondents in a valuation study; in general, valuation samples are representative of the underlying population (since it is taxpayers who fund health care insurance) using either standard gamble or time trade-off. When the descriptive system is administered to study participants (usually patients) their responses are replaced by the item values from the valuation study sample, and a combination rule (either multiplicative or additive) is used to recombine the item values into a HRQOL index utility score. One of the most commonly used rating scale instruments is the EQ-5D, with five dimensions and three levels for each dimension.

The crucial difference between these and other measures of HRQOL is that the weights used to score them have been obtained using one of the preference elicitation techniques as described above (TTO or VAS).[29] Furthermore, the MAUs scales produce a score of 1 or less, where 1 is equivalent to *full health* and 0 is *death*. Scores may take a negative value for health states regarded as *worse than death*. The most common questionnaires to evaluate preferences are listed in Table 12-4 and briefly described. For a detailed description of psychometric criteria, including practicality, internal consistency, reliability, validity, and responsiveness to change in health, we refer to recent publications.[19,30] The relevance to PD patients is discussed for each scale and is summarized in Table 12-4.

Direct measurements

STANDARD GAMBLE

The standard gamble approach (SG) is the classic method of measuring preferences in economics based on the research by von Neumann and Morgenstern in the early 1940s.[31] The SG uses hypothetical lotteries as a means of measuring people's preferences. These lotteries involve a choice between two alternatives: the certainty of one outcome and a gamble with two possible outcomes.

It must be noted that only the SG provides a true measure of utility according to the theory described by von Neumann and Morgenstern. Analyses of health status using SG have been performed in patients with Parkinson's disease[32] Furthermore, it has been tested clinimetrically, but validation data in PD specifically still needs to be performed to establish its place as a pertinent rating measure. Whilst fulfilling criteria

Table 12-4. Generic Instruments Used to Evaluate Patients' Preferences in Patients With Parkinson's Disease (Adapted from Brazier et al.[19] and Hawthorne et al.[42])

GENERIC INSTRUMENTS	NUMBER OF ITEMS	DIMENSIONS	VALUING METHOD	HEALTH STATES	COST/ AVAILABILITY/ LANGUAGE AVAILABILITY	ADMINISTRATION TIME▲/ ADMINISTRATION	DOMAINS OF HRQOL COVERED BY SCALE	USED IN PD	COUNTRY
Quality of Well-being Scale	32		VAS	1,170	Free/	15–35 min (short version:15 min)/ Interview-based/ Training required	Mobility, physical activity, social functioning 27 symptoms/ problems	−	USA
SF-6D	6	6	SG	18,000	See SF-36 Review sheet/	10 min/See the SF-36 Review Sheet/	Physical functioning, role limitations, social functioning, pain, mental health, vitality	+	UK
EuroQol (EQ-5D; EQ-VAS)	5	3	TTO	243	Free/A copy can be ordered from the EQ-5D webpage	2–5 min/Multiple languages available/ Self-administered. Can also be administered by interviewer and over the telephone.	Pain/discomfort; mobility; usual activities; self-care; anxiety/depression	+	UK
15D questionnaire (15D)	15	4–5	VAS	billions	Free/A copy can be found in Sintonen[84]	5–10 min/Self-administered. Can also be administered by interviewer and over the telephone/ Multiple languages available	Mobility, vision, hearing, breathing, sleeping, eating, speech, elimination, usual activities, mental function, discomfort and symptoms, depression, distress, vitality, sexual activity.	+	Finland

(continued)

Table 12-4. (continued)

GENERIC INSTRUMENTS	NUMBER OF ITEMS	DIMENSIONS	VALUING HEALTH STATES METHOD	HEALTH STATES	COST/ AVAILABILITY/ LANGUAGE AVAILABILITY	ADMINISTRATION TIME▲/ ADMINISTRATION	DOMAINS OF HRQOL COVERED BY SCALE	USED IN PD	COUNTRY
Health Utility Index (HUI-II)	15	3–5	TTO	24,000			Sensation, mobility, emotion, cognition, self-care, pain, and fertility.		Canada
Health Utility Index (HUII-III)	17	5–6	VAS/SG	972,000	CAN$4,000/ Order a copy at www. healthutilities. com/hui3.htm/.	5–10 min/multiple languages available Self-administered. Can also be administered by interviewer and over the telephone.	Vision, hearing, speech, ambulation, dexterity, emotion, cognition, and pain.	+	Canada
Rosser classification	2	8 (Disability) 4 (distress)	ME	29	Free/Copy can be found in Kobelt.	?/training required	Disability, distress.	–	UK
Assessment of Quality of Life (AQoL)	15	5	TTO		Free/A copy can be found in[43]./ English, Danish.	Self-administered. Can also be administered by interviewer and over the telephone./5–10 min.	Illness, independent living, social relationships, physical senses, psychological well-being.	–	Australia

HS: health status; ME: magnitude estimation; VAS: visual analogue scale; TTO: time-trade-off; SG: standard gamble;
▲ Data were mainly taken from refs. 46, 120.

Table 12-5. Utility Measurements Used in Patients With Parkinson's Disease

INSTRUMENT	AUTHORS	SAMPLE SIZE	DIAGNOSIS	FEMALE/ MALE RATIO	UPDRS	DEMENTIA EVALUATED	DEPRESSION EVALUATED	EXAMINER	MULTIVARIATE ANALYSES APPLIED	CONCLUSION
EQ-5D*	Marras 2004[121]	301	Early PD	96/205	yes	n.r.	n.r.	Neurologist	Multiple linear regression	Recommended (with some limitations)
	Siderowf 2002[61]	100	Idiopathic PD	33/67	Yes	Within PDQ-39	Within PDQ-39	Physician	yes	
	Schrag 2000[59]	124	UK Brain Bank Criteria	47/50	yes	MMSE PDQ-39	BDI	Neurologist	no	
HUI-III	Kleiner–Fisman 2010[69]	68	UK Brain Bank Criteria	Only men	UPDRS II + III	Assessment of pharmacotherapy for dementia		Neurologist	yes	Recommended but requires validation in PD
	Pohar 2009[122]	261 PD patients 111,707 respondents without PD							ANCOVA for comorbidities	
	Jones 2009[123]	259 patients with self-reported PD					Yes, self-reported			
HUI-II	Siderowf 2002[61]	100	Idiopathic PD	33/67	Yes	Within PDQ-39	Within PDQ-39	Physician	yes	Recommended but requires validation in PD
SF-6D	Vossius 2009[81]	199 patients 172 controls	Newly diagnosed PD	61/104	yes	n.r.	n.r.	n.r. neurological examination	yes	Recommended but requires validation in PD
15D	Haapaniemi 2004[88]	260 PD patients and matched controls	Idiopathic PD	137/122	yes	Within PDQ-39	Within PDQ-39		yes	Recommended but requires validation in PD
	Isacson 2008[124]	25	Advanced, idiopathic PD, motor fluctuations and dyskinesia	6/19	yes	Yes, exclusion criterion PDQ-39	Within PDQ-39		yes	Recommended but requires validation in PD

*Only selected studies assessing utilities in Parkinson's disease, n.r. = not reported.

for a "Recommended" instrument for analyses, because of this latter weakness, it meets this designation with those limitations.

TIME TRADE-OFF

This approach to valuation is intended to determine the amount of time in better health the person would accept as equivalent to a fixed period of time in an impaired health state. After considering a certain health state (e.g., the current health state or a probable health state), it is valued using a TTO by offering subjects a choice between two options.[33] One option allows the subject to live in the health state under consideration for a certain number of years. The second option allows the subject to live in the best (or better) health state, but for fewer years. The time that the subject must trade (i.e., give up), to live in the best health state is varied systematically until the subject is indifferent between living in the health state for a certain number of years and living in the best health state. This is then taken as the approximation for the utility value of a certain health state. Currently, two studies were identified applying TTO for patients with PD.[34,35] In spite of validation outside of the PD population, only limited clinimetric information is available for use in patients with PD. Therefore, the measurement is classified as "Recommended" but with limitations.

VISUAL ANALOGUE SCALE

Subjects are asked to mark where they would classify their health state on a scale in which 0 represents the worst imaginable health state and 100 represents the best imaginable health state.[20,36] This scale may be displayed as a vertical line, a feeling thermometer, or a horizontal line of predefined longitude. The value for the health state is then estimated as the measured distance between 0 and the respondent's mark. There are several VASs available; the most common is used as (an optional) part of the EQ-5D[37] (see below). This VAS together with the EQ-5D has been applied in a large number of studies with PD involving.[32] The use of VASs to elicit utilities, however, is controversial.[38,39] VASs do not require participants to make decisions under uncertainty; rather they ask that participants rate health states. For this reason, it has been argued that VASs should never be used to elicit utilities without first undergoing transformation.[18,19,38,40] However, these transformations have been shown to be unsatisfactory. (For further reading see reference 41.) As VAS is mostly applied as part of the EQ-5D, its ratings will be discussed below. Table 12-5 summarizes the studies that utilized direct utility measurements and the recommendations for the instruments used.

INDIRECT MEASUREMENTS

The indirect utility measurements are summarized in Table 12-6. Multi-attribute utility instruments are explicitly designed to be used in CU evaluations. No published papers were found applying the AQoL, QWB, or the Rosser classification in PD patients. The next sections provide an overview of the leading multi-attribute utility scales and assess them against issues relevant to PD, in alphabetical order (Table 12-7 and Table 12-8).

ASSESSMENT OF QUALITY OF LIFE (AQOL)

This instrument was developed for use in prioritizing healthcare spending in Australia.[42–44] The purpose of the instrument is to assist with the measurement of HRQOL, and it was specially designed for use in cost-utility analysis. It holds a classification with five "major" dimensions (illness [not used in utility computation], independent living, social relationships, physical senses, and psychological well-being) with each of three items (total of 15 items with four levels). It takes approximately five to ten minutes for self-completion. A stratified sample representative of the Australian adult population completed TTOs based on a 10-year time frame to provide the utility weights. A multiplicative model is used to compute the utility index. The upper boundary is 1.00, and the lower boundary is −0.04: it permits health state values "worse than death."

It has been named the Australian Multi-Attribute Utility Instrument, and more

Table 12-6. Indirect Utility Measurements Used in Patients With Parkinson's Disease and Recommendation According to the Criteria of the Movement Disorders Task Force

INSTRUMENT	AUTHOR	SAMPLE SIZE	DIAGNOSIS	FEMALE/ MALE RATIO	UPDRS	MULTIVARIATE ANALYSES APPLIED	USE IN PD	USE BEYOND ORIGINAL DEVELOPERS	SUCCESSFUL CLINIMETRIC TESTING	SUCCESSFUL CLINIMETRIC TESTING IN PD	CONCLUSION**
EQ-5D*	Marras 2004[21]	301	Early PD	96/205	yes	Multiple linear regression	X	X	X	X needs more validation in PD	Recommended (with some limitations)
	Siderowf 2002[61]	100	idiopathic PD	33/67	Yes	yes					
	Schrag 2000[58,59]	124	UK Brain Bank Criteria	47/50	yes	yes					
SF-6D	Vossius 2009[1]	199 patients 172 controls	Newly diagnosed PD	61/104	yes	yes	X	X	X	–	Recommended but requires validation in PD
15D	Haapaniemi 2004[88]	260 PD patients and matched controls	Idiopathic PD	137/122	yes	yes	X	X	X	–	Recommended but requires validation in PD
	Isacson 2008[24]	25	Advanced, idiopathic PD, motor fluctuations and dyskinesia	6/19	yes	yes					
HUI-III	Kleiner–Fisman 2010[69]	68	UK Brain Bank Criteria	Only men	UPDRS II + III	yes	X	X	X	–	Recommended but requires validation in PD
	Pohar 2009[22]	261 PD patients, 111,707 respondents without PD				ANCOVA for Comorbidities					
	Jones 2009[23]	259 patients with self-reported PD									
HUI-II	Siderowf 2002[61]	100	idiopathic PD	33/67	Yes	yes	X	X	X	–	Recommended but requires validation in PD

*Only selected studies assessing utilities in Parkinson's disease; n.r. not reported.

Table 12-7. Comparison of Preference-Based Instruments in Regard to Their Psychometric Properties (Adapted in Part from Refs. 44, 48)

INSTRUMENTS

	QWB scale		HUI (HUI-III)		EQ-5D		15D		Rosser Index		AQoL		SF-6D	
	General Population	PD	General population	PD	General population	PD	General population	PD	General population	PD	General population	PD	General Population	PD
Conceptual and measurement model (general)	+++	–	+++	–	++	–	+++	–	–	–	+++	–	++	–
Reliability	++	–	++	–	++	–	++	–	–	–	++	–	++	–
Validity	+++	–	++	–	++	++	++	–	–	–	++	–	++	–
Respondent and administrative burden[a]	+	–	++	–	++(+)	++	++	–	++	–	++	–	++	–
Alternative forms	+	–	+++	–	+	–	++	–	–	–	++	–	++	–
Cultural and language adaptations	+	–	++	–	+++	–	++	–	–	–	+	–	++	–

– not tested; +, limited; ++, adequate; +++, extensive; n.a.: not applicable

a + high; ++ medium/small burden

Table 12-8. Generic Instruments Used to Evaluate Patients' Preferences in Patients with Parkinson's Disease (Adapted from Refs. 19, 42)

GENERIC INSTRUMENTS	NUMBER OF ITEMS	DIMENSIONS	VALUING METHOD	HEALTH STATES	COST/ AVAILABILITY/ LANGUAGE AVAILABILITY	ADMINISTRATION TIME▲/ ADMINISTRATION	DOMAINS OF HRQOL COVERED BY SCALE	USED IN PD	COUNTRY
Australian multi-attribute utility instrument (AQoL)	15	5	TTO		Free/A copy can be found in[43]./ English, Danish.	Self-administered. Can also be administered by interviewer and over the telephone./5–10 min.	Illness, independent living, social relationships, physical senses, psychological well-being.	–	Australia
EuroQol (EQ-5D; EQ-VAS)	5	3	TTO	243	Free/A copy can be ordered from the EQ-5D webpage	2–5 min./multiple languages available/Self-administered. Can also be administered by interviewer and over the telephone.	Pain/discomfort; mobility; usual activities; self-care; anxiety/depression.	+	UK
Health Utility Index (HUI-II)	15	3–5	TTO	24,000			Sensation, mobility, emotion, cognition, self-care, pain, and fertility.		Canada
Health Utility Index (HUII-III)	17	5–6	VAS/SG	972,000	~CAN$4,000/ Order a copy at www. healthutilities. com/hui3.htm./	5–10 min./multiple languages available Self-administered. Can also be administered by interviewer and over the telephone.	Vision, hearing, speech, ambulation, dexterity, emotion, cognition, and pain.	+	Canada

(continued)

Table 12-8. (continued)

GENERIC INSTRUMENTS	NUMBER OF ITEMS	DIMENSIONS	VALUING METHOD	HEALTH STATES	COST/ AVAILABILITY/ LANGUAGE AVAILABILITY	ADMINISTRATION TIME▲/ ADMINISTRATION	DOMAINS OF HRQOL COVERED BY SCALE	USED IN PD	COUNTRY
Quality of Well-being Scale	32		VAS	1,170	Free	15–35 min. (short version:15 min.)/ interview-based/ training required	Mobility, physical activity, social functioning. 27 symptoms/ problems.	–	USA
Rosser classification	2	8 (disability) 4 (distress)	ME	29	Free	?/training required	Disability, distress.	–	UK
SF-6D	6	6	SG	18,000	See SF-36 Review Sheet/	10 min./See the SF-36 Review Sheet/	Physical functioning, role limitations, social functioning, pain, mental health, vitality,	+	UK
15D question- naire (15D)	15	4–5	VAS	billions	Free/A copy can be found in[84]	5–10 min./Self- administered. Can also be administered by interviewer and over the Telephone/multiple languages available	mobility, vision, hearing, breathing, sleeping, eating, speech, elimination, usual activities, mental function, discomfort and symptoms, depression, distress, vitality, sexual activity.	+	Finland

HS: health status; ME: magnitude estimation; VAS: visual analogue scale; TTO: time-trade-off; SG: standard gamble.
▲ Data were mainly taken from refs. 46, 120.

recently, AQoL (Assessment of Quality of Life).[43] Currently, several instruments with different numbers of domains have been developed (8D, 7D, 6D, 4D: Independent Living [all], Life Satisfaction [8D], Mental Health [all], Coping [8D, 7D, 6D], Relationships [8D, 7D, 6D], Self Worth [8D], Pain [8D, 7D, 6D], Senses [all] as well as short assessment instruments.[45]) The available instruments have not yet been used in PD patients. However, it is the most commonly used questionnaire in Australia. As the scale has been well validated outside PD but has not been applied to PD, the questionnaire is currently "Listed" for the use in PD patients.

EQ-5D

This instrument was developed by a multidisciplinary group of researchers from seven centers in five countries.[37] The original version had six dimensions, the EQ-6D, which has been succeeded by the five-dimensional EQ-5D. The patient-reported EQ-5D comprises five questions on mobility, self care, pain, usual activities, and psychological status, with three possible answers for each item (*no problems, moderate problems, severe problems*) defining 243 different health states. Each state is described in the form of a five-digit code ("profile") using the three levels (e.g., state 21321 means moderate problems in mobility, no problems in self-care, severe problems in usual activities, and so on). Recently, a new version using five instead of three levels has been introduced, however, further analysis is necessary and cannot be recommended at that time. (Herdman M, Gudex C, Lloyd A, Janssen M, Kind P, Parkin D, Bonsel G, Badia X. Development and preliminary testing of the new five-level version of EQ-5D (EQ-5D-5L). Qual Life Res. 2011;20(10):1727-36.). Recently, a new version using five instead of three levels has been introduced, however, further analysis is necessary and cannot be recommended at that time. (Herdman M, Gudex C, Lloyd A, Janssen M, Kind P, Parkin D, Bonsel G, Badia X. Development and preliminary testing of the new five-level version of EQ-5D (EQ-5D-5L). *Qual Life Res.* 2011;20(10):1727–36.).

In addition, the patient may mark the subjective impression of his actual health status on a 20-centimeter visual analogue scale (VAS) with endpoints labeled "Worst imaginable health state" and "Best imaginable health state," in which a score of 0 represents the "worst" and 100 the "best imaginable health state." It takes one to two minutes to self-complete.[46] Separate algorithms for the calculation of the EQ-5D available index score are available for different sociodemographic groups.[47] It is important to use the respective algorithms for the sample in question in order to avoid bias. Worldwide, there are several tariff sets for the EQ-5D available, implying that the utility weights used to score may be culture-specific; results from one tariff set may not be directly comparable with those from a different tariff. Where local tariffs are not available, it is recommended that the United Kingdom weights be used.

Three types of data can be displayed from the EQ-5D: (1) a descriptive profile, indicating the extent of problems on each of the five dimensions with three graduations; (2) a population-weighted health score, based on the descriptive data; and (3) a self-rated assessment of perceived health status based on the VAS.

EQ-5D is designed for self-administration (guidelines for observer, telephone, and proxy use are available). It is intended for use in population health surveys or in combination with a condition-specific instrument for assessment to a specific condition (e.g., a spine disorder). The weights—referred to as *tariffs*—were derived using TTO and regression. It has good reliability and validity.[48,49] The EQ-5D is available free of charge for noncommercial uses from the EuroQol Group and is available in more than 30 different languages (http://www.euroqol.org). The EQ-5D has been used in large number of studies to evaluate health status and utilities in PD patients.[50–65] It has shown minor sensitivity to change over a period of 12 months.[57] Currently, it is the most applied utility instrument for PD patients; however, the clinimetric properties of this scale for PD patients are not evaluated in great detail. The scale is ranked "Recommended" (with some limitations) for the evaluation of health status, as all key criteria are fulfilled; however, clinimetric testing requires more validation (Tables 12-3 and 12-4), and studies need to state which tariff set was used in obtaining utilities.

HEALTH UTILITY INDEX (HUI)

The Health Utility Index was devised in Canada.[40] The earliest version (HUI-I) has been superseded by two revised classifications, the HUI-II and HUI-III.[40,66] The latter two systems are independent but complementary[67]; however, they differ considerably from the HUI-I.[68] The HUI-II has seven dimensions: sensation, mobility, emotion, cognition, self-care, pain, and fertility, with three to five dimensions each. The HUI-III is an adaptation of the HUI-II with eight dimensions (vision and hearing as separate dimensions, along with speech, ambulation, dexterity, emotion, cognition, and pain, whilst fertility was removed). The number of response levels has been increased to five and six, respectively. Patients are assigned to the classifications from a 15-item/17-item self-completed questionnaire, from face-to-face interview and/or by telephone (time needed to complete: ~10 min.). Social aspects of HRQOL are not measured. The utility weights were elicited using the VAS, and scores then transformed based on four "corner" health states valued with the SG where a 60-year time frame was used. These results were based on stratified sampling of the Hamilton, Ontario, population. An utility value is obtained by putting weights for each dimension into a multiplicative formula. Utility values for PD patients using the HUI have been assessed by multiple groups outside the original developers of the scale.[61,69] The instrument has been evaluated for validity and reliability for a number of conditions, but only inadequately for PD patients.[48] Therefore, the HUI fulfills criteria as "Recommended," but further validation steps in PD are required.[48,61]

INDEX OF HEALTH RELATED QUALITY OF LIFE

The Index of Health Related Quality of Life (IHQL) was developed from the disability/distress classification.[70,71] In the first stage of its development, distress was subdivided into physical discomfort and emotional distress. 175 composite health states are valued in the three dimensions of disability, discomfort, and distress. The three dimensions have been further divided into seven attributes (dependency, dysfunction, pain/discomfort, symptoms, dysphoria, disharmony, and fulfillment), and these in turn into 44 scales. The scales have been divided into 107 descriptors, which have 225 levels in total. This hierarchical classification of the IHQL defines many millions of states. The three dimensions have been valued using SG and a matrix of health state values published in an edited volume. Self-rated, observer-rated, and relative-rated versions are available. In our literature search, we could not find that this scale was applied to patients with PD. As the scale has been well validated outside PD but has not been applied to PD, the IHQL is therefore "Listed."

ROSSER DISABILITY/DISTRESS SCALE

This classification was developed as a measure of hospital output, and in the 1980s it became the most widely used instrument for deriving QALYs in the United Kingdom.[72,73] The classification has two dimensions, disability and distress, with eight and four levels, respectively. The disability dimension has descriptions for each level. Together the two dimensions define a total of 29 health states (the matrix defines 32 states, but the worst level of disability is unconsciousness, and hence there is no distinction between the four states defined by the different levels of distress). A revised version was released in the early 1990s based on SG procedures and included an additional dimension of discomfort.[74] Administration requires a trained interviewer. The upper boundary is 1.00, and the lower boundary is −1.49; i.e., health states worse than death are allowed. The Rosser Index has given rise to two variants: the Health Measurement Questionnaire (HMG)[75] and the Utility-Based Quality of Life-Heart Questionnaire (UBQ-H).[76] In our literature search we could not identify a study that used the questionnaire in patients with PD. As the scale has been well validated outside PD but has not been applied to PD, the questionnaire, therefore, is "Listed."

SF-6D

Based on the SF-36, a method was devised for deriving a single index value[77] (several other approaches exist for transforming SF-36 scores into utilities[78,79]). The SF-36 descriptive system is US-American, and the SF-6D weights are British. Two different algorithms have been published by deriving preference-based values from the SF-36, referred to as the SF-6D-1 and SF-6D-2. The advantage of the SF-6D procedures is that any patient who completes the SF-36 or the SF-12 can be uniquely classified according to the SF-6D. The SF-6D uses 10 items from the SF-36: three from the physical functioning scale, one from physical role limitation, one from emotional role limitation, one from social functioning, two bodily pain items, two mental health items, and one vitality item. These form six dimensions: physical functioning (PF: 6 levels), role limitation (RL: 4 levels), social functioning (SF: 5 levels), pain (PA: 6 levels), mental health (MH: 5 levels), and vitality (VI: 5 levels). An SF-6D "health state" is defined by selecting one level from each dimension. The SF-6D provides a means for using the SF-36 and SF-12 in economic evaluation by estimating a preference-based single-index measure for health from these data.[80] Values or preference weights for a sample of these health states were obtained from a community sample using a standard gamble technique. The SF-6D preference-based measure can be regarded as a continuous outcome scored on a 0.29 to 1.00 scale, with 1.00 indicating "full health."

A key issue with the SF-6D is that the scoring range is censored at the lower end to 0.29, which raises questions concerning its validity for use in cost-utility analysis. Consistent with this restriction, floor effects have been reported, indicating that SF-6D over-predicts poorer health states compared with the EQ-5D. Good reliability and validity have been reported,[49] but not for a PD population. Only one study was retrieved in our search in patients with Parkinson's disease where the SF-6D was applied.[81] With the current evidence available, the instrument is categorized as "Suggested."

QUALITY OF WELL-BEING SCALE

The American Quality of Well-Being Scale, formerly called the Index of Well-Being, is one of the oldest instruments.[82] This interview-based questionnaire contains two components: three multilevel dimensions relating to function (mobility, physical activity, and social activity), with three to five levels each, and an additional 27 illness symptoms. Combined, these provide an index of "well-life expectancy" of which there are 43 functioning levels. The QWB was designed for interviewer administration (15–35 min.), although a shorter version has been developed that takes about 15 minutes.[83] Interviewer training is required. The preference weights were elicited using VAS scores, which were obtained from a sample of the San Diego, California, population. The upper boundary is 1.00, and the lower boundary is 0.00 (death equivalent), and health states worse than death are not allowed. An overall health state score is calculated by an additive formula.

In our literature search, we could not identify a study that used the scale in patients with PD, therefore we classified this scale as currently "Listed."

15D

This measure was developed by a Finish team and has undergone several revisions since its first presentation.[84,85] The 15D is a generic, standardized, self-administered measure of HRQOL that can be used as a profile and single-index score measure. There are 15 items, each with five levels, measuring mobility, vision, hearing, breathing, sleeping, eating, speech, elimination, usual activities, mental function, discomfort and symptoms, depression, distress, vitality, and sexual activity. It takes approximately five to ten minutes for self-completion.[46] Health-state values are estimated by applying an additive formula, where a value is assigned to each dimension level, and these are multiplied by a weight representing the relative importance of that dimension and summed to derive a single index. The weights came from five random samples of the Finnish population investigated using VAS questions; as such the 15D utilities are subject to the caveats relating to utilities derived from VASs. A limitation of the additive-scoring model is that each health state can only ever contribute a fixed proportion of utility loss; large losses in utility can only occur where all aspects of life are affected. The impact of this restriction is to over-value poor health states when compared with other measures, such as the EQ5D. The scale has nevertheless been established as a feasible instrument and has been used to assess health status among patients with PD.[86–88] This scale therefore fulfills criteria for being "Recommended" but remains to be subjected to appropriate clinimetric testing in the PD population (Table 12-7).

CONCLUSION

Although numerous studies on the costs of PD are available, currently no standardized and validated methodological approach to evaluate the *cost of illness* (COI) in PD has been established. This is in contrast to Alzheimer's disease, where an instrument called *The Resource Utilization Instrument for Dementia (RUD)* was especially designed to evaluate resource use by patients and their caregivers. It has been used widely, validated repeatedly, and has become the standard questionnaire in this indication.[89,90]

Recently, a short version of the RUD has been developed (RUDlight) (Wimo A, Nordberg G, Jansson W, et al. 2000. Assessment of informal services to demented people with the RUD instrument. *Int J Geriatr Psychiatry* 15: 969–971). The currently available instruments for COI in PD analyses have considerable problems. First, none of the questionnaires used in the different studies has been published, thus a formal evaluation is not feasible. Second, there are many methodological differences among the selected studies, both from a clinical point of view (e.g., the cohort investigated) as well as from an economical point of view (included cost, and how cost, charges, and prices have been derived, etc.). Furthermore, most of the studies do not adhere to the national or international guidelines for health economic evaluations, which provide a framework for an appropriate evaluation. All these limitations make a comparison within and particularly between countries and healthcare systems difficult. Thus, a validated instrument would provide more reliable and transparent cost data of patients with PD to better estimate the burden of

the disease, design rational resource allocation, and collect basic data for CE analyses.

Utilities and preference-based outcomes

In the current review of preference-based outcomes, we have determined that most of the direct methods have not been applied in PD patients. In contrast, indirect, questionnaire-based instruments, such as the EQ-5D or the HUI, have been used repeatedly in PD patients.

Currently, the most commonly applied preference-based questionnaire is the EQ-5D. It can be used in a wide range of disease states, including patients with mild to moderate cognitive impairment,[91] is recommended for use in adults, and it displays a good response in PD patients. However, longitudinal data did not show a significant response after twelve months compared to baseline, in contrast to the UPDRS and the PD-specific PDQ-39 scale.[57,92]

In the choice of the instruments for a study, it is important to consider that there is a gold standard neither for the measurement of quality of life nor for evaluating utilities. The selection of the respective questionnaire is dependent on the research question and on a variety of factors that are specific to the given research question but also relate to the characteristics of the population and the environment in which the measurement will be undertaken (e.g., clinical trial, routine visit, cognitively impaired patients, etc.). There are only a few published recommendations. Guyatt et al.[93] considered that "trials should measure HR-QOL using at least one generic instrument, one disease-specific instrument, and one utility (preference-based) instrument." Furthermore, Brazier et al. recommended in their evaluation: "the EQ-5D and HUI are currently the best preference-based health status measurements, and should be considered for inclusion in all trials intended to be used in economic evaluation." From our review of the literature, we found currently the EQ-5D (almost) fulfilling the requests for an instrument to be applicable in the PD population.

There are, however, some important points that should be kept in mind:

1. The concept of *health* varies across the different instruments. For instance, the HUI-II and HUI-III, in contrast to other classification systems, are based on functional capacity without the assistance of corrective devices rather than on performance. For example, the vision subscale is based on the ability of a subject to see without corrective lenses.

2. The scope of the respective instruments may be generic, designed to be used in all patient groups, population-specific, or even condition-specific. Recently, preference-based condition-specific measurements have been developed[94,95] but are currently not available for PD.

3. For most HRQOL and utility instruments, we do not know the exact changes in score that constitute clinically important differences and the longitudinal changes associated with disease progression among PD patients (about 4–6 utility points are considered relevant, but there is no evidence to support these as constituting clinically important differences in PD). This is an area where more research is needed.

4. Different instruments have been shown to generate different health status utility values, even for the same patient, which has distinct consequences for the cost-utility analyses. This problem is partly due to the differences in their descriptive systems (e.g., dimensions and the number and range of levels) and their methods of valuation. This inconsistency may also occur when different population preferences for a subset of health states are used (e.g., different tariffs for the EQ-5D). The instrument of choice and the weights used should therefore be chosen carefully, depending on the aim of the study, study population, and methodology.[75] Final models must be evaluated in appropriate sensitivity analyses and may vary with PD progression.

5. None of the studies addressed the potential variability by several factors, which are due to variation in relation to medication ("on" versus "off" states; DBS on/off) and other PD related factors.

In conclusion, the methods and instruments to evaluate cost of illness and utilities have not been adequately developed for PD patients. Where as several utility measures fulfill criteria for "Recommended," even the scale most

studies in PD, the EQ-5D does not address all issues and have limited sensitivity to change. For Cost of Illness studies, given the very successful resource-utilization instrument used in Alzheimer's disease (RUD), the task force considers the development of a new instrument directly focused on PD to adequately evaluate cost of illness to be an important priority for the Movement Disorder Society. In addition, appropriate validation studies of existing MAUs in PD are needed. As health economics are expected to impact more and more on practice- and health system–level decisions, suitable and validated measures are necessary for an appropriate evaluation of PD patients.

RECOMMENDED SCALES–utility measurments
Standard Gamble
Time trade Off
EQ-5D
HUI
15D
SF-6D

References

1. Bach JP, Ziegler U, Deuschl G, Dodel R. Projected numbers of people with movement disorders in the years 2030 and 2050. *Mov Disord.* 2011;26(12):2286–2290.
2. Dorsey ER, Constantinescu R, Th ompson JP, et al. Projected number of people with Parkinson disease in the most populous nations, 2005 through 2030. *Neurology.* 2007;68(5):384–386.
3. Gold MR, Siegel JE, Russell LB, Weinstein MC. *Cost-Effectiveness in Health and Medicine.* New York: Oxford University Press; 1996.
4. Drummond MF, Sculpher MJ, Torrance GW, O'Brien B, Stoddart GL. *Methods for the Economic Evaluation of Healthcare Programmes.* Oxford: Oxford University Press; 2005.
5. Dams J, Conrads-Frank A, Reese JP, Bornschein B, Siebert U, Dodel R. Modelling the cost effectiveness of treatments for Parkinson's disease: a methodological review. *Pharmacoeconomics.* 2011; 29(12):1025–49
6. Shearer J, Green C, Counsell CE, Zajicek JP. The use of decision-analytic models in Parkinson's disease: a systematic review and

critical appraisal. *Appl Health Econ Health Policy.* 2011;9(4):243–258.

7. Siebert U, Bornschein B, Walbert T, Dodel RC. Systematic assessment of decision models in Parkinson's disease. *Value Health.* 2004;7(5):610–626.

8. The Netherlands Cancer Institute. Assessing health status and quality-of-life instruments: attributes and review criteria. *Qual Life Res.* 2002;11(3):193–205.

9. Terwee CB, Bot SD, de Boer MR, et al. Quality criteria were proposed for measurement properties of health status questionnaires. *J Clin Epidemiol.* 2007;60(1):34–42.

10. Strzelczyk A, Reese JP, Dodel R, Hamer HM. Cost of epilepsy: a systematic review. *Pharmacoeconomics.* 2008;26(6):463–476.

11. von Campenhausen S, Winter Y, Silva AR, et al. Costs of illness and care in Parkinson's disease: an evaluation in six countries. *Eur Neuropsychopharmacol.* 2011;21(2):180–191.

12. Vossius C, Gjerstad M, Baas H, Larsen JP. Drug costs for patients with Parkinson's disease in two different European countries. *Acta Neurol Scand.* 2006;113(4):228–232.

13. Tarricone R. Cost-of-illness analysis. What room in health economics? *Health Policy.* 2006;77(1):51–63.

14. Lopez-Bastida J, Oliva J, Antonanzas F, et al. Spanish recommendations on economic evaluation of health technologies. *Eur J Health Econ.* 2010;11(5):513–520.

15. Walter E, Zehetmayr S. Guidelines for health-economic evaluations in Austria. *Wien Med Wochenschr.* 2006;156(23–24):628–632.

16. Goetghebeur MM, Rindress D. Towards a European consensus on conducting and reporting health economic evaluations—a report from the ISPOR Inaugural European Conference. *Value Health.* 1999;2(4):281–287.

17. Schöffski O, Schulenburg J. Consensus on a framework for European guidelines—declaration of the EUROMET Group. In: Schöffski O, Schulenburg J, eds. *Gesundheitsökonomische Evaluationen.* Berlin: Springer; 2007:485–489.

18. Bennett K, Torrance G. Measuring health state preferences and utilities: rating scale, time trade-off, and standard gamble techniques. In: Spilker B, ed. *Quality of Life and Pharmacoeconomics in Clinical Trials.* Philadelphia, PA: Lippincott-Raven Publishers; 1996:253–265.

19. Brazier J, Deverill M, Green C, Harper R, Booth A. A review of the use of health status measures in economic evaluation. *Health Technol Assess.* 1999;3(9):i–iv, 1–164.

20. Green C, Brazier J, Deverill M. Valuing health-related quality of life. A review of health state valuation techniques. *Pharmacoeconomics.* 2000;17(2):151–165.

21. Gyrd-Hansen D. Willingness to pay for a QALY: theoretical and methodological issues. *Pharmacoeconomics.* 2005;23(5):423–432.

22. Froberg DG, Kane RL. Methodology for measuring health-state preferences—II: scaling methods. *J Clin Epidemiol.* 1989;42(5):459–471.

23. Froberg DG, Kane RL. Methodology for measuring health-state preferences—I: measurement strategies. *J Clin Epidemiol.* 1989;42(4):345–354.

24. Froberg DG, Kane RL. Methodology for measuring health-state preferences—IV: progress and a research agenda. *J Clin Epidemiol.* 1989;42(7):675–685.

25. Froberg DG, Kane RL. Methodology for measuring health-state preferences—III: population and context effects. *J Clin Epidemiol.* 1989;42(6):585–592.

26. Brazier J, Deverill M, Green C. A review of the use of health status measures in economic evaluation. *J Health Serv Res Policy.* 1999;4(3):174–184.

27. Torrance GW. Utility measurement in healthcare: the things I never got to. *Pharmacoeconomics.* 2006;24(11):1069–1078.

28. Torrance GW, Furlong W, Feeny D, Boyle M. Multi-attribute preference functions. Health Utilities Index. *Pharmacoeconomics.* 1995;7(6):503–520.

29. Drummond MF, Stoddart GL, Torrance GW. *Methods for the Economic Evaluation of Health Care Programmes.* Oxford: Oxford University Press; 1987.

30. Nemeth G. Health related quality of life outcome instruments. *Eur Spine J.* 2006;15(suppl 1):S44–S51.

31. von Neumann J, Morgenstern OT. *Theory of Games and Economic Behaviour.* New York: Wiley; 1944.

32. Palmer CS, Schmier JK, Snyder E, Scott B. Patient preferences and utilities for "off-time" outcomes in the treatment of Parkinson's disease. *Qual Life Res.* 2000;9(7):819–827.

33. Torrance GW, Thomas WH, Sackett DL. A utility maximization model for evaluation of health care programs. *Health Serv Res.* 1972;7(2):118–133.

34. Gray A, McNamara I, Aziz T, et al. Quality of life outcomes following surgical treatment of Parkinson's disease. *Mov Disord.* 2002;17:68–75.

35. Morimoto T, Shimbo T, Orav JE, et al. Impact of social functioning and vitality on preference

for life in patients with Parkinson's disease. *Mov Disord.* 2003;18:171–175.

36. Wewers ME, Lowe NK. A critical review of visual analogue scales in the measurement of clinical phenomena. *Res Nurs Health.* 1990;13(4):227–236.

37. The EuroQol Group. EuroQol—a new facility for the measurement of health-related quality of life. *Health Policy.* 1990;16:199–208.

38. Robinson A, Dolan P, Williams A. Valuing health status using VAS and TTO: what lies behind the numbers? *Soc Sci Med.* 1997;45(8):1289–1297.

39. Parkin D, Devlin N. Is there a case for using visual analogue scale valuations in cost-utility analysis? *Health Econ.* 2006;15(7):653–664.

40. Torrance GW, Boyle MH, Horwood SP. Application of multi-attribute utility theory to measure social preferences for health states. *Oper Res.* 1982;30(6):1043–1069.

41. Hawthorne G, Richardson J. Measuring the value of program outcomes: a review of multiattribute utility measures. *Expert Rev Pharmacoecon Outcomes Res.* 2001;1(2):215–228.

42. Hawthorne G, Richardson J, Day NA. A comparison of the Assessment of Quality of Life (AQoL) with four other generic utility instruments. *Ann Med.* 2001;33(5):358–370.

43. Hawthorne G, Richardson J, Osborne R. The Assessment of Quality of Life (AQoL) instrument: a psychometric measure of health-related quality of life. *Qual Life Res.* 1999;8(3):209–224.

44. Hawthorne G & Richardson J. (2001). Measuring the value of program outcomes: a review of multiattribute utility measures. *Expert Review of Pharmacoeconomics Outcomes Research.* 1 (2): 215–228.

45. Hawthorne G. Assessing utility where short measures are required: development of the short Assessment of Quality of Life-8 (AQoL-8) instrument. *Value Health.* 2009;12(6):948–957.

46. Nord E. *A Review of Synthetic Health Indicators.* Oslo: National Institute of Public Health for the OECD Directorate for Education, Employment, Labour and Social Affairs; 1997.

47. Greiner W, Weijnen T, Nieuwenhuizen M, et al. A single European currency for EQ-5D health states. Results from a six-country study. *Eur J Health Econ.* 2003;4(3):222–231.

48. Coons SJ, Rao S, Keininger DL, Hays RD. A comparative review of generic quality of life instruments. *Pharmacoeconomics.* 2000;17: 13–35.

49. Petrou S, Hockley C. An investigation into the empirical validity of the EQ-5D and SF-6D based on hypothetical preferences in a general population. *Health Econ.* 2005;14(11): 1169–1189.

50. A'Campo LE, Spliethoff-Kamminga NG, Macht M, Roos RA. Caregiver education in Parkinson's disease: formative evaluation of a standardized program in seven European countries. *Qual Life Res.* 2010;19(1):55–64.

51. Cheung YB, Tan LC, Lau PN, Au WL, Luo N. Mapping the eight-item Parkinson's disease questionnaire (PDQ-8) to the EQ-5D utility index. *Qual Life Res.* 2008;17(9):1173–1181.

52. Clarke CE, Furmston A, Morgan E, et al. Pilot randomised controlled trial of occupational therapy to optimise independence in Parkinson's disease: the PD OT trial. *J Neurol Neurosurg Psychiatry.* 2009;80(9):976–978.

53. Litvinenko IV, Odinak MM, Mogil'naia VI, Sologub OS, Sakharovskaia AA. Direct switch from conventional levodopa to stalevo (levodopa/carbidopa/entacapone) improves quality of life in Parkinson's disease: results of an open-label clinical study. *Zh Nevrol Psikhiatr Im S S Korsakova.* 2009;109(1):51–54.

54. Luo N, Low S, Lau PN, Au WL, Tan LC. Is EQ-5D a valid quality of life instrument in patients with Parkinson's disease? A study in Singapore. *Ann Acad Med Singapore.* 2009;38(6):521–528.

55. Noyes K, Dick AW, Holloway RG. Pramipexole versus levodopa in patients with early Parkinson's disease: effect on generic and disease-specific quality of life. *Value Health.* 2006;9(1):28–38.

56. Noyes K, Dick AW, Holloway RG. The implications of using US-specific EQ-5D preference weights for cost-effectiveness evaluation. *Med Decis Making.* 2007;27(3): 327–334.

57. Reuther M, Spottke EA, Klotsche J, et al. Assessing health-related quality of life in patients with Parkinson's disease in a prospective longitudinal study. *Parkinsonism Relat Disord.* 2007;13(2):108–114.

58. Schrag A, Jahanshahi M, Quinn N. How does Parkinson's disease affect quality of life? A comparison with quality of life in the general population. *Mov Disord.* 2000;15(6):1112–1118.

59. Schrag A, Selai C, Jahanshahi M, Quinn NP. The EQ-5D—a generic quality of life measure-is a useful instrument to measure quality of life in patients with Parkinson's disease. *J Neurol Neurosurg Psychiatry.* 2000;69(1):67–73.

60. Schrag A, Spottke A, Quinn NP, Dodel R. Comparative responsiveness of Parkinson's disease scales to change over time. *Mov Disord.* 2009;24(6):813–818.

61. Siderowf A, Ravina B, Glick HA. Preference-based quality-of-life in patients with Parkinson's disease. *Neurology.* 2002;59(1):103–108.

62. Siderowf AD, Werner RM. The EQ-5D—a generic quality of life measure—is a useful instrument to measure quality of life in patients with Parkinson's disease. *J Neurol Neurosurg Psychiatry.* 2001;70(6):817.

63. Winter Y, von Campenhausen S, Popov G, et al. Social and clinical determinants of quality of life in Parkinson's disease in a Russian cohort study. *Parkinsonism Relat Disord.* 2010;16(4):243–248.

64. Visser M, van Rooden SM, Verbaan D, Marinus J, Stiggelbout AM, van Hilten JJ. A comprehensive model of health-related quality of life in Parkinson's disease. *J Neurol.* 2008;255(10):1580–1587.

65. Visser M, Verbaan D, van Rooden S, Marinus J, van Hilten J, Stiggelbout A. A longitudinal evaluation of health-related quality of life of patients with Parkinson's disease. *Value Health.* 2009;12(2):392–396.

66. Feeny D, Furlong W, Boyle M, Torrance GW. Multi-attribute health status classification systems. Health Utilities Index. *Pharmacoeconomics.* 1995;7(6):490–502.

67. Horsman J, Furlong W, Feeny D, Torrance G. The Health Utilities Index (HUI): concepts, measurement properties and applications. *Health Qual Life Outcomes.* 2003;1:54.

68. Furlong WJ, Feeny DH, Torrance GW, Barr RD. The Health Utilities Index (HUI) system for assessing health-related quality of life in clinical studies. *Ann Med.* 2001;33(5):375–384.

69. Kleiner-Fisman G, Stern MB, Fisman DN. Health-related quality of life in Parkinson disease: correlation between Health Utilities Index III and Unified Parkinson's Disease Rating Scale (UPDRS) in U.S. male veterans. *Health Qual Life Outcomes.* 2010;8:91.

70. Rosser RM, Cottee M, Rabin R, Selai C. Index of health-related quality of life (IHQL). In: Hopkins A, ed. *Measures of the Quality of Life and the Uses to Which Such Measures May Be Put.* New York: Royal College of Physicians of London; 1992:81–89.

71. Rosser RM. A health index and output measure. In: Walker SR, Rosser RM, eds. *Quality of Life: Assessment and Application.* Lancaster, England: MTP Press; 1988.

72. Rosser RM, Watts VC. The measurement of hospital output. *Int J Epidemiol.* 1972;1(4): 361–368.

73. Rosser R, Kind P. A scale of valuations of states of illness: is there a social consensus? *Int J Epidemiol.* 1978;7(4):347–358.

74. Rosser R. A health index and output measure. In: Walker S, Rosser R, eds. *Quality of Life Assessment: Key Issues in the 1990s.* Dordrecht, The Netherlands: Kluwer Academic Publishers; 1993.

75. Gudex C, Kind P, van Dalen H, Durand M, Morris J, Williams A. Comparing Scaling Methods for Health State Valuations—Rosser Revisited. Discussion Paper. Report 107. York: University of York; 1993.

76. Martin A, Glasziou P, Simes RA. *Utility-Based Quality of Life Questionnaire for Cardiovascular Patients: Reliability and Validity of the UBQ-H(eart) Items.* Sydney: University of Sydney; 1996.

77. Brazier J, Usherwood T, Harper R, Thomas K. Deriving a preference-based single index from the UK SF-36 health survey. *J Clin Epidemiol.* 1998;51(11):1115–1128.

78. Nichol MB, Sengupta N, Globe DR. Evaluating quality-adjusted life years: estimation of the health utility index (HUI2) from the SF-36. *Med Decis Making.* 2001;21(2):105–112.

79. Hawthorne G, Densley K, Pallant JF, Mortimer D, Segal L. Deriving utility scores from the SF-36 health instrument using Rasch analysis. *Qual Life Res.* 2008;17(9):1183–1193.

80. Brazier J, Roberts J, Deverill M. The estimation of a preference-based measure of health from the SF-36. *J Health Econ.* 2002;21(2):271–292.

81. Vossius C, Nilsen OB, Larsen JP. Health state values during the first year of drug treatment in early-stage Parkinson's disease: a prospective, population-based, cohort study. *Drugs Aging.* 2009;26(11):973–980.

82. Kaplan RM, Anderson JP, Wu AW, Mathews WC, Kozin F, Orenstein D. The Quality of Well-being Scale. Applications in AIDS, cystic fibrosis, and arthritis. *Med Care.* 1989;27 (3 suppl):S27–S43.

83. Kaplan RM, Sieber WJ, and Ganiats TG. The quality of well-being scale: Comparison of the interviewer-administered version with a self-administered questionnaire. *Psych Health.* 1997;12:783–791.

84. Sintonen H. The 15D instrument of health-related quality of life: properties and applications. *Ann Med.* 2001;33(5):328–336.

85. Sintonen H. Health-related quality of life measures. *Sairaanhoitaja.* 1993(4):17–19.

86. Kristiansen IS, Bingefors K, Nyholm D, Isacson D. Short-term cost and health consequences of duodenal levodopa infusion in advanced Parkinson's disease in Sweden: an exploratory study. *Appl Health Econ Health Policy.* 2009;7(3):167–180.

87. Nyholm D, Nilsson Remahl AI, Dizdar N, et al. Duodenal levodopa infusion monotherapy vs oral polypharmacy in advanced Parkinson disease. *Neurology.* 2005;64(2):216–223.

88. Haapaniemi TH, Sotaniemi KA, Sintonen H, Taimela E. The generic 15D instrument is valid and feasible for measuring health related quality of life in Parkinson's disease. *J Neurol Neurosurg Psychiatry.* 2004;75(7):976–983.

89. Wimo A, Jonsson L, Zbrozek A. The Resource Utilization in Dementia (RUD) instrument is valid for assessing informal care time in community-living patients with dementia. *J Nutr Health Aging.* 2010;14(8):685–690.

90. Wimo A, Wetterholm A, Mastey V, et al. Evaluation of the resource utilization and caregiver time in anti-dementia drug trials: a quantitative battery. In: Wimo A, Jönsson B, Karlsson G, eds. *The Health Economics of Dementia.* London: John Wiley & Sons; 1988:465–499.

91. Naglie G, Tomlinson G, Tansey C, et al. Utility-based quality of life measures in Alzheimer's disease. *Qual Life Res.* 2006;15(4):631–643.

92. Martinez-Martin P, Jeukens-Visser M, Lyons KE, et al., Health-related quality-of-life scales in Parkinson's disease: critique and recommendations. *Mov Disord.* 2011;26(13):2371–2380.

93. Guyatt GH, Jaeschke RJ. Reassessing quality-of-life instruments in the evaluation of new drugs. *Pharmacoeconomics.* 1997;12(6):621–626.

94. Revicki DA, Leidy NK. Integrating patient preferences into health outcomes assessment: the multiattribute Asthma Symptom Utility Index. *Chest.* 1998;114:998–1007.

95. Marra CA, Woolcott JC, Kopec JA, et al. A comparison of generic, indirect utility measures (the HUI2, HUI3, SF-6D, and the EQ-5D) and disease-specific instruments (the RAQoL and the HAQ) in rheumatoid arthritis. *Soc Sci Med.* 2005;60(7):1571–1582.

96. von Campenhausen S, Winter Y, Gasser J, et al. Cost of illness and health services patterns in Morbus Parkinson in Austria. *Wien Klin Wochenschr.* 2009;121(17–18):574–582.

97. Guttman M, Slaughter PM, Theriault ME, DeBoer DP, Naylor CD. Burden of parkinsonism: a population-based study. *Mov Disord.* 2003;18:313–336.

98. Wang G, Cheng Q, Zheng R, et al. Economic burden of Parkinson's disease in a developing country: a retrospective cost analysis in Shanghai, China. *Mov Disord.* 2006;21(9):1439–1443.

99. Winter Y, von Campenhausen S, Brozova H, et al. Costs of Parkinson's disease in eastern Europe: a Czech cohort study. *Parkinsonism Relat Disord.* 2010;16(1):51–56.

100. Keranen T, Kaakkola S, Sotaniemi K. Economic burden and quality of life impairment increase with severity of PD. *Parkinsonism Relat Disord.* 2003;9:163–168.

101. LePen C, Wait S, Moutard-Martin F, Dujardin M, Ziegler M. Cost of illness and disease severity in a cohort of French patients with Parkinson's disease. *Pharmacoeconomics.* 1999;16:59–69.

102. Barth F, Baum B, Bremen D, Meuser T, Jost WH. Indirect costs in idiopathic Parkinson's disease. *Fortschr Neurol Psychiatr.* 2005;73(4):187–191.

103. Dengler I, Leukel N, Meuser T, Jost WH. Prespektive Erfassung der direkten und indirekten Kosten des idiopathischen Parkinson-Syndroms. *Nervenarzt.* 2006;77(10):1204–1209.

104. Dodel RC, Singer M, Kohne-Volland R, et al. The economic impact of Parkinson's disease: an estimation based on a 3-month prospective analysis. *Pharmacoeconomics.* 1998;14(3):299–312.

105. Ehret R, Balzer-Geldsetzer M, Reese JP, et al. Direct costs for Parkinson's treatment in private neurology practices in Berlin. *Nervenarzt.* 2009;80(4):452–458.

106. Reese JP, Winter Y, Balzer-Geldsetzer M, et al. Parkinson's disease: cost-of-illness in an outpatient cohort. *Gesundheitswesen.* 2010;73(1):22–29.

107. Spottke AE, Reuter M, Machat O, et al. Cost of illness and its predictors for Parkinson's disease in Germany. *Pharmacoeconomics.* 2005;23:817–836.

108. Winter Y, Balzer-Geldsetzer M, Spottke A, et al. Longitudinal study of the socioeconomic burden of Parkinson's disease in Germany. *Eur J Neurol.* 2010;17(9):1156–1163.

109. Winter Y, Balzer-Geldsetzer M, von Campenhausen S, et al. Trends in resource utilization for Parkinson's disease in Germany. *J Neurol Sci.* 2010;294(1–2):18–22.

110. Ragothaman M, Govindappa ST, Rattihalli R, Subbakrishna DK, Muthane UB. Direct

costs of managing Parkinson's disease in India: concerns in a developing country. *Mov Disord.* 2006;21(10):1755–1758.

111. Winter Y, von Campenhausen S, Reese JP, et al. Costs of Parkinson's disease and antiparkinsonian pharmacotherapy: an Italian cohort study. *Neurodegener Dis.* 2010;7(6):365–372.

112. Winter Y, von Campenhausen S, Popov G, et al. Costs of illness in a Russian cohort of patients with Parkinson's disease. *Pharmacoeconomics.* 2009;27(7):571–584.

113. Cubo E, Martinez Martin P, Gonzalez M, Frades B. Impact of motor and non-motor symptoms on the direct costs of Parkinson's disease. *Neurologia.* 2009;24(1):15–23.

114. Hagell P, Nordling S, Reimer J, Grabowski M, Persson U. Resource use and costs in a Swedish cohort of patients with Parkinson's disease. *Mov Disord.* 2002;17:1213–1220.

115. Findley L, Aujla M, Bain PG, et al. Direct economic impact of Parkinson's disease: a research survey in the United Kingdom. *Mov Disord.* 2003;18:1139–1145.

116. McCrone P, Allcock LM, Burn DJ. Predicting the cost of Parkinson's disease. *Mov Disord.* 2007;22(6):804–812.

117. Huse DM, Schulman K, Orsini L, Castelli-Haley J, Kennedy S, Lenhart G. Burden of illness in Parkinson's disease. *Mov Disord.* 2005;20(11):1449–1454.

118. Leibson CL, Long KH, Maraganore DM, et al. Direct medical costs associated with Parkinson's disease: a population-based study. *Mov Disord.* 2006;21(11):1864–1871.

119. Noyes K, Liu H, Li Y, Holloway R, Dick AW. Economic burden associated with Parkinson's disease on elderly Medicare beneficiaries. *Mov Disord.* 2006;21(3):362–372.

120. Thomas S, Nay R, Moore K, et al. *Continence Outcomes Measurement Suite Project* [final report]. Sydney: Australian Government Department of Health and Ageing; 2006.

121. Marras C, Lang A, Krahn M, Tomlinson G, Naglie G. Quality of life in early Parkinson's disease: impact of dyskinesias and motor fluctuations. *Mov Disord.* 2004;19(1):22–28.

122. Pohar SL, Allyson Jones C. The burden of Parkinson disease (PD) and concomitant comorbidities. *Arch Gerontol Geriatr.* 2009;49(2):317–321.

123. Jones CA, Pohar SL, Patten SB. Major depression and health-related quality of life in Parkinson's disease. *Gen Hosp Psychiatry.* 2009;31(4):334–340.

124. Isacson D, Bingefors K, Kristiansen IS, Nyholm D. Fluctuating functions related to quality of life in advanced Parkinson disease: effects of duodenal levodopa infusion. *Acta Neurol Scand.* 2008;118(6):379–386.

125. Schöffski O, v. Schulenburg JM. *Gesundheitsökonomische Evaluationen.* Berlin: Springer; 2007.

PART 3

NON-MOTOR DOMAINS OF PARKINSON'S DISEASE

13

APATHY AND ANHEDONIA

Albert F. G. Leentjens and Sergio E. Starkstein

Summary

Apathy is a common condition in Parkinson's disease (PD) and is generally defined as a disorder of motivation, characterized by reduced activities, cognition, and emotion. *Anhedonia* is defined as the inability to experience pleasure and can be a symptom of apathy as well as other syndromes. Apathy and anhedonia rating scales can be used to assess and quantify these phenomena. Scales that have either been validated or used in studies with PD patients include the Apathy Evaluation Scale (AES), the Apathy Scale (AS), the Apathy Inventory (AI), and the Lille Apathy Rating Scale (LARS). In addition, item 4 (motivation/initiative) of the Unified Parkinson's Disease Rating Scale (UPDRS), and item 7 (apathy) of the Neuropsychiatric Inventory (NPI) are used as measures of apathy.

Anhedonia scales that have been validated or used in studies with PD patients include the Snaith-Hamilton Pleasure Scale (SHAPS) and the Chapman scales for physical and social anhedonia. Based on criteria of the MDS Task Force on Parkinson's Disease Rating Scales, both the AS and the LARS are classified as "Recommended" scales to assess apathy in PD. Although item 4 of the UPDRS also meets the criteria to be classified as "Recommended," it should be considered for screening only because of the obvious limitations of a single-item construct. For the assessment of anhedonia, no scale meets the criteria to be designated as "Recommended," and only the SHAPS meets the criteria of "Suggested" scales.

Even though the apathy and anhedonia scales have been classified according to the criteria of the MDS, detailed clinimetric properties have not been studied extensively for any of them. Information on the validity of apathy scales is almost absent, because of the lack of consensus on diagnostic criteria for these conditions. Recently formulated proposed consensus criteria may, however, be used for further validation of these scales.

INTRODUCTION

Apathy and anhedonia are commonly observed in patients with neurodegenerative disorders such as Parkinson's disease (PD). Neither of these clinical phenomena is well defined, and both lack generally accepted diagnostic criteria.

The lack of such criteria also implies that there is no gold standard against which existing apathy and anhedonia rating scales can be validated. This dilemma is a serious limitation for research concerning the epidemiology, symptomatology, pathophysiology, and treatment of these disturbances.[1]

In an attempt to overcome this problem, in 2008, a consensus meeting was held by representatives from the European Psychiatric Association (EPA), the European Alzheimer's Disease Consortium (EADC), the Association Française de Psychiatrie Biologique (AFPB), as well as invited experts from Europe, Australia, and North America. The intention of this meeting was to agree on diagnostic criteria for apathy as a syndrome.[2] Based on earlier proposals by individual researchers,[3-5] *apathy* was defined as a syndrome of reduced motivation, characterized by a deficiency in three symptom domains: activities, cognition, and emotion.[2] The diagnostic criteria proposed by this work group have recently been validated in 306 patients suffering from a range of neuropsychiatric diseases, including Alzheimer's disease (AD), mixed dementia, mild cognitive impairment (MCI), Parkinson's disease, schizophrenia, and "major depressive episode."[6] In this study, the criteria were shown to have good acceptability, inter-rater reliability, and known-groups validity. Subsequently, these criteria were validated in a population of 122 PD patients and showed good acceptability and internal consistency, as well as a good concurrent validity with the Lille Apathy Rating Scale (LARS) and the apathy section of the Neuropsychiatric Inventory (NPI). The discriminant validity of the criteria with measures for depression was moderate to good.[1] As such, the criteria provide a valid basis for the syndromal diagnosis of apathy.

Anhedonia is less well defined and has been used in many different ways since the term was coined by the French psychologist Théodule Ribot in 1897.[7] In earlier literature, the terms "apathy" and "anhedonia" were often used interchangeably. Currently, "anhedonia" is used to describe the "reduced ability to experience pleasure," which may occur in a variety of different syndromes that include apathy, but also depressive disorder, schizophrenia, and substance-abuse disorders. Thus, anhedonia is considered a symptom, while apathy is considered a syndrome.

Apathy is one of the most common neuropsychiatric syndromes in PD. Frequencies of 17 to 70% have been reported, depending on the population characteristics and assessment procedures.[8-10] In PD, apathy is associated with more severe cognitive deficits, more severe depressive symptoms, and a decreased quality of life.[11-13] To date, there is no effective treatment for apathy.[14]

OVERVIEW OF SCALES

A systematic review of apathy and anhedonia rating scales, commissioned by the Movement Disorders Society (MDS), included all scales that have been designed to assess apathy and anhedonia, and that have either been validated or used in studies with PD patients.[15] Multidimensional scales that are used to screen more broadly for different psychiatric and neuropsychological symptom areas were considered to be beyond the scope of the review, even though some of these scales have been used in the assessment of apathy and anhedonia in PD, such as the Brief Psychiatric Rating Scale (BPRS) and the Frontal Systems Behavior Scale (FSBS, previously known as the Frontal Lobe Personality Scale).[16,17] Scales assessing momentary mood states, such as the Profile of Moods States Questionnaire (POMS) were also excluded.[18] Because of its special status in the assessment of PD patients, as well as its widespread use, an exception was made for Item 4 (motivation) of Part I of the Unified Parkinson's Disease Rating Scale (UPDRS).[19] Another exception was made for the Apathy section of the NPI, because of the frequency with which this scale is used to assess psychiatric symptoms of patients with neurodegenerative diseases.[20] With respect to the lack of operational criteria for apathy at the time the scales were validated or used in research, the task force committee did not adhere to a restrictive or specified definition of apathy, but instead included all scales and articles referring to apathy in whatever definition the authors had used.

Four apathy rating scales and two anhedonia rating scales that have been validated or used in PD were identified. These scales include the Apathy Evaluation Scale (AES), an abbreviated version of the AES known as the Apathy Scale (AS), the Apathy Inventory (AI), and the LARS.[3,21-23] Although the AI was specifically designed and validated to assess apathy in PD, no subsequent studies involving the scale were identified. All the other apathy scales discussed here have been used in several studies with PD patients.

Two anhedonia scales were identified and included in the review: the Snaith-Hamilton Pleasure Scale (SHAPS) and the Chapman scales for physical and social anhedonia.[24,25] For an overview of the general properties of the apathy and anhedonia scales: see table 13.1; for an overview of the classification of scales according to the MDS criteria: see table 13.2.

Apathy Evaluation Scale (AES)[3]

DESCRIPTION

The AES consists of 18 items, with scores ranging from 1 to 4 points for each item, and a total score ranging from 18 to 72 points. Higher scores indicate more severe apathy. Scale items include behavioral, cognitive, and emotional items, some of which rate the intensity of a feature, while others rate the frequency. According to the instructions for administration, subjects should be "primed" with two questions regarding general interests, activities, and daily routines before the actual assessment starts. The time frame is defined as "the past four weeks." Clinician-rated, patient-rated, and caregiver-rated versions

are available. The most commonly used version is the clinician-rated one, which is not only clinician-rated, but also includes four self-evaluation items (items 3 [starting chores], 8 [interest in finishing chores], 13 [interest in meeting friends] and 16 [interest in doing things]). Item 15 [self-awareness] requires the rater to evaluate the patient's insight.

A number of items overlap with potential symptoms of PD (items 2 [finishing chores], and 9 [being involved in activities]), depression [items 1 [interests], 6 [poor effort], 7 [intensity of life], 9 [being involved in activities], 13 [interest in meeting friends], 14 [getting excited], 17 [initiative] and 18 [motivation]), and cognitive decline (items 5 [learning], 9 [being involved in activities], 10 [needing guidance] and 15 [self-awareness]). It takes 10 to 20 minutes to administer the scale.

KEY EVALUATION ISSUES

The AES has been used by multiple authors and has been validated in a mixed population including 123 patients with AD and other dementias, stroke, and major depression,[26] and among 121 patients with dementia.[27] In these populations, the AES demonstrated good internal consistency, inter-rater and test-retest reliability, and moderate item-total correlations. The informant- and

Table 13-1. General Description and Properties of Scales.

SCALE	RATED BY	ADMINISTRATION TIME (MINUTES)	RELIABILITY IN PD	VALIDITY IN PD	SENSITIVITY TO CHANGE
AES	clinician	15	?		?
AS	patient	10	?	?	+
AI	clinician patient	5	?		
LARS	clinician	15	+	+	
UPDRS item 4	clinician	1	+	+	?
NPI section 7	informant	1–10	?		
SHAPS	patient	5	?		+
Chapman	patient	10			−

Abbreviations: AES = apathy evaluation scale, AS = apathy scale, AI = apathy inventory, LARS = Lille apathy rating scale, UPDRS = Unified Parkinson's Disease Rating Scale, NPI = neuropsychiatric inventory, SHAPS = Snaith Hamilton anhedonia rating scale.
+ = good, − = poor, ? = not reported completely, or based on studies with serious limitations. Further explanations: see text.

Table 13-2. Classification of Apathy Scales. For an Explanation of the Classifying Groups, see Chapter 6.

SCALE	USED IN PD	USED BEYOND ORIGINAL DEVELOPERS	SUCCESSFUL CLINIMETRIC TESTING	CLASSIFICATION
AES	X	X	0	Suggested
AS	X	X	X	Recommended
AI	X	0	0	Listed
LARS	X	X	X	Recommended
UPDRS item 4	X	X	X	Recommended**
NPI section 7	X	X	0	Suggested
SHAPS	X	X	0	Suggested
Chapman	X	*	0	Listed

* Although the Chapman scales were used in PD patients in one study beyond their original developers, this study concluded that the scale was not useful. Hence the scale was classified as "Listed."

** As a single-item construct, item 4 of the UPDRS cannot be considered a "scale," and its use is advised only for crude screening purposes.

patient-based versions have a good convergent validity, but concurrent validity with the NPI apathy subscore is weak.[9,27] Discriminant validity with depression and anxiety is adequate.[9]

In PD patients, the scale has shown good internal consistency, with a Cronbach's alpha of 0.92, and good test-retest reliability (r = 0.85).[9] The convergent validity of patient- and informant-rated versions was high (r = 0.74), but, importantly, convergent validity with other apathy scales has not been assessed. The AES was shown to be sensitive to change in one study with methylphenidate to treat apathy, and it was also able also detect changes in levels of apathy after deep brain stimulation.[28,29] However, many clinimetric properties are unknown, among them, the cutoff score for screening and diagnosis of apathy in PD.

STRENGTHS AND WEAKNESSES

Advantages of the AES are several. This scale has been used in different populations over the past 20 years. It is in the public domain and has been translated into several languages. Face validity is good, since its items cover the core criterion as well as the three different symptom domains of the recently formulated diagnostic criteria for apathy (motivation, behavior, cognition, and emotion).

Disadvantages are the fact that this scale has not been properly validated in PD, and during the rating procedure, some of the items require clinical judgement.

FINAL ASSESSMENT

The AES meets the criteria for "Suggested scale." In PD, only information on reliability, but not on validity, is available. The scale may be useful to screen for and to assess the severity of apathetic symptoms, and may also be used to follow changes in apathy during treatment.

The Apathy Scale (AS)[21]

DESCRIPTION OF THE SCALE

The AS is presented as an abridged and modified version of the AES. The AS is a patient-based assessment consisting of 14 items. In the original patient-based version, questions are read aloud to the patient by the examiner, but a caregiver-rated version is also available.[30] Each item is formulated as a question. The patient has to choose his answer from four possibilities: *not at all, slightly, some, a lot.* The score range varies from 14 to 56. The time frame was defined as "four weeks." The scale was developed specifically for patients with PD because the AES was considered too demanding.

Some of the items overlap with those of Parkinsonism (item 8 [energy]), depression (items 1 [interest], 2 [interest], 4 [putting effort into things], 6 [plans for the future], 7 [motivation], 8 [energy], 12 [difficulty getting started], 13 [emotional blunting], 14 [insight]) or with those of cognitive decline (items 6 [plans for the future], 9 [tell what to do]). It takes about 10 minutes to administer the scale.

KEY EVALUATION POINTS

The AS has been used by multiple authors and in PD patients. The AS it has good face validity since it covers the core criteria and three symptom domains of apathy. In addition, it was shown to have good internal consistency, with a Cronbach's alpha of 0.76.[21] Inter-rater reliability (r = 0.81) and test-retest reliability (r = 0.90) have been assessed in 11 PD patients only, and were good.[21] For screening purposes, a cutoff score of 13/14 was recommended, with scores of 14 or higher indicating clinically relevant levels of apathy. Using this cutoff, the scale has a high specificity (100%), but rather low sensitivity of 66% when item 4 of the UPDRS Part I (motivation) is used as the gold standard.[21] No other studies assessing the validity of the AS have been performed. The scale has demonstrated sensitivity to change during pharmacological treatment[31] or treatment by deep brain stimulation.[28,32,33] Although the AS was developed for patients with PD, it has subsequently been used also in patients with Alzheimer's disease and stroke.

STRENGTHS AND WEAKNESSES

The advantages of the AS are that this scale was especially designed to measure apathy in PD patients and has been used in a moderate number of studies involving PD patients. It is easy to use and does not require much time to administer. It is in the public domain and available in several languages. Although the clinimetric validation is limited, there is not only information on reliability, but also limited information on the validity, including a recommended cutoff for screening. Specificity may be probably high.

A disadvantage is that the scale relies on self-assessment by the patient, which requires insight. This makes the scale less appropriate for patients with more severe cognitive decline. In these cases, the caregiver-rated version should be used.

FINAL ASSESSMENT

The AS meets the criteria for a "Recommended" scale. It is recommended to screen for and to assess the severity of apathy in PD patients. Given its use in patients with AD, it can probably be used in patients with *mild* dementia associated with PD as well. It has proven to be sensitive to change and may be used in treatment studies.

The Apathy Inventory (AI)[22]

DESCRIPTION OF THE SCALE

Two versions of the AI are available: a patient-based version and an informant-based version, both consisting of three items. In both versions, the three items address emotional blunting, lack of initiative, and lack of interest. Each item follows the same structure: two or three questions ask whether behavior has changed in a specified time frame. If the response is positive, the frequency (1 to 4) and the severity (1 to 3) of this change is assessed by two additional questions. The item score is the product of frequency times severity, and total scores range from 0 to 36. The time frame is not specified and left open for the rater to define.[22] There is no overlap with motor symptoms of PD, but all three items may overlap with depression. The scale takes five minutes to administer.

KEY EVALUATION POINTS

The original validation study of the AI included 60 patients with AD, 24 with MCI," 12 PD patients, and 19 healthy volunteers. In this study, the AI showed good internal consistency, with a Cronbach's alpha of 0.84 across all diagnostic groups. Inter-rater reliability (kappa = 0.99) and test-retest reliability (kappa = 0.96) were high.[22] Except for the 12 PD patients included in the original validation study, the scale has not been used or validated in other studies involving PD patients. No information on the validity of the AI is available. The scale has been used in some studies involving patients with MCI and AD.

STRENGTHS AND WEAKNESSES

The AI is in the public domain. The advantages of the AI are that the scale is very short and easy to administer; in addition it can be used in patients with dementia. The main disadvantage is that there are hardly any clinimetric data available for a PD population. In addition, the score distribution is non-linear and non-continuous, since the only possible scores are 1, 2, 3, 4, 6, 8, 9, and 12. This potentially weights the scale towards milder overall ratings and also has implications for data-analysis. Floor effects have been observed in patients with MCI and healthy control subjects.[22]

FINAL ASSESSMENT

Because it has not been used by multiple authors nor clinimetrically examined in detail, the AI is classified as "Listed." The brevity of the scale would make it an attractive instrument, but it should be better validated and used more extensively in a PD population, so that its clinimetric properties may become better known.

The Lille Apathy Rating Scale (LARS)[23]

DESCRIPTION OF THE SCALE

The LARS is a recently developed scale that consists of 33 items divided into nine domains. It is administered to the patient as a structured interview. The first three questions are scored on a 5-point Likert scale, whereas the remaining items are answered as *yes* or *no*. The LARS assesses four aspects of apathy that do not readily follow the diagnostic criteria (which were formulated after the scale was developed): action initiation,

emotion, intellectual curiosity and self-awareness. The LARS total score ranges from −36 to +36 points, with positive scores indicating more severe apathy. The time frame is defined as "the past four weeks." Some of the items overlap with symptoms of Parkinsonism (item 1 [productivity]), depression (items 1 [productivity], 2 [interests], 3 [initiative], 4 [novelty seeking], 5 [motivation], [social life], and 9 [self-awareness]) and cognitive decline (items 1 [productivity], 2 [interests], 3 [initiative], 4 [novelty seeking], 5 [motivation], 8 [social life] and 9 [self-awareness]).[23] Although this scale is the longest of all the apathy scales, it only takes about 15 minutes to administer.

KEY EVALUATION POINTS

The LARS was especially designed for patients with PD, and was validated in a group of PD patients with and without dementia. It has a good internal consistency, with a Cronbach's alpha of 0.80. Test-retest reliability (r = 0.95) and inter-rater reliability (r = 0.98) were good, and item-total correlations acceptable (average 0.65; range 0.52 to 0.81). Concurrent validity with the AES was high (r = 0.87). Validated against a clinical judgement of apathy, it showed a high sensitivity (89%) and specificity (92%) with a high accuracy index (81%). Based on expert judgement, a cutoff of −16/−17 was recommended for clinically relevant levels of apathy. The four subscales (see above) were identified on the basis of a factor analysis.

In a recently published study, this scale was used as an external standard for validation of the proposed diagnostic criteria for apathy.[1] The correlation (as a measure of concurrent validity) between the diagnostic criteria of apathy and the LARS was good (r = 0.72). In addition, the percentage of agreement between the diagnosis of apathy based on a cutoff score on the LARS of ≥ −16 and the diagnostic criteria for apathy was high (81%). The scale has been used by different groups in studies involving PD patients,[34] but not yet in other populations.

STRENGTHS AND WEAKNESSES

The LARS provides a comprehensive assessment of apathy in a structured interview in a reasonable amount of time. It is well validated and the only scale that has been subject to factor analysis. The scale is validated for PD patients and available in the public domain. Disadvantages are that it requires insight by the patient and may thus not be suitable for patients with more severe cognitive decline. In frail patients, the scale may be too demanding. The score range, from negative to positive scores, is not very easy to apprehend, and special expertise is required for statistical analyses involving this scale.

FINAL ASSESSMENT

The LARS meets the criteria for a "Recommended" scale. It was specifically designed for PD patients, has been used by multiple authors, and has demonstrated good clinimetric properties. The scale is suitable to study the phenomenology, etiology, and correlations with potential biological markers of apathy in patients with mild or moderate PD.

Item 4 (motivation/initiative) of the Unified Parkinson's Disease Rating Scale (UPDRS)[19]

DESCRIPTION OF THE SCALE

Item 4 of the UPDRS is a single item of a comprehensive scale. However, it is often used as an indicator of apathy in studies involving PD patients. The UPDRS is the most widely used multimodal assessment scale in PD. It is clinician-rated and consists of four sections. Part I assesses mood, mentation, and behavior, and includes four items. Items 1 through 3 assess intellectual impairment, thought disorder, and depression; while item 4 assess motivation and initiative and can be used as an indicator of apathy. The item is scored on a 5-point scale ranging from 0 to 4, with increasing scores indicating more severe loss of motivation and/or initiative.[19] The item is particularly related to *activities* and does not capture the cognitive and emotional concomitants of apathy. Moreover, the item is not specific for apathy as an isolated syndrome, but overlaps with depression and cognitive decline. The time frame for the UPDRS is usually "one week," but other time frames may be applied.

KEY EVALUATION ISSUES

Although the full UPDRS is often used in studies with PD patients, the apathy question has been used by multiple authors in studies of apathy in PD. For item 4, inter-rater reliability is fair, with kappa values ranging from 0.71 to 0.75.[35,36] Test-retest reliability is moderate (kappa 0.57, reported in one study).[37] One study found acceptable sensitivity (73%) and specificity (65%) in relation to the diagnosis of apathy (based on an algorithm applied to the AS), when a cutoff of 2/3 was applied, with an Area under the ROC curve (AUC) of 76%. For moderate to severe PD, this threshold should probably be increased to 3/4, which would give a sensitivity of 61% and a specificity of 89%, and an AUC of 80%.[38] The concurrent validity with the AS is moderate (r = 0.55).[21,38]

STRENGTHS AND WEAKNESSES

The UPDRS is in the public domain and available in many languages. Being a single item, item 4 of the UPDRS Part I, it hardly takes any time to administer and is often used as part of routine clinical practice. It has been used in many studies involving PD. Being a single item, however, means it will not capture the different dimensions of the apathy syndrome, and has limited ability to quantify severity and changes in severity.

FINAL ASSESSMENT

Formally, the UPDRS item 4 is classified as "Recommended" in the MDS system of appraisal of rating scales, because it has been used in PD assessments in reports other than the original scale description and has successfully undergone at least some clinimetric testing. However, being a single item, it provides limited information. Therefore, this item may only be considered as a crude initial screening measure for apathy.

Item 7 (Apathy) of the Neuropsychiatric Inventory (NPI)[20]

DESCRIPTION OF THE SCALE

The NPI was developed as a structured interview conducted by the clinician to assess 10 behavioral disorders that may occur in patients with dementia, including delusions, hallucinations, agitation/aggression, depression, anxiety, euphoria/elation, apathy, disinhibition, irritability/lability, and aberrant motor behavior.[20] Subsequently a 12-section version was developed that also includes sleep and appetite disturbances. Other versions have subsequently been developed, including a nursing-home version (NPI-NH), a version for use in general practice settings (the NPI-Questionnaire, NPI-Q), and the Caregiver Administered NPI (CGA-NPI).

Only Section 7 (apathy) of the 12-item version is assessed here. This version is clinician-rated, based on a structured interview with an informant who is familiar with the patient's behavior. Four initial scripted screening questions assess the presence of apathy symptoms that represent changes from premorbid behaviors. If the screening probe is endorsed positively, the interviewer asks an additional set of eight scripted questions that address more specific features about behaviors, cognitions, and emotions related to apathy. These topics cover the core criterion and symptom domains of apathy. The frequency and the severity of the various apathetic behaviors are rated separately. The frequency is scored on a 4-point scale with clear anchors (1–*occasionally*, less than once per week; 2–*often*, about once per week; 3–*frequently*, several times per week but less than every day; or 4–*very frequently*, nearly always present). The severity score is rated on a 3-point scale (1–*mild*, 2–*moderate*, or 3–*severe*). A symptom subscale score is the product of the frequency score multiplied by the severity score. As such, the subscale score distribution is nonlinear and has a score ranging from 0 to 12. The time frame is usually "the last four weeks," though different time frames have been applied.

Some of the eight items of the apathy section overlap with symptoms of Parkinsonism (items 1 [less spontaneous or active], 2 [less conversational], 3 [less emotional] and 4 [less contributory to chores]) and cognitive decline (item 2 [less conversational]). The apathy section does not include a question on mood, although all 8 sub-items may also be present in depression. The scale takes about ten minutes to administer.

KEY EVALUATION ISSUES

The full NPI, including the apathy section, has been used in a large number of studies involving different populations, including patients with Alzheimer's disease, frontotemporal dementia, Huntington's disease, progressive supranuclear palsy (PSP), multiple sclerosis, and head injury. It has a good internal consistency (Cronbach's alpha 0.88), inter-rater agreement (89.4 to 97.9%) and test-retest reliability (r = 0.74) in patients with AD.[20] In PD patients, the apathy subscale has been used by multiple authors, but the clinimetric issues have not been well studied in PD. No information about internal consistency or test-retest reliability are available. Inter-rater reliability and inter-rater agreement, although based on a single study with 12 patients, were good (ICC = 0.84).[20] No additional information on reliability or validity of the NPI apathy section in PD patients is available.

STRENGTHS AND WEAKNESSES

The main advantage of the apathy section of the NPI is that it constitutes a brief screening measure that is easy to administer and has clear instructions and anchor points. The use of probing questions reduces the administration time in patients without apathetic symptoms. The NPI is in the public domain, widely used and translated into many languages. It is a caregiver-based interview, and hence applicable in patients with dementia. The disadvantages are that its clinimetric properties remain to be better studied in patients with PD. In addition, its score has a non-linear and non-continuous distribution, which has implications for data-analysis.

FINAL ASSESSMENT

Section 7 of the NPI can be considered a "Suggested" scale, because its clinimetric properties are still poorly defined in PD. The *full* NPI is frequently used to screen and assess the severity of neuropsychiatric symptoms, including apathy, in neurodegenerative disorders, and has also been used to study the phenomenology and clinical correlations of apathy in PD populations.

The Snaith-Hamilton Pleasure Scale (SHAPS)[24]

DESCRIPTION OF THE SCALE

The SHAPS is a self-rated instrument that assesses the presence and severity of anhedonia. The scale consists of 14 items rated on a 4-point Likert scale. All 14 items refer to the inability to experience pleasure. Although there are four answering options (*definitely agree, agree, disagree,* and *strongly disagree*), scoring is reduced to two alternatives. Following the method of the General Health Questionnaire, both *agree* options score 0 points and both *disagree* options score 1 point (except in a Dutch validation study in which a 1–4 score option is used).[39,40] The order of responses (in increasing or decreasing severity) varies from item to item. Thus, the total score range is 0 to 14. The time frame is "the past few days" and thus not well defined. Some of the items may overlap with symptoms of PD (items 4 [enjoy meal], 6 [enjoy nice smells], 10 [enjoy favorite drink], and 13 [enjoy helping others]), or cognitive decline (items 1 [enjoy radio or television program], and 9 [enjoy reading]). Since anhedonia may be a symptom of depression, all items may be part of a depressive disorder. Scale administration takes about five minutes.

KEY EVALUATION ISSUES

In non-PD patients, the SHAPS has a good face validity, internal consistency, item-total correlation, and test-retest correlation.[24] Only one study provides information on the internal consistency of the SHAPS (Cronbach's alpha equals 0.90 and 0.92 in depressed and non-depressed patients, respectively). The same study provides a factor analysis of the SHAPS, documenting significant loading on a single factor, explaining 75% of the variance.[41] No study has reported on the clinimetric properties of the SHAPS in PD patients, although this is probably the most widely used scale to assess anhedonia in the PD population.[9,41–45] The scale has been used to assess the level of anhedonia in PD patients and to evaluate the effect of (pharmacological) treatment of motor symptoms of PD on hedonic symptoms. It has proven to be sensitive to changes in hedonic tone.

STRENGTHS AND WEAKNESSES

The SHAPS has the advantage of being brief and easy to apply. It has been used in a fair number of studies involving PD patients and has shown to be sensitive to change. Disadvantages are the absence of validation studies in PD and the ambiguous time frame.

FINAL ASSESSMENT

The SHAPS is classified as a "Suggested" scale, because it has been used in PD by multiple authors, but its clinimetric properties are insufficiently defined in PD patients. It is probably suitable for assessing levels of hedonic tone and for studying the epidemiology, etiology, and treatment of anhedonia.

The Chapman Scales for Physical and Social Anhedonia[25]

DESCRIPTION OF THE SCALES

The Chapman Scales for Physical and Social Anhedonia are probably the most widely used instruments to measure anhedonia in patients with psychiatric diseases, such as schizophrenia and depressive disorder. The original scale is a patient-rated instrument that consists of 88 true/false questions, divided over two subscales: a subscale for physical anhedonia consisting of 40 items, and another for social anhedonia consisting of 48 items. Higher scores indicate more severe anhedonia, except in the Italian translation, which is reverse-scored with higher scores indicating less severe anhedonia.[25,46] The scale for physical anhedonia was revised to include 61 items and is often used independently from the social anhedonia scale. The time frame is not defined.

Some of the items overlap with symptoms of PD (items P4 [muscle strength], P5 and P41 [dancing], P7 and P29 [taste and smell], P8 [physical activities], P11 [vigorous activity], P34, P45, and P60 [taking walks], and S29 [long discussions]), or cognitive impairment (items S23 [talking with others] and S26 [listening attentively]). Since anhedonia may be part of depression, all individual items may also overlap with depression. Completing the scale may take ten minutes.

KEY EVALUATION ISSUES

The scale lacks face validity as it focuses on long-standing characteristics, rather than on current feelings. Many items refer to aspects of apathy rather than anhedonia (e.g., items referring to social withdrawal, loss of interest, and lack of motivation). In addition, many items are sensitive to personal opinions, preferences, and habits. Some items are unsuitable to ask older people or patients with PD (e.g., items referring to sexual activities [P1, P9, P40, P53], rides in an amusement park [P19], flying a kite [P54], moving to a new city [P20], etc). Nevertheless, it has good internal consistency and item-total correlation in non-PD patients.[25] Reliability in PD patients has not been assessed. The scale was used in one study with PD patients, but in that study, the researchers highlighted the shortcomings and impracticability of the scale.[47]

STRENGTH AND WEAKNESSES

In the opinion of the authors, this scale cannot be recommended for use in PD. It is too long for the assessment of a single symptom and lacks face and content validity.

FINAL ASSESSMENT

The Chapman Scales are classified as "Listed." It has been used in only one study of PD patients and lacks content validity.

CONCLUSIONS

Apathy scales

A number of apathy and anhedonia scales are available for clinical use. Three of the scales

are classified as "Recommended"; for the other scales, limited clinimetric information is available. Of the "Recommended" scales, both the AS and the LARS were specifically developed for and validated in patients with PD. The LARS is the best-studied scale, and the only one that has been subjected to factor analysis and validated against the recently proposed diagnostic criteria. Although item 4 of the UPDRS also classifies as "Recommended," this single item should be considered for initial screening only.

For most scales, only some aspects of reliability have been assessed. In the absence of an external gold standard, it is difficult to establish sensitivity and specificity of scales. With the recent proposal of diagnostic criteria for apathy, further validation studies of these scales may be conducted. Minimally clinically important change and minimal clinically relevant incremental difference have not been assessed for any of the scales. The influence of the overlap of apathy with symptoms of Parkinson's disease, depression, and cognitive decline on the clinimetric performance of apathy rating scales has not yet been established.

Anhedonia scales

For the assessment of anhedonia, two scales are available, but because neither has been validated in PD, no scale can be designated as recommended. The Chapman Scales for Physical and Social Anhedonia cannot be recommended for use given its lack of content validity and its length. The SHAPS is the most frequently used scale to assess anhedonia in the PD population, but it has not been validated in PD patients.

Clinical perspectives

All apathy and anhedonia rating scales show overlap with symptoms of PD to some extent. The clinimetric properties of rating scales may depend on the extent of this overlap. Scales may be rated using the exclusive, inclusive, substitution, or attribution approach. In a recent critique of *depression* rating scales, the inclusive approach was recommended.[48] This approach requires all symptoms to be scored, irrespective of the fact that they may also be attributable to PD ("rate what you see"). This approach was thought to be more consistent with the definition of depression as a syndrome (i.e., a constellation of symptoms without reference to a specific etiology), and it may also be expected to result in a higher inter-rater agreement. For the same reasons, an inclusive approach is recommended when administering apathy or anhedonia rating scales. When using patient-rated scales, the patient should be explicitly instructed to score every symptom according to its severity or frequency, irrespective of its presumed etiology.

None of the available scales is specifically suited to assessing apathy or anhedonia in the different phases of motor fluctuations ("on" versus "off" states). Since the time frame specified in the scales exceeds the duration of "on" or "off" states, the timing of assessment should not be a relevant issue. Nevertheless, the state of mind of patients during the different phases may have an impact on the way they perceive their feelings and actions, and produce different results. Therefore, it is recommended that the assessment of apathy and anhedonia in PD be performed only during the "on" period, which is also in line with the advice of the task force on depression rating scales.[48] Given the recent formulation of diagnostic criteria for apathy, symptoms that are only reported during "off states" would not count for the diagnosis of apathy as a syndrome.

RECOMMENDED SCALES
Lille apathy rating scale (LARS)
Apathy Scale (AS)
UPDRS item 4

References

1. Drijgers RL, Dujardin K, Reijnders JSAM, Defebvre L, Leentjens AFG. Validation of diagnostic criteria for apathy in Parkinson's disease. *Parkinsonism Relat Disord.* 2010;16(10):656–660.
2. Robert P, Onyike CU, Leentjens AFG, et al. Proposed diagnostic criteria for apathy in Alzheimer's disease and other neuropsychiatric disorders. *Eur Psychiatry.* 2009;66:531–535.
3. Marin RS. Apathy, a neuropsychiatric syndrome. *J Neuropsychiatry Clin Neurosci.* 1991;3:243–254.
4. Starkstein SE. Apathy and withdrawal. *Int Psychogeriatr.* 2000;12(suppl 1):135–138.
5. Starkstein SE, Leentjens AFG. The nosological position of apathy. *J Neurol Neurosurg Psychiatry.* 2008;79:1088–1092.
6. Mulin E, Leone E, Dujardin K, et al. Diagnostic criteria for apathy in clinical practice. *Int J Geriatr Psychiatry* [accepted].
7. Berrios GE. *The History of Mental Symptoms.* Cambridge: Cambridge University Press; 1996.
8. Dujardin K, Sockeel P, Devos D, et al. Characteristics of apathy in Parkinson's disease. *Mov Disord.* 2007;22:778–784.
9. Pluck GC, Brown RG. Apathy in Parkinson's disease. *J Neurol Neurosurg Psychiatry.* 2002;73:636–642.
10. Starkstein SE, Merello M, Jorge R, Brockman S, Bruce D, Power B. The syndromal validity and nosological position of apathy in Parkinson's disease. *Mov Disord.* 2009;24:1211–1216.
11. Oguru M, Tachibana H, Toda K, Okuda B, Oka N. Apathy and depression in Parkinson disease. *J Geriatr Psychiatry Neurol.* 2010;23(1):35–41.
12. Pedersen KF, Larsen JP, Alves G, Aarsland D. Prevalence and clinical correlates of apathy in Parkinson's disease: a community-based study. *Parkinsonism Relat Disord.* 2009;15(4):295–299.
13. Pedersen KF, Alves G, Aarsland D, Larsen JP. Occurrence and risk factors for apathy in Parkinson disease: a 4-year prospective longitudinal study. *J Neurol Neurosurg Psychiatry.* 2009;80(11):1279–1282.
14. Drijgers RL, Aalten P, Winogrodzka A, Verhey FR, Leentjens AFG. Pharmacological treatment of apathy in neurodegenerative diseases: a systematic review. *Dement Geriatr Cogn Disord.* 2009;28(1):13–22.
15. Leentjens AFG, Dujardin K, Marsh L, et al. Apathy and anhedonia rating scales in Parkinson's disease: critique and recommendations. *Mov Disord.* 2008;23(14):2004–2014.
16. Overall J, Gorham D. Brief psychiatric rating scale. *Psychol Rep.* 1962;10:799–812.
17. Grace J, Stout JC, Malloy PF. Assessing frontal lobe behavioral syndromes with the frontal lobe personality scale. *Assessment.* 1999;6:269–284.
18. McNair DM, Lorr M, Droppleman LF. *Manual for the Profile of Mood States.* San Diego: Educational and Industrial Testing Service; 1971.

19. Fahn S, Elton RL; and members of the UPDRS committee. Unified Parkinson's Disease Rating Scale. In: Fahn S, Marsden CD, Goldstein M, Calne DB, eds. *Recent Developments in Parkinson's Disease.* New Jersey: MacMillan Health Care; 1987:153–163.

20. Cummings JL, Mega M, Gray K, Rosenburg-Thompson S, Carusi DA, Gornbein J. The Neuropsychiatric Inventory: comprehensive assessment of psychopathology in dementia. *Neurology.* 1994;44:2308–2314.

21. Starkstein SE, Mayberg HS, Preziosi TJ, Andrezejewski P, Leiguarda R, Robinson RG. Reliability, validity, and clinical correlates of apathy in Parkinson's disease. *J Neuropsychiatry Clin Neurosci.* 1992;4(2):134–139.

22. Robert PH, Clairet S, Benoit M, et al. The Apathy Inventory: assessing apathy and awareness in Alzheimer's disease, Parkinson's disease and mild cognitive impairment. *Int J Geriatr Psychiatry.* 2002;17:1099–1105.

23. Sockeel P, Dujardin K, Devos D, Deneve C, Destee A, Defebvre L. The Lille apathy rating scale (LARS), a new instrument for detecting and quantifying apathy: validation in Parkinson's disease. *J Neurol Neurosurg Psychiatry.* 2006;77:579–584.

24. Snaith RP, Hamilton M, Morley S, Humayan A, Hargreaves D, Trigwell P. A scale for the assessment of hedonic tone: the Snaith-Hamilton Pleasure Scale. *Br J Psychiatry.* 1995;167:99–103.

25. Chapman LJ, Chapman JP, Raulin ML. Scales for physical and social anhedonia. *J Abnorm Psychol.* 1976;85(4):374–382.

26. Marin RS, Biedrycki RC, Firiciogullari S. Reliability and validity of the Apathy Evaluation Scale. *Psychol Res.* 1991;38(2): 143–162.

27. Clarke DE, Van Reekum R, Simard M, Streiner DL, Freedman M, Conn D. Apathy in dementia: an examination of the psychometric properties of the Apathy Evaluation Scale. *J Neuropsychiatry Clin Neurosci.* 2007;19:57–64.

28. Drapier D, Drapier S, Sauleau P, et al. Does subthalamic nucleus stimulation induce apathy in Parkinson's disease. *J Neurol.* 2006;253:1083–1091.

29. Padala PR, Burke WJ, Bhatia SC, Petty F. Treatment of apathy with methylphenidate. *J Neuropsychiatry Clin Neurosci.* 2007;19:81–83.

30. Starkstein SE, Ingram L, Garau ML, Mizrahi R. On the overlap between apathy and depression in dementia. *J Neurol Neurosurg Psychiatry.* 2005;76:1070–1074.

31. Czernicki V, Pillon B, Houeto JL, Pochon JB, Levy R, Dubois B. Motivation, reward, and Parkinson's disease: influence of dopatherapy. *Neuropsychologia.* 2002;40:2257–2267.

32. Czernecki V, Pillon B, Houeto JL, et al. Does bilateral stimulation of the subthalamic nucleus aggravate apathy in Parkinson's disease? *J Neurol Neurosurg Psychiatry.* 2005;76(6):775–779.

33. Funkiewiez A, Ardouin C, Cools R, et al. Effects of levodopa and subthalamic nucleus stimulation on cognitive and affective functioning in Parkinson's disease. *Mov Disord.* 2006;21(10):1656–1662.

34. Reijnders JSAM, Scholtissen B, Weber WEJ, Aalten P, Verhey FRJ, Leentjens AFG. Neuroanatomical correlates of apathy in Parkinson's disease: a magnetic resonance imaging study using voxel-based morphometry. *Mov Disord.* 2010;25(14):2318–2325.

35. Martínez-Martín P, Gil-Nagel A, Morlán Gracia J, et al. Unified Parkinson's Disease Rating Scale characteristics and structure. *Mov Disord.* 1994;9:76–83.

36. Louis ED, Lynch T, Marder K, Fahn S. Reliability of patient completion of the historical section of the Unified Parkinson's Disease Rating Scale. *Mov Disord.* 1996;11:185–192.

37. Siderowf A, McDermott M, Kieburtz K, et al. Test-retest reliability of the UPDRS in patients with early Parkinson's disease: results of a multicenter clinical trial. *Mov Disord.* 2002;17:758–763.

38. Starkstein SE, Merello M. The Unified Parkinson's Disease Rating Scale: validation study of the mentation, behavior, and mood section. *Mov Disord.* 2007;22(15):2156–2161.

39. Goldberg D. *The Detection of Psychiatric Illness by Questionnaire.* London: Oxford University Press; 1972.

40. Franken IHA, Rassin E, Muris P. The assessment of anhedonia in clinical and non-clinical populations: further validation of the Snaith-Hamilton Pleasure Scale (SHAPS). *J Affect Disord.* 2007;99:83–89.

41. Lemke MR, Brecht HM, Koester J, Kraus PH, Reichmann H. Anhedonia, depression, and motor functioning in Parkinson's disease during treatment with pramipexole. *J Neuropsychiatry Clin Neurosci.* 2005;17(2):214–220.

42. Reichmann H, Brecht HM, Kraus PH, Lemke MR. Pramipexol bei der Parkinson-Krankheit. Ergebnisse einer Anwendungsbeobachtung. *Nervenarzt.* 2002;73:745–750.

43. Reichmann H, Brecht MH, Köster J, Kraus PH, Lemke MR. Pramipexole in routine

clinical practice: a prospective observational trial in Parkinson's disease. *CNS Drugs.* 2003;17(13):965–973.

44. Lemke MR, Brecht HM, Koester J, Reichmann H. Effects of the dopamine agonist pramipexole on depression, anhedonia and motor functioning in Parkinson's disease. *J Neurol Sci.* 2006;248:266–270.

45. Witt K, Daniels C, Herzog J, et al. Differential effects of L-dopa and subthalamic stimulation on depressive symptoms and hedonic tone in Parkinson's disease. *J Neuropsychiatry Clin Neurosci.* 2006;18(3):397–401.

46. Isella V, Appolonio I, Meregalli L, et al. [Normative data for the Italian version of the apathy and anhedonia scale]. *Archivio di Psicologia, Neurologia e Psichiatria.* 1998;59:356–375.

47. Isella V, Iurlaro S, Piolti R, Ferrarese C, Frattola L, Appolonio I. Physical anhedonia in Parkinson's disease. *J Neurol Neurosurg Psychiatry.* 2003;74:1308–1311.

48. Schrag A, Barone P, Brown RG, et al. Depression rating scales in Parkinson's disease: critique and recommendations. *Mov Disord.* 2007;22(8):1077–1092.

14

ANXIETY

Laura Marsh and Amber L. Bush

Summary

Prevalence of anxiety disorders in patients with Parkinson's Disease (PD) ranges between 30% and 40%. Valid and reliable measurement tools for PD patients with anxiety are needed to improve its recognition and guide treatment through screening and symptom monitoring. This chapter reviews and evaluates 7 anxiety measures that have been used and investigated psychometrically in PD: the Beck Anxiety Inventory, the Hospital and Depression Scale—Anxiety subscale (HADS-A) , the Self-Rating Anxiety Scale, the Anxiety Status Inventory, the State Trait Anxiety Inventory, the Hamilton Anxiety Rating Scale (HARS), and the Neuropsychiatric Inventory—Anxiety subscale. The clinimetric properties of each measure both outside of and within PD populations were varied and did not receive unanimous support. Therefore, each of the reviewed scales has shortcomings and cannot be unequivocally recommended for use in PD populations. However, of the measures evaluated, the HADS-A appears to be the most suitable as a screening tool and the HARS most suitable as a symptom rating tool in those with PD who have known anxiety disturbances. A better characterization of anxiety disturbances in PD, including PD-specific presentations, will allow for optimal evaluation of existing anxiety rating scales or the development of a PD-specific anxiety rating scale.

INTRODUCTION

Several recent studies have addressed assessment and measurement of anxiety symptoms or disorders in patients with Parkinson's Disease (PD). This is a significant advance, given the high prevalence of anxiety disturbances in PD, including before formal diagnosis of the movement disorder.[1] Cross-sectional studies using the *Diagnostic and Statistical Manual, 4th edition, Text Revision* (DSM-IV-TR) diagnostic criteria[2] estimate the prevalence of anxiety disorders in PD populations ranges between 30% and 40%; lifetime prevalence approaches 50%.[3,4] Rates of clinically significant anxiety symptoms in the absence of formal diagnostic exams are comparable.[5] However, valid and reliable approaches to diagnosing and evaluating anxiety disorders in PD are lacking.

Several challenges affect assessment of anxiety disorders and anxiety phenomena in PD. First, many patients have clinically significant anxiety disturbances that are specific to PD. Others fail to experience all the symptoms needed to meet criteria for a typical DSM anxiety diagnosis. In the general population, as well as in PD, anxiety disorders comprise a heterogeneous group of disturbances that involve persistent anxiety in some cases and episodic phenomena in others. A mixture of emotional, cognitive, and somatic features further characterize the different anxiety disorder diagnoses based on DSM-IV-TR criteria; i.e., generalized anxiety disorder (GAD), panic disorder, agoraphobia, specific phobias, social phobia, post-traumatic stress disorder, and obsessive-compulsive disorder.[2] Whereas anxiety disturbances in PD frequently meet criteria for one of the typical anxiety disorders, current diagnostic approaches do not account for "atypical" or PD-specific anxiety disturbances. Examples of such "atypical" anxiety disorders include recurrent panic attack–like episodes, often associated with fluctuating motor effects related to anti-Parkinsonian therapy, or extreme situational anxiety associated with akinesia or freezing of gait.[3] Specific diagnostic criteria and methods to assess PD-specific anxiety disturbances would facilitate their recognition and investigations of treatments.[4]

The coexistence of depressive and anxiety symptoms in PD poses another challenge for symptom assessment.[6,7] In the general population as well as in PD, individuals with anxiety disorders commonly experience comorbid depressive disorders, though depressive disorders can also be accompanied by a high level of anxiety symptoms.[5] Overlap in the symptoms of depressive and anxiety disturbances; e.g., insomnia, muscle tension, or agitation, impacts diagnostic accuracy, particularly when patients have dementia and may be less able to communicate their affective state. Rating scales for anxiety will include items that overlap with depressive disorder phenomena, but may not distinguish anxiety from depression. However, since depression rating scales are inadequate for identifying anxiety diagnoses in patients with PD, valid and reliable measurement tools for PD-anxiety are needed to improve its recognition and guide treatment through screening and symptom monitoring.[8]

Even when features of a typical anxiety disorder are evident in a patient with PD, the DSM diagnostic criteria pose a quandary with respect to symptom attribution. At issue is whether features of a typical anxiety disorder might be regarded as "secondary to a general medical condition" in a patient with PD, or as non-pathological. Inclusive diagnostic approaches have been recommended for depressive disorders in PD,[9] such that all symptoms, regardless of possible etiology, are considered to be related to the psychiatric diagnosis; it is assumed that the same recommendations should pertain to anxiety disorders in PD. However, current DSM criteria permit certain symptoms to be regarded as non-pathological when a comorbid medical condition or medication side-effect might provide a meaningful explanation for the symptoms. A specific example is provided in the DSM for social phobia; i.e., that the fear of being observed does not meet criteria as a symptom if it is "solely" accounted for by tremor in patients with PD. However, it cannot be resolved as to whether such a fear is psychopathological versus an appropriate reaction. Accordingly, an inclusive approach to symptom attribution provides a more reliable route to a diagnosis that has greater sensitivity without sacrificing specificity.[10] A similar approach is recommended for symptom rating scales to achieve greater reliability.

Altogether, a limited number of studies have used anxiety rating scales in studies of PD populations, but the essential clinimetric properties of most measures were not thoroughly evaluated until recently.[11–13] In February of 2007, the Movement Disorder Society formed a task force to critique existing anxiety rating scales for their use in PD.[14] Since then, rigorous clinimetric testing has been conducted in PD populations for some of the identified anxiety tools (see, e.g., Ref. 13). The seven anxiety rating measures the Task Force identified in 2007 as having been used, if not additionally validated, in PD are discussed in this chapter: the Beck Anxiety Inventory (BAI),[15] the Hospital Anxiety and Depression Scale–anxiety subscale (HADS-A),[16] the Self-Rating Anxiety Scale (SAS),[17] the Anxiety Status Inventory (ASI),[17] the State Trait Anxiety Inventory (STAI),[18] the Hamilton Anxiety Rating Scale (HARS),[19] and the Neuropsychiatric Inventory–anxiety subscale (NPI-A).[20] This chapter also includes more recent findings from clinimetric evaluations of these anxiety measures conducted in PD samples since 2007. Table 14-1 lists descriptive characteristics of each measure.

BECK ANXIETY INVENTORY (BAI)

The BAI[15] was developed to assess the severity of somatic, affective, and cognitive symptoms associated with GAD and panic attacks in psychiatric populations. It is a self-report measure that consists of 21 items (each representing a symptom), each rated on a four-point Likert scale from 0 to 3. Scores to individual items are summed such that total scores range from 0 to 63, with higher scores indicating more severe anxiety symptoms. Scores between 0 and 9 indicate normal or no anxiety, 10 to 18 mild to moderate anxiety, 19 to 29 moderate to severe anxiety, and 30 to 63 severe anxiety. The measure is brief and takes approximately five minutes

to complete. However, the measure is not in the public domain and is copyrighted.

Outside of PD populations, the BAI demonstrates high internal consistency, good test-retest reliability[15] and is sensitive to change following pharmacological and psychotherapeutic treatment. It also has good face validity and construct validity, but only for panic disorder.[21]

In a multicenter study of 342 patients with idiopathic PD, the BAI demonstrated good acceptability (i.e., very little missing data), test-retest reliability, and known-groups validity.[13] Specifically, PD patients with anxiety disorders or those suffering from more severe anxiety scored higher on the BAI relative to those without anxiety disorders or those suffering from less severe anxiety. However, the BAI had low inter-item correlations, unsatisfactory convergent validity with other anxiety scales, and extremely skewed item distributions that precluded evaluation of its factor structure.[13] Examination of the discriminatory power of the BAI revealed

Table 14-1. Descriptive Characteristics of Each of the Scales Assessed.

SCALE	RATER	NUMBER OF ITEMS	TIME TO ADMINISTER	DISCRIMINATES BETWEEN ANXIETY AND DEPRESSION	TYPES OF ANXIETY
BAI	self-report	21	5 minutes	Yes	Panic and GAD
HADS-Anxiety	self-report	7	1–2 minutes	Overall scale: Yes Anxiety subscale: No	Panic and GAD
Zung SAS	self-report	20	5 minutes	Not known	Mostly panic and GAD
Zung ASI	observer-rated	20	5 minutes	Not known	Mostly panic and GAD
STAI	self-report	40 (20 state and 20 trait)	10 minutes	Not known	Panic and GAD (but not all symptoms)
HARS	clinician-rated	14	15–20 minutes	No	GAD
NPI Anxiety*	clinician-rated	1 (based on frequency x severity from 3 screeners and 7 items)	5 minutes	No	Less likely to detect episodic anxiety disturbances

*Note the NPI Anxiety Item is not a formal scale, but a single item from the Neuropsychiatric Inventory.

moderate overall diagnostic accuracy. The ideal cutoff of 12/13 had moderate ability to correctly identify those without anxiety (specificity), but poor ability to correctly identify those with anxiety (sensitivity), potentially leading to under-recognition of anxiety. Largely because of good face and construct validity, the BAI may be a preliminary means of screening for panic attacks in PD. However, its low sensitivity suggests a high likelihood of misclassification, such that individuals with anxiety may not be detected and subsequently not followed up or referred to treatment.

THE HOSPITAL ANXIETY AND DEPRESSION SCALE—ANXIETY SUBSCALE (HADS-A)

The HADS[16] is a self-report measure designed to screen for mood disorders in general (non-psychiatric) medical outpatients. The HADS consists of 14 items that can be broken down into an anxiety subscale (HADS-A) and a depression subscale (HADS-D), which each consist of seven items. The anxiety subscale has three items that refer to panic symptoms and four that refer to GAD symptoms, each rated on a four-point Likert scale from 0 to 3. Responses to items are summed (after reversal where appropriate) such that scores range from 0 to 21, with higher scores reflecting greater anxiety. The HADS is copyrighted. It takes only a few minutes to complete.

In non-PD samples, the HADS-A demonstrates satisfactory internal consistency reliability and test-retest reliability, good sensitivity and specificity for detecting any anxiety disorder, GAD, panic disorder, and social phobia.[22,23] It also has some evidence of construct validity, given its fair correlations with other anxiety measures.[22] However, the item content of the HADS-A does not clearly reflect defined anxiety symptoms or diagnostic criteria, leading to questionable face validity.

The clinimetric properties of the HADS-A have recently been studied somewhat extensively within PD populations. It has good acceptability and known-groups validity,[13] demonstrates satisfactory internal consistency and test-retest reliability,[24] and is inversely associated with quality of life.[25,26] Furthermore, it has decent construct validity and is not related to demographic characteristics or clinical features of PD.[11] Rasch models within item response theory revealed that the HADS-A is a unidimensional construct with no differential item functioning and good reliability.[12] These strengths have led some to conclude that the HADS-A is an acceptable patient-reported anxiety measure (see, e.g., endnotes 11, 12). Despite these strengths, the HADS-A has not been used as an outcome measure in treatment studies in PD. Furthermore, it has unsatisfactory inter-item correlations, unsatisfactory construct validity with some anxiety measures,[13] and cannot discriminate between anxiety and depression in PD patients.[27] Although the HADS-A has low overall diagnostic accuracy within PD patients, the ideal cutoff of 6/7 has a moderate ability to correctly identify those without anxiety (specificity), and good ability to correctly identify those with anxiety (sensitivity). Therefore, the HADS-A is suggested primarily as a screening tool for anxiety in PD.

SELF-RATING ANXIETY SCALE (SAS)

The Zung SAS[17] is a self-rated measure of the severity of anxiety, based on intensity, frequency, and duration of symptoms. The measure was developed for use in rating anxiety severity in patients with known anxiety disorders. It consists of 20 items with symptoms mostly relating to GAD and panic disorder. Responses are made on a four-point Likert scale (1–4) and an index is derived by summing the raw scores (after reversal where appropriate) and dividing this sum by the maximum possible score of 80, converted to a decimal point and multiplied by 100. Higher scores reflect greater anxiety. Scores above 44 are considered to have clinical significance.

Outside of PD, the SAS has adequate internal consistency, good item-total correlations and test-retest reliability,[28,29] but little evidence of convergent validity.[17] The SAS has been used in descriptive studies on the epidemiology of anxiety in PD (see, e.g., references 5, 30). However, it has not been validated within PD samples or used in treatment studies involving PD. Therefore, it is only "Listed" for measuring anxiety in PD populations.

ANXIETY STATUS INVENTORY (ASI)

The ASI[17] is the observer-rated equivalent to the SAS. It consists of the same 20 items, with responses made on a four-point Likert scale (1–4). The same index as with the SAS is derived for the ASI by summing the raw scores (after reversal where appropriate) and dividing this sum by the maximum possible score of 80, converted to a decimal point and multiplied by 100. Higher scores reflect greater anxiety.

Outside of PD, the ASI has good internal consistency in older adults but has unsatisfactory convergent validity.[17] As with the SAS, the ASI has been used in epidemiological studies of anxiety in PD,[31] but it has not been validated within PD patients or used in treatment studies involving PD. Therefore, the ASI can only be "Listed" for measuring anxiety in PD populations.

STATE TRAIT ANXIETY INVENTORY (STAI)

The STAI[18] is a self-report measure of anxiety severity and frequency that exists in two versions: one developed in the 1960s (STAI-X)[32] and a revised version developed in 1983 (STAI-Y).[18] Although the revised version has improved psychometric properties,[33] both are commonly used. The STAI has 40 items: 20 that assess state anxiety and 20 that assess trait anxiety. The state subscale assesses anxiety "right now" and reflects intensity of anxiety, whereas the trait subscale assesses anxiety during an undefined time frame and reflects frequency of anxiety. Respondents rate items on four-point Likert scales where 1 = *not at all* and 4 = *very much so* for the state scale and 1 = *almost never* and 4 = *almost always* for the trait scale. Some symptoms of GAD and panic disorder are not included in the state scale.

The trait anxiety subscale of the STAI has good construct validity, internal consistency, reliability, and test-retest reliability outside of PD.[18] In addition, the STAI appears to be sensitive to change. However, the trait scale has poor diagnostic accuracy, with low sensitivity and specificity at all cut-points.[34]

Within PD, some evidence for construct validity exists, given high correlations with the HADS-A and HARS.[11] Furthermore, there is known-groups validity for the STAI in that PD patients diagnosed with a current anxiety disorder had higher STAI state scores than those who did not have an anxiety disorder.[35] Similarly, although PD patients and healthy spouse controls had similar mean scores on the trait subscale, PD patients had higher state anxiety scores.[30] The STAI trait and state scales were not sensitive to change following deep brain stimulation of the subthalamic nucleus in 72 PD patients.[36] Therefore, the STAI is "Suggested" for measuring anxiety in PD populations.

HAMILTON ANXIETY RATING SCALE (HARS)

The HARS[19] is a clinician-rated instrument designed to quantify the severity of anxiety symptoms. Although several versions exist, the most frequently used is the 14-item measure, which consists of 13 questions and one observational rating of the patient's behavior during the interview. Each item is rated on a five-point Likert scale (from 0 to 4), where higher scores reflect more severe anxiety. The scale was developed to determine the severity of anxiety in individuals with known anxiety. Thus, a score less than 17 is generally thought to represent milder anxiety, and scores over 25 indicate severe anxiety. The questions are not structured, and patients may need additional inquiry to rate a given item. The measure takes approximately 15 to 30 minutes to administer and is not copyrighted, making it accessible, free, and within the public domain.

The HARS has received much clinimetric support outside of PD, allowing newer work to be anchored by published results. It has good internal consistency, test-retest reliability, and construct validity.[37,38] It also has good diagnostic utility, as it can distinguish between those with and without an anxiety disorder. Furthermore, the HARS is the most widely used anxiety measure in pharmacotherapy studies of anxiety, has been used to monitor treatment outcomes, and is sensitive to change with treatment. However, it does not clearly distinguish anxiety from depression.

The clinimetric properties of the HARS within PD have recently been tested in abundance. The HARS has good acceptability, known-groups validity, inter-rater reliability, and inter-item correlations,[13] as well as good internal consistency.[39] However, it has mixed evidence of construct validity in PD.[11,13] Although the HARS has good diagnostic utility in predicting GAD,[39] it has low diagnostic utility in predicting any anxiety disorder.[13] Specifically, at the optimal cutoff of 12/13, the HARS does a moderate to good job accurately identifying those without an anxiety disorder (specificity) and a fair job identifying those with an anxiety disorder. The HARS is "Suggested" for use in PD populations, especially as a rating tool.

THE NEUROPSYCHIATRIC INVENTORY—ANXIETY SUBSCALE (NPI-A)

The NPI-A[20] is a clinician-rated instrument designed to assess behavioral manifestations of the emotional and somatic symptoms of anxiety in patients diagnosed with dementia. The NPI is based on a structured interview with an informant familiar with the patient and assesses 12 psychiatric disturbances that occur in dementia, including anxiety. Administration of the NPI-A involves three questions that serve as screening probes to assess the presence of anxiety symptoms. If one question screens positive, seven additional questions are asked that address more specific features about behaviors associated with worry. Based on responses to these seven questions, overall frequency (rated on a 1–4 scale) and severity (rated on a 1–3 scale) of the symptoms are rated. Frequency and severity are then multiplied to create the total NPI-A score, with higher scores reflecting greater anxiety.

In non-PD samples, the NPI-A demonstrates good internal consistency and inter-rater

agreement, fair construct validity, and fair to moderate test-retest reliability.[20] In studies with Alzheimer's patients, the NPI-A has demonstrated sensitivity to change following treatment with cognition-enhancing drugs.[40]

Although evaluation of the NPI-A within PD is limited, a study of 12 PD patients revealed good inter-rater reliability.[41] Although the NPI-A has been used as an outcome measure in treatment studies of dementia in PD patients, there is no evidence that the NPI-A is sensitive to change.[42] Furthermore, in a multicenter study of 342 patients with idiopathic PD, the NPI-A demonstrated low to moderate convergent validity, based on its associations with other anxiety measures.[13] Although only consisting of one item, the NPI-A can be "Suggested" for use in PD.

FINAL ASSESSMENT

The study of anxiety disturbances in PD and their treatment is an evolving area of research. There remains a need for better characterization of anxiety disturbances in PD, including the PD-specific presentations. That accomplishment will set the stage for optimal assessment of existing anxiety rating scales or the development of a PD-specific anxiety rating scale. Table 14-2 provides conclusions regarding scale status for measuring anxiety in PD. Each of the seven measures reviewed in this chapter has been employed or evaluated in PD populations, but none has achieved unanimous clinimetric support within this group. Noting their respective limitations, the HADS-A appears to be most suitable as a screening tool for an anxiety diagnosis in PD. It is a commonly used self-report anxiety scale that is quick to administer, mostly validated in PD samples, and also useful in detecting persistent anxiety symptoms (i.e., it has good test-retest reliability). Furthermore, it has good sensitivity and a cut-point of 6/7 accurately identified those with an anxiety diagnosis. The HARS has received much attention in PD, but it is not especially viable as a screening or diagnostic tool in PD patients, as it does only a fair job identifying those with any anxiety disorder and requires valuable clinician time. Given

Table 14-2. Overview of the Scales Assessed and their Key Evaluation Points and Final Designation.

SCALE	APPLIED IN PD	APPLIED BEYOND ORIGINAL AUTHORS	CLINIMETRIC TESTING IN PD	ADEQUATE CLINIMETRIC PERFORMANCE IN PD	FINAL MEASURE DESIGNATION
BAI	X	X	X	0	Suggested
HADS-Anxiety	X	X	X	0	Suggested, as screening tool
Zung SAS	X	X	0	0	Listed
Zung ASI	X	X	0	0	Listed
STAI	X	X	X	0	Suggested
HARS	X	X	X	0	Suggested, as rating tool
NPI Anxiety	X	X	X	0	Suggested

Measures are considered **Listed** if they have been applied to but not tested in PD populations. Measures are considered **Suggested** if they have been both applied to and tested in PD populations. Note that none of the scales is fully **Recommended** as none has demonstrated a uniformly successful clinimetric performance, and limitations of each must be considered.

its widespread use in pharmacotherapy trials for anxiety disorders, its sensitivity to change, and its accessibility, the HARS appears most suitable as a symptom rating tool in individuals with known anxiety disturbances.

In spite of the above suggestions, each of the reviewed scales has shortcomings and cannot be considered ideal for use in PD populations. The measures of construct validity may be influenced by the extent to which the different anxiety scales emphasize the somatic, cognitive, or emotional aspects of anxiety, as well as variations in the pattern of these symptoms across the different anxiety disorders. There is also a need to include the atypical PD-specific anxiety disturbances in analyses of scale performance or, at least, to capture the intensity or severity of that particular phenomenon. However, the absence of standardized diagnostic approaches for delineating cases with PD-specific disturbances hampers progress in that area. Additionally, the influence of cognitive status and comorbid anxiety or depressive disorders on scale performance has not been examined. Accordingly, until these considerations are addressed, it is premature to recommend development of a new anxiety scale.

Acknowledgments

Support provided by NIH RO1-MH069666 and the Department of Veterans Affairs.

RECOMMENDED SCALES
None

References

1. Shiba M, Bower JH, Maraganore DM, et al. Anxiety disorders and depressive disorders preceding Parkinson's disease: a case-control study. *Mov Disord.* 2000;15:669–677.
2. American Psychiatric Association. *Diagnostic and Statistical Manual of Mental Disorders. 4th edition, text revision (DSM-IV-TR).* Washington, DC: American Psychiatric Association; 2000.
3. Pontone GM, Williams JR, Anderson KE, et al. Prevalence of anxiety disorders and anxiety subtypes in patients with Parkinson's disease. *Mov Disord.* 2009;24:1333–1338.
4. Leentjens AF, Dujardin K, Marsh L, Martinez-Martin P, Richard IH, Starkstein SE. Symptomatology and markers of anxiety disorders in Parkinson's disease: a cross-sectional study. *Mov Disord.* 2011;26:484–492.
5. Menza MA, Robertson-Hoffman DE, Bonapace AS. Parkinson's disease and anxiety:

comorbidity with depression. *Biol Psychiatry.* 1993;34:465–470.

6. Brown RG, Landau S, Hindle JV, et al. Depression and anxiety related subtypes in Parkinson's disease. *J Neurol Neurosurg Psychiatry.* 2011;82:803–809.

7. Negre-Pages L, Grandjean H, Lapeyre-Mestre M, et al. Anxious and depressive symptoms in Parkinson's disease: the French cross-sectional DoPaMiP study. *Mov Disord.* 2010;25:157–166.

8. Calleo J, Bush AL, Williams JR, et al. Screening accuracy of comorbid anxiety and depression in Parkinson's disease. *Mov Disord.* 2011;26:I–IX [twenty-fifth annual symposium on etiology, pathogenesis, and treatment of Parkinson's disease and other movement disorders].

9. Marsh L, McDonald WM, Cummings J, Ravina B. Provisional diagnostic criteria for depression in Parkinson's disease: report of an NINDS/NIMH Work Group. *Mov Disord.* 2005;21:148–158.

10. Koenig HG, George LG, Peterson BL, Pieper CF. Depression in medically ill hospitalized older adults: prevalence, characteristics, and course of symptoms according to six diagnostic schemes. *Am J Psychiatry.* 1997;154:1376–1383.

11. Mondolo F, Jahanshahi M, Grana A, Biasutti E, Cacciatori E, Di Benedetto, P. Evaluation of anxiety in Parkinson's disease with some commonly used rating scales. *Neurol Sci.* 2007;28:270–275.

12. Rodriguez-Blazquez C, Frades-Payo B, Forjaz MJ, de Pedro-Cuesta J, Martinez-Martin P. Psychometric attributes of the Hospital Anxiety and Depression Scale in Parkinson's disease. *Mov Disord.* 2009;24:519–525.

13. Leentjens AF, Dujardin K, Marsh L, Richard IH, Starkstein SE, Martinez-Martin P. Anxiety rating scales in Parkinson's disease: a validation study of the Hamilton anxiety rating scale, the Beck anxiety inventory, and the hospital anxiety and depression scale. *Mov Disord.* 2011;26:407–415.

14. Leentjens AF, Dujardin K, Marsh L, et al. Anxiety rating scales in Parkinson's disease: critique and recommendations. *Mov Disord.* 2008;23:2015–2025.

15. Beck AT, Epstein N, Brown G, Steer RA. An inventory for measuring clinical anxiety: psychometric properties. *J Consult Clin Psychol.* 1988;56:893–897.

16. Zigmond AS, Snaith RP. The hospital anxiety and depression scale. *Acta Psychiatr Scand.* 1983;67:361–370.

17. Zung WWK. A rating instrument for anxiety disorders. *Psychosomatics.* 1971;122:371–379.

18. Spielberger CD, Gorsuch RL, Lushene R, Vagg PR. *A Manual for the State-Trait Anxiety Inventory (Form Y).* Palo Alto, CA: Consultant Psychologist Press; 1983.

19. Hamilton M. The assessment of anxiety states by rating. *Br J Med Psychol.* 1959;32:50–55.

20. Cummings JL, Mega M, Gray K, Rosenberg-Thompson S, Carusi DA, Gornbein J. The Neuropsychiatric Inventory: comprehensive assessment of psychopathology in dementia. *Neurology.* 1994;44:2308–2314.

21. Leyfer OT, Ruberg JL, Woodruff-Borden J. Examination of the utility of the Beck Anxiety Inventory and its factors as a screener for anxiety disorders. *J Anxiety Disord.* 2006;20:444–458.

22. Bjelland I, Dahl AA, Haug TT, Neckelmann D. The validity of the Hospital Anxiety and Depression Scale. An updated literature review. *J Psychosom Res.* 2002;52:69–77.

23. Bunevicius A, Peceliuniene J, Mickuviene N, Valius L, Bunevicius R. Screening for depression and anxiety disorders in primary care patients. *Depress Anxiety.* 2007;24:455–460.

24. Marinus J, Leentjens AF, Visser M, Stiggelbout AM, Van Hilten JJ. Evaluation of the hospital anxiety and depression scale in patients with Parkinson's disease. *Clin Neuropharmacol.* 2002;25:318–324.

25. Havlikova E, van Dijk JP, Nagyova I, et al. The impact of sleep and mood disorders on quality of life in Parkinson's disease patients. *J Neurol.* 2011;258:2222–2229.

26. Quelhas R, Costa M. Anxiety, depression, and quality of life in Parkinson's disease. *J Neuropsychiatry Clin Neurosci.* 2009;21:413–419.

27. Leentjens AFG, Lousberg R, Verhey FRJ. Markers for depression in Parkinson's disease. *Acta Psychiatr Scand.* 2002;106:196–201.

28. Jegede RO. Psychometric attributes of the Self-Rating Anxiety Scale. *Psychol Rep.* 1977;40:303–306.

29. Olatunji B, Deacon B, Abramowitz J, Tolin D. Dimensionality of somatic complaints: factor structure and psychometric properties of the Self-rating Anxiety Scale. *J Anxiety Disord.* 2006;20:543–561.

30. Henderson R, Kurlan R, Kersun JM, Como P. Preliminary examination of the comorbidity of anxiety and depression in Parkinson's disease. *J Neuropsychiatry Clin Neurosci.* 1992;4:257–264.

31. Stein MB, Heuser IJ, Juncos JL, Uhde TW. Anxiety disorders in patients with Parkinson's disease. *Am J Psychiatry.* 1990;147:217–220.

32. Spielberger CD, Gorsuch RL, Lushene R, Vagg PR, Jacobs GA. *Manual for the State-Trait Anxiety Inventory (Self-examination Questionnaire, Form X).* Palo Alto, CA: Consulting Psychologists Press, Inc.; 1970.

33. Barnes LLB, Harp D, Jung WS. Reliability generalization of scores on the Spielberger State-Trait Anxiety Inventory. *Educ Psychol Meas.* 2002;62:603–618.

34. Kabacoff R, Segal D, Hersen M, Van Hasselt V. Psychometric properties and diagnostic utility of the Beck Anxiety Inventory and the State-Trait Anxiety Inventory with older psychiatric patients. *J Anxiety Disord.* 1997;11:33–47.

35. Dissanayaka NN, Sellbach A, Matheson S, et al. Anxiety disorders in Parkinson's disease: prevalence and risk factors. *Mov Disord.* 2010;25:838–845.

36. Castelli L, Perozzo P, Zibetti M, et al. Chronic deep brain stimulation of the subthalamic nucleus for Parkinson's disease: effects on cognition, mood, anxiety and personality traits. *Eur Neurol.* 2006;55:136–144.

37. Bruss GS, Gruenberg AM, Goldstein RD, Barber JP. Hamilton Anxiety Rating Scale interview guide: joint interview and test-retest methods for interrater reliability. *Psychiatry Res.* 1994;53:191–202.

38. Riskind JH, Beck AT, Brown G, Steer RA. Taking the measure of anxiety and depression. Validity of the reconstructed Hamilton scales. *J Nerv Ment Dis.* 1987;175:474–479.

39. Kummer A, Cardoso F, Teixeira AL. Generalized anxiety disorder and the Hamilton Anxiety Rating Scale in Parkinson's disease. *Arq Neuropsiquiatr.* 2010;68:495–501.

40. Wynn ZJ, Cummings JL. Cholinesterase inhibitor therapies and neuropsychiatric manifestations of Alzheimer's disease. *Dement Geriatr Cogn Disord.* 2004;17:100–108.

41. Aarsland D, Larsen JP, Cummings JL, Laake K. Prevalence and clinical correlates of psychotic symptoms in Parkinson disease. A community-based study. *Arch Neurol.* 1999;56:595–601.

42. Aarsland D, Hutchinson M, Larsen JP. Cognitive, psychiatric and motor response to galantamine in Parkinson's disease with dementia. *Int J Geriatr Psychiatry.* 2003;18: 937–941.

15

COGNITIVE IMPAIRMENT
SCREENING SCALES

Glenn T. Stebbins

Summary

There are multiple brief cognitive screening measures that can be used in studies of cognitive functioning in PD. These scales supply an adequate assessment of cognitive functioning that can be accomplished within a standard clinical or research visit. From a search of the existing literature, 12 cognitive screening measures were identified that assessed multiple cognitive domains and could be completed within a standard clinical visit (less than one hour). Recommendations for use of the 12 screening measures were based on three separate criteria: use in PD cohorts, wide application of the scale beyond the scale developers, and sufficient clinimetric strength to warrant its use, based on studies in cognitively impaired populations, preferably with PD.

Seven scales can be recommended for use in PD: Addenbrooke's Cognitive Examination; Alzheimer's Disease Assessment Scale–Cognition; Dementia Rating Scale; Montreal Cognitive Examination; Repeatable Battery for the Assessment of Neuropsychological Status; and Scales for Outcomes of Parkinson's Disease–Cognition. Three scales can be suggested for use in PD: Mini-Mental State Examination; Parkinson's Disease Cognitive Rating Scale; and Parkinson Neuropsychometric Dementia Assessment. A number of the other scales with limited information at this time may achieve these designations with future studies. These rankings are offered for individuals deciding on which cognitive screening scale to use in a given clinical or research situation.

INTRODUCTION

Cognitive impairment is a common non-motor feature in patients with Parkinson's disease. The deficits can range from mild difficulties with executive processing to severe dementia with impairments in all domains of cognitive functioning. The prevalence of Parkinson's disease dementia (PDD) in community- and clinic-based samples is common and ranges from 30% to 40%.[1-3] Annual incidence rates of PDD range between 10% and 30% in patients with PD[3,4] and 2% to 5% in the general population.[3,5] Development of dementia appears to be associated with disease duration,[6-8] with some cumulative prevalence rates reaching close to 80% in patients with PD.[8] Although all cognitive domains may be affected in PDD, there are subtle differences in presentation between PDD and the most common form of dementia found in patients with Alzheimer's disease,[9] with PDD demonstrating less impairment in memory and language functioning, but greater impairment in executive, attention, and visuospatial abilities. Because of these phenomenological differences in presentation, efforts have been undertaken by the Movement Disorder Society to establish specific diagnostic criteria for PDD.[10]

Cognitive impairment insufficient for a diagnosis of PDD is common in patients with Parkinson's disease. Mild cognitive impairment in PD (PD-MCI) is often found in the early stages of the disease,[11] and appears to be a risk factor for later development of dementia.[12,13] Although a consensus diagnosis for PD-MCI is not established, the Movement Disorder Society has formed a task force to critically review PD-MCI[14] and a separate task force to develop diagnostic criteria. In the absence of a consensus for diagnostic criteria, most studies define PD-MCI as impairment in one or more cognitive domains compared to normal performance, but not severe enough to warrant a diagnosis of dementia. "Impairment" is usually defined as performance levels 1 to 1 and one-half standard deviation below normative levels.[15,16] Prevalence estimates for PD-MCI suggest that between 20% and 30% of patients with PD manifest PD-MCI.[14] The range of prevalence rates was supported by the results of a large multicenter study ($n = 1346$) that reported a 25.8% prevalence rate.[16] Unlike MCI associated with Alzheimer's disease, where memory problems are most common, this study found that most patients (11.3%) were classified as non-amnestic single-domain MCI.

Various methods of assessing cognitive functioning are employed in studies of cognitive impairment in PD. The most common approach utilized is formal testing of various cognitive abilities. Neuropsychological assessment provides a gold standard for such assessments[17] and offers a quantification of cognitive functioning that can be evaluated in reference to normative performance.

Two important aspects define the utility of neuropsychological testing. The first is the clinimetric rigor employed during the development of the tests. As discussed in Chapter 2 *Statistics*

for the Scale Developer, the two most important clinimetric properties of any scale are reliability and validity. "Reliability" refers to the degree to which a given test score represents differences in the behavior of interest as opposed to error associated with the measurement tool. Reliability measures assess the degree to which a test is internally consistent (split-half reliability, Cronbach's alpha); the degree to which a test provides consistent information across alternate forms (alternate-form reliability); and the degree to which a test provides consistent scores across different time points (test-retest reliability; intra-rater reliability) or different examiners (inter-rater reliability). A "valid" test is one that measures what it is purported to measure. This clinimetric property is never fully established, but rather is examined in an ongoing manner. Validity measures include the degree to which the items of the test cover the relevant domain of interest but not other domains (content validity); the degree to which the test agrees with either a gold standard of the domain of interest or another test designed to measure the same domain (concurrent validity); the degree to which a test does not agree with another test designed to measure a different domain (discriminant validity); and the degree to which a test measures the theoretical construct under study (construct validity). The relationship between reliability and validity is statistically constrained,[18] such that validity scores cannot exceed the square of reliability scores. Thus, it is possible for a test to be highly reliable but invalid, but according to clinimetric theory, a test cannot be valid but unreliable.

Another important aspect to neuropsychological assessment is the adequacy with which the testing covers relevant cognitive abilities. The cognitive domains typically assessed in full neuropsychological testing include attention/orientation, executive/frontal lobe function, verbal and visual memory, language and visuospatial abilities, praxis and motor skills.[17] The standard practice is to use more than one test to measure each domain, so that issues of measurement error and subject fatigue can be mitigated. This redundancy increases the accuracy of the assessment, but can make the testing overly time-consuming and burdensome to patients and healthcare staff. The length of a full neuropsychological examination can require multiple testing sessions, often extending across several clinic visits. Because most clinic and research settings afford limited time for assessing cognitive functioning, the use of full neuropsychological testing is constrained. To meet the needs of cognitive assessment within a limited clinic visit, cognitive screening measures have been developed.

The intended use of cognitive screening measures is similar to that of full neuropsychological testing, but accomplished in a much shorter time frame. Typically, cognitive screening measures are brief enough to be used in typical clinic and research settings. Some measures are very brief, on the order of 10 to 15 minutes, while others require more extensive testing time. Regardless of the time requirements, the screening measures are designed to accomplish the same goal as full testing: to assess cognitive functioning in multiple domains and provide reliable and valid assessments. Therefore, a useful cognitive screening measure needs to assess multiple cognitive domains and have acceptable clinimetric properties.

The purpose of this chapter is to review the existing cognitive rating scales that have been used in the context of cognitive assessment in PD. Following the template established by the larger MDS effort to critique scales covering all clinically pertinent domains of PD involvement (see Chapter 2:6, scales for cognition are included only if they assess multiple domains of cognitive functioning to provide a robust measure of cognitive abilities and if they can be administered within the time limitations of clinical and research settings. Unlike other chapters in this volume, the information in this chapter has not yet been evaluated by the MDS Task Force on Cognitive Rating Scales in Parkinson's Disease. Therefore slight changes in the reviews presented below may occur. Each screening measure is reviewed for clinimetric strengths and weaknesses and its applicability to PD, and recommendations are provided as to the scale's utility. Recommendations are based on the following criteria: (1) A scale is considered "Recommended" if it has undergone clinimetric testing, has been used by groups other than the scale's developers, and has been applied to PD samples. Specific clinimetric testing in PD samples is noted when conducted. (2) A scale is considered "Suggested" if it has been applied to PD samples and one of the other criteria applies. (3) A scale is considered "Listed" if it has been used in PD, and none of the other criteria apply.

To accomplish this evaluation, the existing literature on cognitive assessment in patients with PD was reviewed. A literature search of PubMed was conducted using the following search terms for studies involving human subjects: *cognition* OR *cognitive assessment* OR *cognitive testing* OR *cognitive scales* OR *neuropsychological assessment* OR *neuropsychological testing* OR *neuropsychological scales*; *clinimetric* OR *psychometric* OR *validation* OR *reliability* OR *validity*; and *Parkinson's disease* OR *Parkinson disease* OR *Parkinson*. The results from search terms 1, 2, and 3 were combined. From this search 290 citations were identified. Each citation was reviewed for cognitive screening measures that met inclusion criteria (administration time within clinical and research limits, and assessment of multiple cognitive domains). Each scale was reviewed for the recommendation criteria. In total, 12 scales were identified that met the inclusion criteria (Table 15-1)—seven developed for generic use or use in other diseases: Addenbrooke's Cognitive Examination (ACE, ACE-R),[19,20] Alzheimer's Disease Assessment Scale–Cognition (ADAS-Cog),[21] Cambridge Cognitive Assessment (CAMCOG),[22] Dementia Rating Scale (DRS, DRS-2),[23] Mini-Mental State Examination (MMSE),[24] Montreal Cognitive Assessment (MoCA),[25] Repeatable Battery for the Assessment of Neuropsychological Status (RBANS)[26]; and five developed specifically for the assessment of cognition in PD: Mini-Mental Parkinson (MMP),[27] Parkinson's Disease Cognitive Rating Scale (PD-CRS),[28] Parkinson's Disease Dementia–Short Screen (PDD-SS),[29] Parkinson Neuropsychometric Dementia Assessment (PANDA),[30] Scales for Outcomes of Parkinson's Disease–Cognition (SCOPA-Cog[31]).

Table 15-1. Cognitive Screening Instruments Identified in the Literature Review

SCALE NAME	ADMINISTRATION TIME	ASSESSED COGNITIVE DOMAINS
Addenbrooke's Cognitive Examination (Revised)—ACE (R)	<20 min	Attention/orientation, memory, fluency, language, visuospatial
Alzheimer's Disease Assessment Scale–Cognition (ADAS-Cog)	~30 min	Memory, language, praxis
Cambridge Cognitive Assessment (Revised)—CAMCOG (R)	~25 min	Orientation, language, memory, attention, praxis, calculations, abstract reasoning, perception
Dementia Rating Scale (2nd edition)/Mattis Dementia Ratings Scale–DRS (2)	~30 min	Attention, initiation/perseveration, construction, conceptualization, memory
Mini-Mental Parkinson (MMP)	~15 min	Orientation, attention, fluency, visual registration, visual memory, set-shifting, conceptualization
Mini-Mental State Examination (MMSE)	~10 min	Orientation, verbal registration and recall, attention, naming and repetition, verbal comprehension, praxis, visuospatial
Montreal Cognitive Assessment (MoCA)	~10 min	Orientation, attention, memory, naming, fluency, verbal repetition, visuospatial/executive
Parkinson's Disease Cognitive Rating Scale (PD-CRS)	~15–30 min	Attention, working memory, fluency (alternating and action), naming, visuospatial, immediate and delayed memory
Parkinson's Disease Dementia–Short Screen (PDD-SS)	~7 min	Immediate and delayed verbal recall, alternating verbal fluency, visuospatial
Parkinson Neuropsychometric Dementia Assessment (PANDA)	~10 min	Attention/working memory, immediate and delayed recall, alternating verbal fluency, visuospatial
Repeatable Battery for the Assessment of Neuropsychological Status (RBANS)	~ 30 min	Attention, language, visuospatial/construction, immediate memory, delayed memory
Scales for Outcomes of Parkinson's Disease–Cognition (SCOPA - Cog)	~15 min	Attention, memory, executive function, delayed recall, visuospatial

ADDENBROOKE'S COGNITIVE EXAMINATION (ACE AND REVISED ACE-R)[19,20]

Scale description

The ACE and ACE-R were developed as an extended version of the Mini-Mental State Examination, expanding testing for memory, language, visuospatial ability, and adding a test of verbal fluency. The test assesses six cognitive domains including orientation, attention, memory, verbal fluency, language, and visuospatial abilities. The total maximum score is 100, and the test can be administered in approximately 20 minutes. The revised ACE (ACE-R)[20] modified the content of the scale, addressed some issues of ceiling and floor effects, developed two alternate forms, and created subscores for the cognitive domains of attention/orientation, memory, fluency, language, and visuospatial ability. Similar to the ACE, the ACE-R requires approximately 20 minutes for administration and has a total maximum score of 100. Because the scale is an expanded version of the MMSE, a MMSE score can be obtained from the ACE-R. The scale may be obtained from the corresponding author of the manuscript describing the development and initial clinimetric examination of the scale.[20]

Key evaluation issues

The clinimetric properties of the ACE-R[20] have not been firmly established in some key areas for cognitive assessment of both non-PD and PD populations. It appears adequate for internal consistency (Cronbach's alpha = 0.80), and the total score correlated significantly with the Clinical Dementia Rating,[32] suggesting concurrent validity. The ACE-R total score and domain scores provided differentiation between normal controls, patients with mild cognitive impairment, and patients with Alzheimer's disease. Diagnostic differentiation between normal cognition and dementia had 94% sensitivity and 89% specificity using a cut-off score of 88/89.

The Addenbrooke's scale has been used in multiple studies of patients with PD, and the clinimetric properties are similar to those noted in non-PD samples. Adequate concurrent validity is seen in the significant correlations between the ACE and ACE-R to MMSE, DRS, and SCOPA-Cog (all r's < 0.84).[33] The scale's diagnostic utility appears good for differentiating PD dementia from non-dementia with sensitivity (80%) and specificity (82%) using a total score cutoff of 83/84.[34] The diagnostic utility of the ACE-R for differentiating PD mild cognitive impairment from non-impaired patients, however, is poor with sensitivity at 61% and specificity at 64%, using a cutoff of 92/93 total scale points.[35]

Strengths and weaknesses

The ACE-R is easy to administer and is relatively short, requiring approximately 20 minutes for administration. The clinimetric profile appears adequate for reliability and some aspects of validity (e.g., concurrent validity). Additional clinimetric studies in PD samples are needed. The diagnostic utility for differentiating demented from non-demented PD patients is good, but differentiation of PD mild cognitive impairment from normal is poor. Although the scale appears to be sensitive to levels of cognitive impairment, there is no evidence on its sensitivity to changes in cognitive functioning.

Final assessment

Recommended—The ACE-R has established clinimetric properties for some aspects of reliability and reliability, and it has been used in studies of cognitive functioning in patients with PD. Information on its sensitivity to change in cognitive functioning in PD needs to be gathered. The diagnostic utility of the ACE-R for differentiation of normal cognition from dementia appears to be good in PD samples, but its ability to differentiate normal cognition from mild cognitive impairment in PD is poor.

ALZHEIMER'S DISEASE ASSESSMENT SCALE–COGNITION (ADAS-COG)[21]

Scale Description

The ADAS-Cog was developed specifically to assess selected aspects of cognitive functioning in patients with Alzheimer's disease. The scale is in widespread use for clinical studies in dementia treatment and consists of 11 items with a maximum score of 70. Three cognitive domains are assessed, including memory, language, and praxis. There are no alternate forms of the ADAS-Cog, but it has been translated and validated in various languages. The original scoring methods were not well defined, but a standard administration and scoring manual is available at

www.dementia-assessment.com.au/cognitive/
ADAS_Packet.pdf or from Prepress Type
(PrepressType@cox.net).[36] The average time
required for administration is 30 minutes, and
formal training is advised.

Key evaluation issues

Clinimetric examinations of the ADAS-Cog
indicate acceptable levels of internal consistency (Cronbach's alpha $\leq$ 0.80), test-retest reliability with correlations in the 0.90 to 0.93
range, inter-rater reliability ranging between
0.65 and 0.99, and concurrent validity (range
r = -0.63 to r = -0.82 with the Mini-Mental State
Examination).[21,37,38] However, ceiling effects, or
lack of sensitivity to higher levels of cognitive
functioning, were noted for seven of the 11 items
in one meta-analysis of three clinical trials.[37] The
scale has demonstrated sensitivity to change[39]
with a reliably detected individual change of
seven points.[36] Although the ADAS-Cog is considered the "gold standard" for assessment of
cognitive functioning in Alzheimer's disease,
the concurrent validity has been criticized for
a lack of attention- and information-processing
assessments.[40]

The ADAS-Cog has been used to assess cognitive functioning in PD. In one validation study,
the ADAS-Cog was found to have good test-
retest reliability (range r = 0.65–0.71, depending on dementia severity), acceptable sensitivity
to dementia (Cohen's effect size d = 0.80), and
concurrent validity to the MMSE (r = -0.60). It
has been used in multiple clinical trials for anti-
dementia medications in PD.[41-44]

Strengths and weaknesses

The strengths of the ADAS-Cog include its use
in many clinical trials for anti-dementia medications. It is the adopted cognitive screening
measure of the Alzheimer's Disease Cooperative
Study, and is considered a gold standard of cognitive assessment. There are specific administration instructions, and training in administration
is recommended. The clinimetric profile of the
scale is acceptable for reliability and some aspects

of validity. Additionally, it has been validated in
PD samples and applied in multiple clinical trials involving demented and cognitively impaired
PD patients. Its limitations include possible ceiling effects for some items and incomplete assessments of attention- and information-processing.
Specific to PD, the scale may put too much
emphasis on memory and language function
and too little emphasis on cognitive functions
affected by PD (e.g., executive function, working memory, visuospatial abilities).

Final assessment

Recommended—Because the ADAS-Cog has
acceptable clinimetric properties, has been used
by groups other than the original developers,
and has been used in PD samples for both clinimetric examinations as well as clinical trials,
this scale is "Recommended" for use. However,
the presence of possible ceiling effects and
weaknesses in assessing cognitive impairments
specific to PD are major limitations to use of the
ADAS-Cog in patients with PD.

CAMBRIDGE COGNITIVE ASSESSMENT (CAMCOG AND CAMCOG-R)[22]

Scale description

The Cambridge Cognitive Assessment scale is
a subsection of the Cambridge Examination
of Mental Disorders (CAMDEX).[22] It assesses
eight cognitive domains including orientation,
language, memory, attention, praxis, calculations, abstract reasoning, and perception. There
is a total of 65 items, with a maximum score of
105. Embedded within the CAMCOG are all the
items from the Mini-Mental State Examination,
so one can obtain an MMSE when administering the CAMCOG. The total administration
time is approximately 25 minutes. There are no
alternate forms available, but the scale has been
translated and validated in various languages.
The scale is not in the public domain, and
Cambridge University Press is the copyright
holder.

Key evaluation issues

The CAMCOG has demonstrated clinimetric properties with acceptable estimates of internal consistency (Cronbach's alpha ≥ 0.90).[45,46] The scale has shown good concurrent validity with other measures of cognitive functioning such as the Clinical Global Impression, MMSE, ADAS-Cog, and Raven's Progressive Matrices (all r's ≥ 0.70).[46,47] Sensitivity to change has been demonstrated,[48,49] and diagnostic cutoff scores of 79 to 80 show sensitivity and specificity greater than 85%.[45,50-53] Item response theory testing has shown a common dimensionality of the CAMCOG to assessing dementia.[54]

The CAMCOG has been studied in patients with PD by multiple authors. Hobson and Meara (1999)[55] reported excellent sensitivity and specificity for diagnosing dementia (both > 90%) using a cutoff of 80 points in a sample of 126 community-dwelling PD patients. This result was superior to that obtained using the MMSE. Sensitivity to change has also been demonstrated in PD[56] with an average decline of 16.5 points in demented PD patients compared to a 1.5 point decline in non-demented patients over a four-year period.[57] Performance on the CAMCOG appears to be related to age and gender[55] and may be a confounding factor for assessments.

Strengths and weaknesses

The major strengths of the CAMCOG are its breadth of coverage of cognitive functioning in different domains, its clinimetric properties for reliability and validity, as well as its diagnostic specificity and sensitivity. These strengths have been demonstrated in both PD and non-PD samples. The major weakness of the scale is possible confounding of performance on the assessment with age and gender. No adjustments for these possible confounds have been developed.

Final assessment

Recommended—Because the CAMCOG has acceptable clinimetric properties, has been used by groups other than the original developers, and has been used in PD samples for both clinimetric examinations as well as epidemiological studies, this scale is "Recommended" for use.

DEMENTIA RATING SCALE (MATTIS DEMENTIA RATING SCALE; MDRS, DRS, DRS-2)[58]

Scale description

The Mattis Dementia Rating Scale (DRS and DRS-2) provides a brief assessment of five cognitive domains, including attention (8 items), initiation/perseveration (11 items), construction (6 items), conceptualization (6 items), and memory (5 items). There is a total of 36 items, and 32 stimuli cards are used for administration of selected items. The maximum score is 144. The revised version, DRS-2, uses the original 36 items and 32 stimuli items, but provides an expanded normative table, reformatted designs, and expanded reference material. The scale has an alternate form for repeat testing. Performance on the DRS has been shown to be influenced by age and education level.[59,60] Therefore, demographic adjustments to domain and total score are suggested. Scoring is facilitated by a manual that includes normative information on score adjustments for age based on the Mayo's Older American Normative Study (MOANS). Age-based normative adjustments provide scale scores and percentiles for each domain as well as for the total score. Adjustments for educational level can be made only to the total DRS-R MOANS adjusted scale score. Use of the assessment is reserved for individuals 55 years and older. An alternate form for the DRS-2 is provided for repeat testing. The DRS require approximately 15 to 30 minutes for administration, although this time may increase when testing patients who are cognitively impaired. The scale is available from Psychological Assessment Resources (www4.parinc.com).

Key evaluation issues

This scale has been used extensively by multiple authors studying PD populations with various levels of cognitive dysfunction. The

DRS demonstrates acceptable levels of internal consistency (Cronbach's alpha range 0.65–0.95).[61-63] Test-retest reliability is good for both the original form (correlations rage 0.61–0.94) and the alternate form (r = 0.93).[64] Concurrent validity appears acceptable, with correlations to the Wechsler Adult Intelligence Scale (WAIS) ranging between 0.57 and 0.73.[61] Sensitivity to change has been established in non-PD samples.[61]

In studies with PD patients, the DRS has also shown diagnostic sensitivity and specificity in differentiating among Alzheimer's disease, mild cognitive impairment, PD dementia, and PD mild cognitive impairment, and healthy controls.[65] Additional diagnostic differentiation between Alzheimer's disease and PD dementia has been demonstrated in multiple community-based and clinic-based studies.[66-68] A small sample study demonstrated 72% sensitivity and 86% specificity between PD and PD with mild cognitive impairment using a cutoff score of 138.[69] The DRS demonstrates concurrent validity by both correlational analyses and discrimination analyses for mild impairments in activities of daily living in PD. Two studies have found the scale to be sensitive to changes in both mild and moderate cognitive impairment in PD samples.[70,71] The DRS has been used as an outcome measure in randomized clinical trials for ravistigmine[72] and deep brain stimulation.[73]

Strengths and weaknesses

The major strengths of the DRS are its strong clinimetric properties and its broad coverage of different cognitive domains. The scale has demonstrated utility in both PD and non-PD samples, and appears to provide useful diagnostic differentiation between demented and non-demented PD patients. Its utility in differentiating PD from PD with mild cognitive impairment is suggested, but the sample size for that study was limited.[69] Additional strengths include the recent development of age-based normative adjustment to the scoring. The major weakness of the DRS is in the length of time required for administration. In demented samples, the administration time might exceed 45 minutes.

Final assessment

Recommended—Because the DRS has acceptable clinimetric properties assessed in both PD and non-PD samples, has been used by groups other than the original developers, and has been used in PD samples for both epidemiological examinations as well as clinical trials, this scale is "Recommended" for use.

MINI-MENTAL PARKINSON (MMP)[27]

Scale description

The Mini-Mental Parkinson (MMP) scale was derived from the Mini-Mental State Examination (see below), and was designed to provide a rapid assessment of mental status specifically for patients with PD.[27] The scale provides brief assessments of orientation, attention, visual registration and recall, fluency, set-shifting, and conceptualization and has a total maximum score of 32. There are no alternate forms, and the test can be administered in less than 15 minutes. The scale is not in the public domain.

Key evaluation issues

The MMP has been used by many authors studying cognition in PD. However, there is very limited clinimetric information available on the scale. In the description of the development of the instrument, the MMP correlated highly with the Mini-Mental State Examination (r −0.93). Diagnostic accuracy of dementia in PD was reported to be good for sensitivity (100%), but low for specificity (70%), although diagnostic agreement between the MMP and MMSE was high (kappa = 0.85).[27] High sensitivity and low specificity were also demonstrated in a non-PD sample of 201 patients in a dementia clinic.[74] In a larger study with PD patients (n = 123), MMP demonstrated minimally acceptable levels for internal consistency (Cronbach's alpha = 0.755), and moderate concurrent validity with the MMSE and the SCOPA-Cog.[75] There are no reports of internal consistency, sensitivity to change measures, or use in clinical trials.

Strengths and weaknesses

The strengths and weaknesses of the MMP are difficult to assess at this point, as there is little evidence available for review. It appears that the scale has some clinimetric attributes that would justify its use, but this has not been put to an empirical test.

Final assessment

Listed—With a lack of detailed clinimetric results or objective findings on the use of the MMP, it is difficult to recommend its use at this time.

MINI-MENTAL STATE EXAMINATION (MMSE)[24]

Scale description

The Mini-Mental State Examination (MMSE) was designed to provide a brief "bedside" cognitive assessment. It is composed of 16 items for a total maximum score of 30. The scale assesses five cognitive domains: orientation; registration and recall; attention/calculations; language (repetition, naming, writing); and visuospatial abilities. There are no official alternate forms, although many unofficial versions exist. Total testing time is approximately 10 minutes. The scale is not in the public domain and may be purchased from Psychological Assessment Resources at www4.parinc.com.

Key evaluation issues

Although the MMSE is one of the most frequently used cognitive screening measures, widely used by multiple authors reporting on cognitive decline in PD, its clinimetric properties are not very compelling. Both age and education are known confounds for performance on the scale,[76] and although normative adjustments for these confounding variables have been developed, they are often not used. As early as 1990,

problems were noted with the validity of the subsections.[77] Specific problems include ceiling effects for high-functioning individuals and use of a cutoff score for defining dementia. The effect of the ceiling effects on diagnostic accuracy of the MMSE was noted in a study comparing the MMSE to the Montreal Cognitive Assessment in a sample of 132 PD patients.[78] Additionally, in many comparisons of the diagnostic accuracy of different cognitive screening measures, the MMSE is found to be inferior to other screening instruments in both general populations[79] as well as in PD-specific studies.[78,80]

Strengths and weaknesses

The major strengths of the MMSE as a screening measure are its brevity in administration and its history. Although other screening measures may be as brief as the MMSE, none has its extensive history of use. Because of this history, the MMSE can provide the clinician and investigator a common metric by which the level of cognitive impairment is measured. The weaknesses of the MMSE relate to its use in non-PD samples as well as in PD patients. Ceiling effects on many individual items, as well as the total score, make assessment of mild levels of cognitive impairment difficult. Added to this, the effects of age and education on performance are often not corrected, so that the score may be confounded by these demographic variables. Finally, the diagnostic ability of the MMSE is usually found to be inferior to that of other cognitive screening measures.

Final assessment

Suggested—Because of the limited clinimetric strengths of the MMSE and its demonstrated inferiority to other cognitive screening measures, it is difficult to recommend its use. However, the one situation that may suggest the use of the MMSE is that of placing the cognitive performance of a sample within a historical context. Because of its extensive use in the literature, the MMSE can provide a common metric for the assessment of cognitive functioning.

MONTREAL COGNITIVE ASSESSMENT (MOCA)[25]

Scale description

The MoCA was originally developed to provide a screening measure for mild cognitive impairment in the general population. The scale assesses seven cognitive domains, including visuospatial/executive, naming, memory/delayed recall, attention, language, abstraction, and orientation, for a total maximum score of 30. The administration time is approximately 10 minutes, and the scale has been translated into more than 30 languages. Alternate forms are available for French and English, and other language alternate forms are being developed. A normative adjustment for low education (≤12 years) adds one point to the total score. The test is not in the public domain and is available at www.mocatest.org. There is no usage charge for clinical, educational, or not-for-profit research use, although prior permission is required. Use by for-profit entities requires prior approval and licensing fees.

Key evaluation issues

This scale has been utilized widely by many authors studying cognition in PD. Basic clinimetric properties of the MoCA were examined in the initial validation study.[25] Adequate internal consistency (Cronbach's alpha = 0.83) and test-retest reliability (r = 0.92) were found. A cutoff score of 25/26 on MoCA demonstrated a diagnostic sensitivity of 90% for individuals diagnosed with mild cognitive impairment and 100% for individuals diagnosed with Alzheimer's disease. Specificity at the same cutoff was good for identifying individuals with normal cognition (87%).

The clinimetric properties of the MoCA have been studied in patients with PD. One small-sample-size (n = 38) study found adequate test-retest reliability in a subset of patients as well as adequate inter-rater reliability (both ICCs ≥ 0.79). Concurrent validity was demonstrated by a significant correlation (r = 0.72) between the MoCA and a composite score of a neuropsychological battery assessing memory,

executive function, working memory, interference inhibition, IQ, and fluency.[81] In PD, the diagnostic utility of the MoCA has been compared to that of the MMSE, with demonstrated superiority of the MoCA. In a sample of 132 patients with PD, a cutoff score of 24/25 on the MoCA provided 70% sensitivity and 75% specificity for identifying any cognitive impairment compared to 20% sensitivity and 99% specificity for the MMSE cutoff score of 24/25. Identification of PD dementia was also superior for the same cutoff scores on the MoCA and the MMSE (MoCA sensitivity = 82%, specificity = 75%; MMSE sensitivity = 29%, specificity = 99%).[78] The sensitivity of the MoCA to the presence of cognitive impairment appears to be greater than that of the MMSE. In a cohort of PD patients who scored within a previously defined normal range on the MMSE, MoCA scores identified approximately 50% of the sample as cognitively impaired as represented by a score of less than 26.[82] The authors of this study also noted an underlying relationship to MoCA performance with age and gender, suggesting a possible confound. Indeed, age- and gender-adjusted norms to the MoCA have been developed, although their use is not widespread.[83]

Strengths and weaknesses

The major strengths of the MoCA include its widespread availability in multiple languages, ease of administration, broad range coverage of multiple cognitive domains, assessment of cognitive domains specifically germane to PD (e.g., executive function), superior sensitivity as a screening instrument for mild cognitive impairment or dementia, and accessibility for clinical use and use by not-for-profit organizations. The major weaknesses of the MoCA include a possible ceiling effect for higher-functioning patients and the lack of adequate age- and gender-normative data.

Final assessment

Recommended—Because the MoCA has acceptable clinimetric properties assessed in both PD and non-PD samples, has been used by groups other than the original developers, and has been used in PD samples with acceptable diagnostic utility, this scale is "Recommended" for use.

PARKINSON'S DISEASE COGNITIVE RATING SCALE (PD-CRS)[28]

Scale description

The PD-CRS was originally developed to provide a comprehensive cognitive screening for patients with PD. The items included in the scale were selected to assess both subcortical and cortical functions. Items contributing to the subcortical function assessment include immediate-recall verbal memory, sustained attention, working memory, clock drawing, delayed-recall verbal memory, alternating verbal fluency, and action fluency. The maximum subcortical score is 114. Items contributing to the cortical function assessment include naming and clock drawing. The maximum cortical score is 20. The subcortical and cortical scores are summed to produce a total maximum score of 134. The total administration time is between 15 minutes to 30 minutes, with greater testing time required for cognitively impaired subjects. The scale is available at www.movementdisorders.org/publications/rating_scales/; however, it is not in the public domain and the Movement Disorder Society holds the copyright.

Key evaluation issues

This scale has not been widely used, and two of the three available studies were authored by the scale developers. Basic clinimetric properties of the PD-CRS were examined in the original description of development of the scale.[28] The final version of the scale demonstrated good internal consistency (Cronbach's alpha = 0.82), as well as good test-retest and inter-rater reliability (IC range 0.75–0.94). The total scale score correlated highly with the DRS (ICC = 0.87), demonstrating an acceptable level of concurrent validity. Diagnostic utility appears to be good, with a sensitivity and specificity of 94% when using a cutoff score of 64/65 to identify PD dementia versus PD with normal cognition, and a sensitivity of 73% and specificity of 84% using the same cutoff score to differentiate PD with mild cognitive impairment from PD with normal cognition. No floor effects were noted in this validation sample, but ceiling effects were found for the clock drawing item in PD patients with normal cognition. Some of these findings were replicated in an independent examination of the clinimetric properties of the PD-CRS using 50 PD subjects. This study found acceptable internal consistency and concurrent validity with the SCOPA-Cog and MMSE.[84] There was also an inverse relationship between the PD-CRS total score and education, suggesting that this variable may confound performance on the scale.

Strengths and weaknesses

One of the major strengths of the PD-CRS is its assessment of multiple domains of cognitive functioning with particular emphasis on the domains most pertinent to PD. The clinimetric properties appear adequate for internal consistency, concurrent validity, and diagnostic sensitivity across two studies. However, both validation studies have somewhat limited sample sizes, particularly for PD patients with dementia. One of the major weaknesses of PD-CRS is its limited use in published studies. Only three published reports have used the PD-CRS, and two of those were from the originators of the scale. As more studies are published, a better sense of the scale's clinical utility can be attained. Additionally, some items may be too easy, and ceiling effects may occur in PD patients with normal cognition. Finally, there is some indication that there may be a confounding effect of low education on performance, but further studies will be required to address this possibility.

Final assessment

Suggested—The clinimetric properties of the PD-CRS appear to be acceptable, and the scale has been used by one group outside of the originators of the scale. However, because of a lack of published studies utilizing the PD-CRS, it is difficult to judge its clinical utility. This limitation is likely to change in the near future as more publications appear.

PARKINSON'S DISEASE DEMENTIA–SHORT SCREEN (PDD-SS)[29]

Scale description

The PDD-SS is designed as a very brief cognitive screening measure that can be administered in less than 10 minutes. The scale assesses five cognitive domains, including immediate verbal memory, delayed verbal memory, alternating verbal fluency, visuospatial abilities (clock drawing). The PDD-SS has a total maximum score of 22. The scale is not in the public domain, and the Movement Disorder Society holds the copyright to the scale.

Key evaluation issues

Although this scale is specifically focused on PD-related dementia, it has not been widely used by multiple authors. The clinimetric properties of the PDD-SS are presented in the description of the scale.[29] The scale appears to have good internal consistency (Cronbach's alpha = 0.82); acceptable test-retest reliability (ICC = 0.91); good inter-rater reliability (ICC = 0.86; and acceptable diagnostic utility with a sensitivity of 90% and specificity of 89% using a cutoff score of 11/12 for the diagnosis of PD dementia.

Strengths and weaknesses

The PDD-SS is newly developed, and there is very limited information available on its clinical utility. More studies will be required to fully understand the scale's strengths and weaknesses. The preliminary clinimetric results from the scale's developers are encouraging, however.

Final assessment

Listed—Because of the limited information available on the PDD-SS, it is difficult to advise its use based on currently available information. This conclusion may change as more information becomes available.

PARKINSON NEUROPSYCHOMETRIC DEMENTIA ASSESSMENT (PANDA)[30]

Scale description

The PANDA was developed to provide a brief screening tool for the assessment of cognitive functions typically impaired in PD and include a brief assessment of depressive symptoms. The scale includes five items: immediate and delayed recall of paired-associate word lists, alternating verbal fluency, visuospatial imagery, and a digit-ordering task for working memory assessment. The depression questionnaire consists of three questions assessing mood, interest, and drive. Scoring is adjusted for age and is scaled to a maximum of 30 points for the cognitive screening and nine points for the mood questionnaire. Total administration time is approximately 10 minutes. There are no alternate forms available, but the scale has been translated into French. The scale is not in the public domain and is available from the lead author of the scale.

Key evaluation issues

This scale has been used in PD, but multiple authors have not published data utilizing the measure. Furthermore, the clinimetric profile for this scale is not well established. Basic clinimetric properties of the PANDA were examined in the original publication on the development of the scale.[30] The scale appears to have adequate test-retest reliability (r = 0.93) and acceptable inter-rater reliability (r = 0.95) for the five cognitive questions. The cognitive score on the PANDA correlated significantly with the MMSE, and the mood score correlated significantly with another measure of depression, suggesting some level of concurrent validity. Diagnostic utility assessment revealed 90% sensitivity and 91% specificity for the classification of PD dementia when using a cutoff score of 17/18 points on the cognitive scale. Sensitivity and specificity decreased slightly when PD patients with mild cognitive impairments were included in the analysis. A cutoff score of 4 on the mood portion of the scale resulted in 80% sensitivity and 92% specificity for classification patients with or without depressive symptoms. The PANDA was used in a subset of a large epidemiological study of PD in Germany. The results of this study suggested that the PANDA was more sensitive to cognitive impairment than the MMSE but may overestimate diagnosed dementia rates in PD.[85] The results of this study also suggested there could be a confounding effect on performance on the PANDA by gender, with males typically scoring higher than females.

Strengths and weaknesses

The major strength of the PANDA is its brevity. The scale appears to have adequate clinimetric properties, but there is limited evidence of this in the published literature. There appear to be three major weaknesses to the PANDA. First, there is a lack of published studies utilizing the scale, so its clinical utility is difficult to assess. Second, the cognitive section of the scale assesses a limited number of cognitive domains, focusing mostly on executive processing, and it appears to overestimate dementia rates. Third, there is the possibility of a gender effect that could confound performance measures.

Final assessment

Listed—The PANDA has been used in PD, but the limited clinimetric studies and lack of use by individuals not involved in its development make it difficult to recommend its use. The overemphasis on assessment of executive function may underestimate impairments in other cognitive domains.

REPEATABLE BATTERY FOR THE ASSESSMENT OF NEUROPSYCHOLOGICAL STATUS (RBANS)[26]

Scale description

The RBANS was developed to provide a brief screening measure of cognitive functioning in adults. The scale assesses functioning in five cognitive domains, including immediate memory, visuospatial/construction, language, attention, and delayed memory. The scale includes 12 items and has a total maximum score of 160. Summary scores for each domain are available. There is an alternate form for repeat testing. The total administration time is approximately 30 minutes. The RBANS score is adjusted for age, based on United States population normative data. The scale is not in the public domain and is available from Pearson Assessment and Information at pearsonassessments.com.

Key evaluation issues

The clinimetric properties of the RBANS have been extensively studied in populations outside the PD cohort. In the technical manual for the test,[26] the basic reliability and validity results are presented. The RBANS appears to have adequate internal consistency with a split-half reliability (similar to a Cronbach's alpha) of 0.94 for the total score and ranges between 0.82 and 0.88 for the domain scores. Test-retest reliability has been established over an approximately 40-week interval ($r = 0.88$) with no practice effects noted. Concurrent validity appears to be adequate for the total score and domain scores as seen by significant correlations with the RBANS and standard neuropsychological measures. Despite age-adjusted norms, there appear to be additional confounding effects from gender,[86] race,[87] and education.[88] Additionally, content validity has been questioned by studies unable to replicate the five-domain structure of the scale.[89,90]

The RBANS has been also been specifically studied in PD samples and was used in a large multicenter study of early PD (the National Institutes of Health Exploratory Trials in Parkinson's Disease [NET-PD]). Clinimetric properties of the scale in PD samples, however, are not as robust as those reported for the general population. Internal consistency was lower than previously reported (Cronbach's alpha = 0.74 for the total score, and ranged between 0.13 and 0.70 for domain scores) and the five-domain factor model could not be replicated.[91] Additionally, sensitivity to changes in cognitive functioning over a 12- to 18-month period was found to be lacking in a large sample of patients with mild PD.[92] In a small sample study, the RBANS was found to provide less than adequate diagnostic accuracy for PD dementia (overall accuracy reported at 78%) or PD with normal cognition (overall accuracy reported at 39%).[93]

Strengths and weaknesses

The major strengths of the RBANS are the extensive development and normative work. The scale has been used in many disease states with good effect and fills a niche in cognitive screening as it covers multiple cognitive domains assessing both cortical and subcortical cognitive functions. The administration time is relatively short, scoring is easy, and a detailed manual facilitates interpretation. In diseases other than PD, it appears that the RBANS provides relevant information on the description of cognitive impairment and differentiating various clinical populations. In PD, however, the scale's sensitivity to changes in cognitive functioning appears to be low, and basic clinimetric properties of internal consistency and content validity appear to be lacking.

Final assessment

Recommended—The RBANS has been used by groups other than the originators, has been applied to PD samples, and has established clinimetric properties in diseases other the PD. However, its relatively poor clinimetric properties reported in large sample studies of PD patients raises concerns about its use in this population.

SCALES FOR OUTCOMES OF PARKINSON'S DISEASE– COGNITION (SCOPA-COG)[31]

Scale description

The SCOPA-Cog was designed specifically to assess cognitive deficits specific to PD and is part of a larger effort to develop scales sensitive to all domains of PD. The scale consists of 10 items assessing four cognitive domains: attention, memory, executive function, and visual spatial function. There is a total maximum score of 43. Administration time is approximately 15 minutes, and there are no alternate forms. The scale is available in multiple languages and can be obtained at www.scopa-propark.eu.

Key evaluation issues

This scale was specifically developed for PD and has been widely utilized in the literature. Basic clinimetric properties of the SCOPA-Cog were examined in the original description of the development of the scale.[31] The final version of the scale demonstrated good internal consistency (Cronbach's alpha = 0.83), as well as good test-retest and inter-rater reliability over a six-week period (ICC for total score = 0.78; kappa range for individual items = 0.40–0.75). The total scale score correlated highly with the CAMCOG (r = 0.83) and the MMSE (r = 0.72), demonstrating an acceptable level of concurrent validity. Differences in SCOPA-Cog performance between control subjects and PD subjects suggests that the scale is sensitive to mild cognitive impairment associated with PD. These clinimetric results were replicated in an independent validation study where the SCOPA-Cog had acceptable internal consistency (Cronbach's alpha = 0.78), moderate concurrent validity with the MMSE (rho = 0.61) and the MMP (rho = 0.50), and little or no floor or ceiling effects.[94] Diagnostic utility of the SCOPA-Cog appears to be good, with a sensitivity of 80% and specificity of 87% for the diagnosis of PD dementia as defined by the Movement Disorder Society recommended criteria,[10] using a cutoff score of 22/23. A similar level of diagnostic accuracy was

Table 15-2. Conclusions Regarding Scale Status to Assess Cognition in Parkinson's Disease

SCALE NAME	GENERIC/OTHER DISEASE/PD SPECIFIC	USED IN PD	USED BY GROUPS OTHER THAN DEVELOPERS	ADEQUATE CLINIMETRICS ESTABLISHED IN NON-PD COHORTS	ADEQUATE CLINIMETRICS ESTABLISHED IN PD COHORTS	RECOMMENDATION
Addenbrooke's Cognitive Examination (Revised)–ACE (R)	Generic	Yes	Yes	Yes	Yes	Recommended*
Alzheimer's Disease Assessment Scale–Cognition (ADAS-Cog)	Other disease	Yes	Yes	Yes	Yes	Recommended*
Cambridge Cognitive Assessment (Revised)–CAMCOG (R)	Generic	Yes	Yes	Yes	Yes	Recommended
Dementia Rating Scale (2nd edition)/Mattis Dementia Ratings Scale–DRS (2)	Generic	Yes	Yes	Yes	Yes	Recommended
Mini-Mental Parkinson (MMP)	PD-specific	Yes	Yes	—	No	Listed
Mini-Mental State Examination (MMSE)	Generic	Yes	Yes	Yes	No	Suggested
Montreal Cognitive Assessment (MoCA)	Generic	Yes	Yes	Yes	Yes	Recommended
Parkinson's Disease Cognitive Rating Scale (PD-CRS)	PD-specific	Yes	No	—	Yes	Suggested
Parkinson's Disease Dementia–Short Screen (PDD-SS)	PD-specific	Yes	No	—	No	Listed
Parkinson Neuropsychometric Dementia Assessment (PANDA)	PD-specific	Yes	No	—	Yes	Suggested
Repeatable Battery for the Assessment of Neuropsychological Status (RBANS)	Generic	Yes	Yes	Yes	Yes	Recommended*
Scales for Outcomes of Parkinson's Disease–Cognition (SCOPA - Cog)	PD-specific	Yes	Yes	Yes	Yes	Recommended

*Meets criteria for "Recommended," but has limitations in clinimetric properties when used in PD samples.

found in an independent study.[80] The scale has been shown to be sensitive to dementia severity with a Cohen's effect size *d* greater than 0.80, and has been used in clinical trials of anti-dementia medications in PDD.[41-44] One study found a differential items function (DIF) for age and gender on some of the items in the SCOPA-Cog,[95] suggesting possible confounds to performance on this scale.

Strengths and weaknesses

The SCOPA-Cog has multiple strengths as a cognitive screening measure. The scale has acceptable clinimetric properties for both reliability and validity, and these findings have been replicated in various studies. There is a history of its use in clinical trails of anti-dementia medication in PD patients with dementia, and it appears to have adequate sensitivity to mild cognitive impairments. As the developers of the scale acknowledge,[31] the SCOPA-Cog focuses on "subcortical" cognitive functioning as distinct from "cortical" cognitive functioning, and this may be a limitation in some settings. The presence of differential item function for age and gender on individual items is a limitation, and some authors suggest revising the scale.[95]

Final assessment

Recommended—The SCOPA-Cog has acceptable clinimetric properties that have been replicated in multiple studies. The scale has been used by many groups beyond the developers, and has been applied to several clinical trials

in PD dementia and cognitive impairment. The one caveat to this recommendation is that the SCOPA-Cog provides sufficient screening for executive or "subcortical" cognitive functions, but does not provide adequate screening for more cortically mediated cognitive functions. This limitation was intended by the developers of the scale.

FUTURE PERSPECTIVES

The evaluation of cognitive screening measures in PD is an ever-evolving endeavor. As new studies using these instruments are published, information on the clinical utility and clinimetric strengths and weaknesses of the screening scales becomes available. The added information from these studies will alter the rankings for the scales in this chapter (see Tables 15-2 and 15-3) such that those that are "Suggested" may be elevated to "Recommended," and those that are "Listed" may move to "Suggested." As new scales are developed, they will be incorporated into the armamentarium of cognitive-assessment measures. All scales used to measure cognitive impairments in PD need to be accompanied by standard definitions of PD dementia and PD mild cognitive impairments. Whereas such recommendations have been the focus of Movement Disorder Society initiatives, the full testing of these criteria for diagnostic classification has not been fully established. Integration of these definitions with the scales reviewed will allow a more comprehensive evaluation of cognitive changes in PD in longitudinal and in treatment studies.

Table 15-3. List of Recommended Cognitive Screening Instruments

1. Addenbrooke's Cognitive Examination (Revised)—ACE (R)
2. Alzheimer's Disease Assessment Scale–Cognition (ADAS-Cog)
3. Cambridge Cognitive Assessment (Revised)—CAMCOG (R)
4. Dementia Rating Scale (2nd edition)/Mattis Dementia Ratings Scale—DRS (2)
5. Montreal Cognitive Assessment (MoCA)
6. Repeatable Battery for the Assessment of Neuropsychological Status (RBANS)
7. Scales for Outcomes of Parkinson's Disease–Cognition (SCOPA-Cog)

References

1. Cummings JL. Intellectual impairment in Parkinson's disease: clinical, pathological, and biochemical correlates. *J Geriatr Psychiatry Neurol.* 1988;1:24–36.

2. Aarsland D, Zaccai J, Brayne C. A systematic review of prevalence studies of dementia in Parkinson's disease. *Mov Disord.* 2005;20: 1255–1263.

3. de Lau LM, Schipper CM, Hoffman A, et al. Prognosis of Parkinson's disease: risk of dementia and mortality: the Rotterdam Study. *Arch Neurol.* 2005;62:1265–1269.

4. Aarsland D. Andersen K, Larsen JP, et al. Risk of dementia in Parkinson's disease: a community-based prospective study. *Neurology.* 2001;56:730–736.

5. Yip AG, Brayne C, Matthews FE. Risk factors for incident dementia in England and Wales: the Medical Research Council Cognitive Function and Ageing Study. A population-based nested case-control study. *Age Ageing.* 2006;35:154–160.

6. Reid WGJ, Hely MA, Morris JGL, et al. A longitudinal study of Parkinson's disease: clinical and neuropsychological correlates of dementia. *J Clin Neurosci.* 1996;3:327–333.

7. Hely MA, Morris JG, Reid WG, et al. Sydney Multicenter Study of Parkinson's disease: non-L-dopa-responsive problems dominate at 15 years. *Mov Disord.* 2005;20:190–199.

8. Aarsland D, Andersen K, Larsen JP, et al. Prevalence and characteristics of dementia in Parkinson's disease: an 8-year prospective study. *Arch Neurol.* 2003;60:387–392.

9. Goetz CG, Emre M, Dubois B. Parkinson's disease dementia: definitions, guidelines, and research perspectives in diagnosis. *Ann Neurol.* 2008;64(suppl 2):S81–S92.

10. Dubois B, Burn D, Goetz C. Diagnostic procedures for Parkinson's disease dementia: recommendations from the Movement Disorder Society Task Force. *Mov Disord.* 2007;22: 2314–2334.

11. Foltynie T, Brayne CEG, Robbins TW, et al. The cognitive ability of an incident cohort of Parkinson's patients in the UK. The CamPaIGN study. *Brain.* 2004;127:550–560.

12. Javin CC, Larsen JP, Aarsland D, et al. Subtypes of mild cognitive impairment in Parkinson's disease: progression to dementia. *Mov Disord.* 2006;21:1343–1349.

13. Williams-Gray CH, Evans JR, Gotis A, et al. The distinct cognitive syndromes of Parkinson's disease: 5 year follow-up of the CamPaIGN cohort. *Brain.* 2009;132:2958–2969.

14. Litvan I, Aarsland D, Adler CH, et al. MDS task force on mild cognitive impairment in Parkinson's disease: critical review of PD-MCI. *Mov Disord.* 2011;26:1814–1824.

15. Aarsland D, Kurz MW. The epidemiology of dementia associated with Parkinson's disease. *Brain Pathol.* 2010;20:633–639.

16. Aarsland D, Bronnick K, Williams-Gray C, et al. Mild cognitive impairment in Parkinson's disease: a multicenter pooled analysis. *Neurology.* 2010;75:1062–1069.

17. Stebbins GT. Neuropsychological testing. In: Goetz CG, ed. *Textbook of Clinical Neurology.* 2nd ed. Philadelphia, PA: Elsevier Science; 2003.

18. Nunnally JC, Bernstein IH. *Psychometric Theory.* 3rd ed. New York, NY: McGraw-Hill; 1994.

19. Mathuranath PS, Nestor PJ, Berrios GE, et al. A brief cognitive test battery to differentiate Alzheimer's disease and frontotemporal dementia. *Neurology.* 2000;55:1613–1620.

20. Mioshi E, Dawson K, Mitchell J, et al. The Addenbrooke's Cognitive Examination Revised (ACE-R): a brief cognitive test battery for dementia screening. *Am J Geriatr Psychiatry.* 2006;21:1078–1085.

21. Rosen WG, Mohs RC, Davis KL. A new rating scale for Alzheimer's disease. *Am J Psychiatry.* 1984;41:1356–1364.

22. Roth M, Huppert FA, Mountjoy CQ, Tym E. *CAMDEX: The Cambridge Examination for Mental Disorders.* Cambridge: Cambridge University Press; 1988.

23. Mattis S. *Dementia Rating Scale Professional Manual.* Odessa, FA: Psychological Assessment Resources; 1988.

24. Folstein MF, Folestine SE, McHugh PR. Mini-mental state. A practical method for grading the cognitive state of patients for the clinician. *J Psychiatry Res.* 1975;12:189–198.

25. Nareddine ZS, Phillips NA, Bedirian V, et al. The Montreal Cognitive Assessment, MoCA: a brief screening tool for mild cognitive impairment. *J Am Geriatr Soc.* 2005;53:695–699.

26. Randolph C. *Repeatable Battery for the Assessment of Neuropsychological Status Manual.* San Antonio, TX: The Psychological Corporation; 1998.

27. Maheux F, Michelet D, Manifacier MJ, et al. Mini-mental Parkinson: first validation study of a new bedside test constructed for Parkinson's disease. *Behav Neurol.* 1995;8:15–22.

28. Pagonabarraga J, Kulisevsky J, Llebaria G, et al. Parkinson's Disease—Cognitive Rating Scale:

a new cognitive scale specific for Parkinson's disease. *Mov Disord.* 2008;23:998–1005.

29. Pagonabarraga J, Kulisevsky J, Llebaria G, et al. PDD-Short Screen: a brief cognitive test for screening dementia in Parkinson's disease. *Mov Disord.* 2010;25:440–446.

30. Kalbe E, Calabrese P, Nils K, et al. Screening for cognitive deficits in Parkinson's disease with the Parkinson neuropsychometric dementia assessment (PANDA) instrument. *Parkinsonism Relat Disord.* 2008;14:93–101.

31. Marinus J, Visser M, Verwey NA, et al. Assessment of cognition in Parkinson's disease. *Neurology.* 2003;61:1222–1228.

32. Morris JC. Clinical Dementia Rating: a reliable and valid diagnostic and staging measure for dementia of the Alzheimer's type. *Int Psychogeriatr.* 1997;9(suppl 1):173–176.

33. Reyes MA, Lloret SP, Gerscovich ER, et al. Addenbrooke's Cognitive Examination validation in Parkinson's disease. *Eur J Neurol.* 2009;16:142–147.

34. Robben SH, Sleegers MJM, Dautzenberg PLJ, et al. Pilot study of a three-step diagnostic pathway for young and old patients with Parkinson's disease dementia: screen, test and then diagnose. *Am J Geriatr Psychiatry.* 2010;25:258–265.

35. Komadina NC, Terpening Z, Haung Y, et al. Utility and limitations of Addenbrooke's Cognitive Examination—Revised for detecting mild cognitive impairment in Parkinson's disease. *Dement Geriatr Cogn Disord.* 2011;31:349–357.

36. Conner DJ, Schafer K. *Administration Manual for the Alzheimer's Disease Assessment Scale.* San Diego, CA: Alzheimer's Disease Cooperative Study; 1998.

37. Cano SJ, Posner HB, Moline ML, et al. The ADAS-Cog in Alzheimer's disease clinical trials: psychometric evaluation of the sum and its parts. *JNNP.* 2010;81:1363–1368.

38. Weyer G, Erzigheit H, Kanowski S, et al. Alzheimer's Disease Assessment Scale: reliability and validity in a multicenter clinical trial. *Int Psychogeriatr.* 1997;9:123–128.

39. Mohs RC, Knopman D, Petersen RC, et al. Development of cognitive instruments for use in clinical trials of antidementia drugs: additions to the Alzheimer's Disease Assessment Scale that broaden its scope. *Alzheimer Dis Assoc Disord.* 1997:11 (suppl 2):S13–S21.

40. Wesnes KA. Assessing change in cognitive function in dementia: the relative utilities of the Alzheimer's Disease Assessment Scale—Cognitive Subscale and the Cognitive Drug Research system. *Neurodegener Dis.* 2008;5:261–263.

41. Emre M, Aarsland D, Albanese A, et al. Rivastigmine for dementia associated with Parkinson's disease. *N Engl J Med.* 2004;351:2509–2518.

42. Litvinenko IV, Odinak MM, Mogil'nava VI, Perstnev SV. Use of memantine (akatinol) for the correction of cognitive impairments in Parkinson's disease complicated by dementia. *Neurosci Behav Physiol.* 2010;40:149–155.

43. Litvinenko IV, Odinak MM, Mogil'naya VI, Emelin AY. Efficacy and safety of galantamine (reminyl) for dementia in patients with Parkinson's disease (an open controlled trial). *Neurosci Behav Physiol.* 2008;38:937–945.

44. Burn D, Emre M, McKeith I, et al. Effects of rivastigmine in patients with and without visual hallucinations in dementia associated with Parkinson's disease. *Mov Disord.* 2006;21: 1899–1907.

45. Huppert FA, Brayne C, Gill C, et al. CAMCOG—a concise neuropsychological test to assist dementia diagnosis: socio-demographic determinants in an elderly population sample. *Br J Clin Psychol.* 1995;34:529–541.

46. Korner A, Lauritzen L, Bech P. A psychometric evaluation of dementia rating scales. *Eur Psychiatry.* 1996;11:185–191.

47. Roth M, Huppert F, Mountjoy C, Tym E. *The Cambridge Examination for Mental Disorders of the Elderly—Revised.* Cambridge: Cambridge University Press; 1999.

48. Ballard C, Patel A, Oyebode F, Wilcock G. Cognitive decline in patients with Alzheimer's disease, vascular dementia and senile dementia of Lewy body type. *Age Ageing.* 1996;25: 209–213.

49. Leeds L, Meara RJ, Woods R, Hobson JP. A comparison of the new executive functioning domains of the CAMCOG-R with existing test of executive function in elderly stroke survivors. *Age Ageing.* 2001;30:251–254.

50. O'Connor DW, Pollitt PA, Jones BJ, et al. Continued clinical validation of dementia diagnosed in the community using the Cambridge Mental Disorders of the Elderly Examination. *Acta Psychiatr Scand.* 1991;83:41–45.

51. Hendrie HC, Hall KS, Brittain HM, et al. The CAMDEX: a standardized instrument for the diagnosis of mental disorder in the elderly: a replication with a US sample. *J Am Geriatr Soc.* 1988;36:402–408.

52. Neri M, Roth M, Mountjoy CQ, et al. Validation of the full and short forms of the CAMDEX interview for diagnosing dementia. *Dementia*. 1994;5:257–265.

53. Lindeboom J, Ter Horst R, Hooyer C, et al. Some psychometric properties of the CAMCOG. *Psychol Med*. 1993;23:213–219.

54. Wouters H, van Gool WA, Schmand B, et al. Three sides of the same coin: measuring global cognitive impairment with the MMSE, ADAS-cog and CAMCOG. *Int J Geriatr Psychiatry*. 2010;25:770–779.

55. Hobson P, Meara J. The detection of dementia and cognitive impairment in a community population of elderly people with Parkinson's disease by use of the CAMCOG neuropsychological test. *Age Ageing*. 1999;28:39–43.

56. Athey RJH, Walker RW. Demonstration of cognitive decline in Parkinson's disease using the Cambridge Cognitive Assessment (Revised) (CAMCOG-R). *Int J Geriatr Psychiatry*. 2006;21:977–982.

57. Hobson P, Meara J. Risk and incidence of dementia in a cohort of older subjects with Parkinson's disease in the United Kingdom. *Mov Disord*. 2004;19:1043–1049.

58. Mattis S. *Dementia Rating Scale Professional Manual*. Odessa, FL: Psychological Assessment Resources, Inc; 1988.

59. Chan AS, Choi MK, Salmon DP. The effects of age, education and gender on the Mattis Dementia Rating Scale performance of elderly Chinese and American individuals. *J Gerontol B Psychol Sci Soc Sci*. 2001;7:535–543.

60. Freidl W, Schmidt R, Stonegger WJ, et al. Sociodemographic predictors and concurrent validity of the Mini Mental State Examination and the Mattis Dementia Rating Scale. *Eur Arch Psychiatry Clin Neurosci*. 1996;246:317–319.

61. Smith GE, Ivnik RJ, Malec JF, et al. Psychometric properties of the Mattis Dementia Rating Scale. *Assessment*. 1994;1:123–132.

62. Vitaliano PP, Breen AR, Russo J, et al. The clinical utility of the Dementia Rating Scale for assessing Alzheimer's disease. *J Chronic Dis*. 1984;37:745–753.

63. Gardner R, Oliver-Munoz S, Fisher L, Empting L. Mattis Dementia Rating Scale: internal reliability study using a diffusely impaired population. *J Clin Neuropsychol*. 1981;3:271–275.

64. Schmidt KS, Mattis PJ, Adams J, Nestor P. Test-retest reliability of the Dementia Rating Scale—2: alternate form. *Dement Geriatr Cogn Disord*. 2005;20:42–44.

65. Matteau E, Dupre N, Langlois M, et al. Mattis Dementia Rating Scale 2: screening for MCI and dementia. *Am J Alzheimers Dis Other Demen*. 2011;26:389–398.

66. Aarsland D, Litvan I, Salmon D, et al. Performance on the Dementia Rating Scale in Parkinson's disease with dementia and dementia with Lewy bodies: comparison with progressive supranuclear palsy and Alzheimer's disease. *J Neurol Neurosurg Psychiatry*. 2003;74:1215–1220.

67. Matteau E, Sinard M, Jean L, et al. Detection of mild cognitive impairment using cognitive screening tests: a critical review and preliminary data on the Mattis Dementia Rating Scale. In: JP Tsai, ed. *Leading-Edge Cognitive Disorders Research*. Hauppauge, NY: Nova Science Publishers Inc.; 2008:9–58.

68. Pablo AM, Troster AI, Glatt SL, et al. Differentiation of the dementias of Alzheimer's and Parkinson's disease with the dementia rating scale. *J Geriatr Psychiatry Neurol*. 1995;8:184–188.

69. Villeneuve S, Rodrigues-Brazete J, Joncas S, et al. Validity of the Mattis Dementia Rating Scale to detect mild cognitive impairment in Parkinson's disease and REM sleep behavior disorder. *Dement Geriatr Cogn Disord*. 2001;31:210–217.

70. Foldi NS, Majerovitz SD, Sheikh K, Rodriguez E. The test for severe impairment: validity with the Dementia Rating Scale and utility as a longitudinal measure. *Clin Neuropsychol*. 1999;13:22–29.

71. Dujardin K, Defebvre L, Duhamel A, et al. Cognitive and SPECT characteristics predict progression of Parkinson's disease in newly diagnosed patients. *J Neurol*. 2004;251:1383–1392.

72. Dujardin K, Devos D, Duhem S, et al. Utility of the Mattis Dementia Rating Scale to assess the efficacy of rivastigmine in dementia associated with Parkinson's disease. *J Neurol*. 2006;253:1154–1159.

73. Schupbach WMM, Chastan N, Welter ML, et al. Stimulation of the subthalamic nucleus in Parkinson's disease: a 5 year follow up. *J Neurol Neurosurg Psychiatry*. 2005;76:1640–1644.

74. Larmer AJ. Mini-mental Parkinson (MMP) as a dementia screening test: comparison with the Mini-mental State Examination (MMSE). *Current Aging Science*. 2011; epub PMID 21834788.

75. Serrano-Duenas M, Calero B, Serrano S, et al. Metric properties of the Mini-mental Parkinson and SCOPA-COG scales for rating cognitive

deterioration in Parkinson's disease. *Mov Disord.* 2010;25:2555–2562.

76. Crum RM, Anthony JC, Bassett SS, Folstein MF. Population-based norms for the Mini-Mental State Examination by age and education level. *JAMA.* 1993;269:2386–2391.

77. Giordani B, Bolvin MJ, Hall AL, et al. The utility and generality of Mini-Mental State Examination scores in Alzheimer's disease. *Neurology.* 1990;40:1894–1896.

78. Hoops S, Nazem S, Siderowf AD, et al. Validity of the MoCA and MMSE in the detection of MCI and dementia in Parkinson's disease. *Neurology.* 2009;73:1738–1745.

79. Damian AM, Jacobson SA, Hentz JG, et al. The Montreal Cognitive Assessment and the mini-mental state examination as screening instruments for cognitive impairment: item analyses and threshold scores. *Dement Geriatr Cogn Disord.* 2011:31:126–131.

80. Dairymaple-Alford JC, MacAskill MR, Nakas CT, et al. The MoCA: well-suited screen for cognitive impairment in Parkinson's disease. *Neurology.* 2010;75:1717–1725.

81. Gill D, Freshman A, Blender JA, Ravina B. The Montreal Cognitive Assessment as a screening tool for cognitive impairment in Parkinson's disease. *Mov Disord.* 2008;23:1043–1046.

82. Nazem S, Siderowf AD, Duda JE, et al. Montreal Cognitive Assessment performance in patients with Parkinson's disease with "normal" global cognitive function according to Mini-Mental State Examination score. *Am J Geriatr Soc.* 2009;57:304–308.

83. Rossetti HC, Lacritz LH, Cullum CM, Weiner MF. Normative data for the Montreal Cognitive Assessment (MoCA) in a population-based study. *Neurology.* 2011;77:1272–1275.

84. Martinez-Martin P, Prieto-Jurczynska C, Frades-Payo B. Psychometric attributes of the Parkinson's Disease—Cognitive Rating Scale. An independent validation study. *Rev Neurol.* 2009;49:393–398.

85. Riedel O, Klotsche J, Spottke A, et al. Cognitive impairment in 873 patients with idiopathic Parkinson's disease results from the German Study on Epidemiology of Parkinson's Disease with Dementia (GEPAD). *J Neurol.* 2008;255:255–264.

86. Duff K, Schoenberg MR, Mold JW, et al. Gender differences on the Repeatable Battery for the Assessment of Neuropsychological Status subtests in older adults: baseline and retest data. *J Clin Exp Neuropsychol.* 2011;33:448–455.

87. Patton DE, Duff K, Schoenberg MR, et al. Performance of cognitively normal African Americans on the RBANS in community dwelling older adults. *Clin Neuropsychol.* 2003;17:513–530.

88. Duff K, Patton D, Schoenberg MR, et al. Age- and education-corrected independent normative data for the RBANS in a community dwelling elderly sample. *Clin Neuropsychol.* 2003;17:351–366.

89. Carlozzi NE, Horner MD, Yang C, Tilley BC. Factor analysis of the Repeatable Battery for the Assessment of Neuropsychological Status. *Appl Neuropsychol.* 2008;15:274–279.

90. Schmitt AL, Livingston RB, Smenoff EN, et al. Factor analysis of the Repeatable Battery for the Assessment of Neuropsychological Status (RBANS) in a large sample of patients with suspected dementia. *Appl Neuropsychol.* 2010;17:8–17.

91. Yang C, Garrett-Mayer E, Schneider JA, et al. Repeatable Battery for the Assessment of Neuropsychological Status in early Parkinson's disease. *Mov Disord.* 2009;24:1453–1460.

92. Schneider JS, Elm JJ, Parashos SA, et al. Predictors of cognitive outcomes in early Parkinson's disease patients: the National Institutes of Health Exploratory Trials in Parkinson's Disease (NET-PD) experience. *Parkinsonism Relat Disord.* 2010;15:507–512.

93. Beatty WW, Ryder KA, Gontkovsky ST, et al. Analyzing the subcortical dementia syndrome of Parkinson's disease using the RBANS. *Arch Clin Neuropsychol.* 2003;18:509–520.

94. Serrano-Duenas M, Calero B, Serrano S, et al. Metric properties of the Mini-Mental Parkinson and SCOPA-COG scales for rating cognitive deterioration in Parkinson's disease. *Mov Disord.* 2010;25:2555–2563.

95. Forjaz MJ, Frades-Payo B, Rodriguez-Blazques C, et al. Should the SCOPA-COG be modified?: a Rasch analysis perspective. *Eur J Neurol.* 2010;17:202–207.

16

DYSAUTONOMIA RATING SCALES IN PARKINSON'S DISEASE: SYMPTOMS OF ORTHOSTATIC HYPOTENSION

Anne Pavy-Le Traon and Stephanie R. Shaftman

Summary

Orthostatic hypotension (OH) is defined by consensus as a fall in blood pressure (BP) of at least 20 mmHg systolic and/or 10 mmHg diastolic within three minutes in an upright position. Several studies have shown that OH increases the risk of all-cause mortality. OH may be symptomatic or asymptomatic, depending on its magnitude and the individual's susceptibility. OH affects up to 50% of patients with Parkinson's disease. Symptoms of OH are generally assessed in scales on wider autonomic or non-motor symptoms. Some scales designed to detect OH-related symptoms provide information on their severity.

Following the guidelines of a larger Movement Disorder Society initiative to evaluate scales covering the gamut of PD impairments, a focused critique on scales to measure symptoms of OH was conducted. In regard to the assessment of OH symptom severity, the SCOPA AUT, the COMPosite Autonomic Symptom Scale (COMPASS), and the Novel Non-Motor Symptoms Scale (NMSS) met criteria for "Recommended" with some limitations; the Orthostatic Grading Scale (OGS) was classified as "Suggested." In regard to screening for the presence or absence of OH symptoms, the NMS Quest was classified as "Recommended," and the UPDRS (OH item) as "Suggested" because of its use beyond its developers (even if limited for screening orthostatic symptoms).

INTRODUCTION

The prevalence of orthostatic hypotension[1,2] increases with age and is reported to occur in 5% to 30% of elderly subjects.[3] OH may lead to syncope and is associated with an increased morbidity and mortality.[4,5] OH affects 20% to 50% of patients with Parkinson's disease.[6–10] The different definitions and assessments of OH may have contributed to discrepancies in reported prevalence estimates.[3] OH mainly results from lesions of sympathetic efferent pathways related to the disease process, and dopaminergic drugs can further worsen it.[7,10–14] OH may be symptomatic or asymptomatic, depending on the magnitude of blood pressure fall, supine BP levels, and individual susceptibility. There is not always good correlation between orthostatic BP drops and symptoms, and several factors are likely to play a role in these discrepancies. First, the BP values at the time of the examination and at other times during the day can vary significantly in patients with autonomic impairment. OH may only occur after eating or immediately after standing in the morning. Second, symptoms of OH other than syncope may not be properly recognized. Some patients with chronic OH may not become symptomatic because of enhanced cerebral autoregulation that maintains cerebral perfusion despite a significant decrease in BP.[15] Symptom-specific scales are necessary to identify symptoms related to OH, to evaluate the effect of therapeutic interventions, and to improve the estimation of OH prevalence in PD. Whereas the "gold standard" of orthostatic BP monitoring involves tilt tables and other complex equipment, this paper evaluates the clinical rating scales that can be applied in a general clinical setting.

METHODS

Following the definitions established by the MDS Task Force on PD Rating Scales (see Chapter 6 of this book), a scale is classified "Recommended" if it has been applied to PD populations, there are data on its use in studies beyond the group that developed the scale, and it has been studied clinimetrically and found valid, reliable, and sensitive to change. The clinimetric criterion could be met by documentation of the scale's sound properties in conditions other than PD, but scales validated in PD itself are considered to be at a higher level. A scale is considered "Suggested" if it has been applied to PD populations, but only one of the other criteria applies. A scale is just "Listed" if it meets only one of the three criteria defined for recommended scales.

DEFINITION AND ASSESSMENT OF ORTHOSTATIC HYPOTENSION

Orthostatic hypotension is defined as a decrease in systolic BP $\geq$ 20 mmHg and/or in diastolic BP (DBP) $\geq$10 mmHg after active or passive (head-up tilt table testing [HUT]) change from supine to upright position, by consensus.[1,2] The period in the supine resting position before the measurement should last five minutes or longer until stabilization of BP and heart rate (HR) values. Three to five minutes in upright position are recommended.[17] In multiple system atrophy (MSA), in which dysautonomia is a key feature of the disease, a more pronounced OH (decrease in SBP $\geq$ 30 mmHg and in DBP $\geq$10 mmHg) is one of the diagnosis criteria.[18] BP can be decreased additionally by fluid depletion, medication intake, food ingestion, increased room temperature, and physical deconditioning.[18] BP measurements have to be repeated if symptoms are probably related to OH. Passive HUT is recommended if the active standing test is negative, especially if the history is suggestive of OH, and/or in patients with severe motor impairment. If available, devices providing non-invasive, automatic heart rate and BP measurements are recommended.[17] Changes in HR induced by the orthostatic maneuver have to be evaluated, and symptoms should be recorded. An autonomic neuropathy will be suspected in case of limited or inappropriate rise in HR. Other disorders known to induce OH, like diabetes mellitus with cardiac autonomic neuropathy,[19] have to be taken into account.

SCALES AND QUESTIONNAIRES

General presentation

Twelve scales or questionnaires were screened for full review. Most were part of larger scales and questionnaires designed to assess non-motor or autonomic symptoms:

- SCOPA-AUT[20]
- Composite Autonomic Symptom Scale (Orthostatic subsection) or COMPASS[21]
- Self-completed Non-Motor Symptoms Questionnaire for Parkinson's disease (NMS Quest)[22,23]
- Non-Motor Symptoms Scale for Parkinson's disease[24]
- MDS-UPDRS Part I[25] and the original UPDRS Part IV
- Freiburg questionnaire[26]

- Autonomic dysfunction in PD Questionnaire[27]
- Hobson et al. Scale[28]

One questionnaire focused only on OH:

- Orthostatic Grading Scale[29]

Other symptom checklists or scales have been used to assess OH symptoms in specific studies[6] or in clinical trials of drugs against OH[30-33].

- Symptoms list used by Senard et al.[6]
- Scale used to assess L-threo-dihydroxyphenylserine (L-Threo DOPS) effects[31]

Some scales provide information on the severity and/or frequency of the OH-related symptoms, while others only look for OH symptoms. However, symptoms per se may also provide information on severity level— for example, syncope is generally induced by severe OH.

Two scales, the UMSARS (Unified Multiple System Atrophy Rating Scale)[34] and the CASS (Composite Autonomic Scoring Scale)[35,36] are not detailed for the following reasons:

- The UMSARS is widely accepted as a validated grading scale in MSA. The Parts I (item 9) and III consider OH. However, the UMSARS has been specifically designed and validated for MSA, not for PD, and it has never been used in PD.
- The CASS (Composite Autonomic Scoring Scale) measures adrenergic and cardiovascular regulation, as well as sudomotor function by performing four tests (tilt, Valsalva, deep breathing, QSART [Quantitative Sudomotor Axon Reflex Test]). However, CASS is a rating tool for objective test results (QSART, HR, and BP responses), but this is not a clinical rating scale for OH-related symptoms. While it is possible that it provides a useful testing paradigm in PD, the CASS does not meet the definition of a clinical rating scale and is therefore not considered further.

A list of symptoms possibly related to OH and their inclusion in the evaluated scales is given in Table 16-1 hereafter.

DETAILED SCALES DESCRIPTION
SCOPA-AUT
DESCRIPTION

The Autonomic Scale for Outcomes in Parkinson's disease (SCOPA-AUT) is a self-administered questionnaire to assess dysautonomia.[20] It is not only focused on orthostatic symptoms. Its development was prompted by the need for a clinically applicable instrument to assess dysautonomia in PD. The SCOPA-AUT consists of 25 items including three cardiovascular (CV) items (orthostatic symptoms), seven gastrointestinal (GI), six urinary, four thermoregulatory, one pupillomotor, and two sexual items, with a frequency score from 0 (*never*) to 3 (*often*). The items are added for a summary score.

Key evaluation issues

USE IN PD AND USE BY MULTIPLE AUTHORS

Verbaan et al.[37] used the SCOPA AUT to evaluate the occurrence of autonomic symptoms in 420 PD patients compared to 150 control subjects. Only 12.9 % of the patients had symptoms in the CV domain. This scale was also used in smaller studies.[38,39] Papapetropoulos et al.[38] used this scale to investigate the correlation between the clinical severity of autonomic symptoms and electrophysiological test abnormalities in advanced PD; they found no correlation. This scale has been used later by Idiaquez et al.[39] to investigate whether there is an association between autonomic failure and cognitive impairment, by comparing 40 PD patients and 30 age-matched controls; the presence of OH did not correlate with the severity of cognitive impairment.

Martinez-Martin et al.[40] studied the characteristics of the caregivers of PD patients and analyzed the association between these characteristics and caregiver burden, perceived health and mood status (289 patient-caregiver pairs). The SCOPA-AUT was one of the numerous scales (motor and non-motor symptoms assessment) used to characterize this population of

Table 16-1. Symptoms of Orthostatic Hypotension Targeted by the Questionnaires

SYMPTOMS ON STANDING SCALES	FAINTNESS OR SYNCOPE	DIZZINESS	LIGHTHEADEDNESS	BLURRED VISION	DIFFICULTY THINKING	WEAKNESS(W)/ FATIGUE (F)	DECREASED HEARING
SCOPA AUT[20]	X		X	X	X		
COMPASS[21]	X	X			X		
NMSQuest[22,23]	Falling	X	X			X (W)	
NMSScale[24]	Falling because of fainting	X	X			X (W)	
UPDRS			X			X (F)	
MDS-UPDRS[25]			X				
Freiburg Questionnaire[26]		X					
Autonomic dysfunction in PD[27]	X	X					
Hobson et al. scale[28]		X					
Orthostatic Grading Scale[29]*	Maximal standing time**						
Senard et al.[6]	X Standing test abortion	X Vertigo, postural instability	X	X		X (W)	X
Matthias et al. (L-threo DOPS)[30,31]	X Maximal standing time**	X	X	X		X (W,F) tiredness, Maximal unassisted walking distance	

*In the OGS, symptoms are not listed (see text). This group used the COMPASS[21] as a scale to assess autonomic symptoms.
**The maximal standing time is a global criterion used in quantitative scales such as the OGS and scales designed to assess drug efficiency.

PD patients. Caregiver scores displayed a weak correlation with patient-related variables; the caregivers' affective status proved the most important factor influencing their burden and perceived health, whereas patient-related variables influenced caregiver burden and mood but not health status.

Oh et al.[41] used the SCOPA AUT together with objective CV measurements using the composite autonomic scoring scale (CASS) to study the relationship between PD stages, cognitive impairment, and autonomic dysfunction in 63 PD patients. They found that autonomic dysfunction might be present from disease onset, whereas the rate of cognitive decline increases with disease progression.

CLINIMETRIC PROPERTIES

Content validity: A postal survey with more than 25 items was administered to 46 PD patients, 21 MSA patients, and eight movement disorder specialists, and items were included based on frequency, burden, and clinical relevance. Redundant items (with inter-item correlation coefficients greater than 0.80) were removed based on the survey results.

Comprehension and ease of readability: The survey was piloted in 10 PD patients, and wording was changed when ambiguous language was pointed out or questions were determined to be misleading.

Construct validity: This questionnaire discriminated well between controls, mild, moderate and severe PD patients.

Test-retest reliability: This was measured and determined to be satisfactory. The intra-class correlation coefficient (ICC) for the total score was 0.87, and the region scores were between 0.65 and 0.90. Stability, based on the kappa statistic, in the items was good. The reliability for individual items was high and ranged from 0.45 to 0.90.

Responsiveness: This validation shows that this instrument may have the potential to indicate changes over time, as (a) the results of this study showed PD patients having higher scores in most regions and most items than non-PD

patients, and (b) within the PD group, those with more severe disease stages (indicated by modified Hoehn and Yahr stages—mild, moderate, severe) also tended to have higher total scores than those in the mild disease stage. However, this needs to be tested further in a longitudinal study.

Time to administer/burden: Only 25 items. The scoring is simple; the items are simply added. The estimated time to complete it is 10 minutes.

Recently an independent validation study has been performed on 387 PD patients; the authors concluded that, despite its heterogeneous content, which determines some weaknesses in the psychometric attributes of its subscales, SCOPA-AUT was an acceptable, consistent, valid, and precise scale.[42,43] In the same way, a Brazilian Portuguese version has been evaluated and found to be an acceptable, reliable, and valid questionnaire.[44] It has also been translated into Spanish and its metric properties have been tested in 100 consecutive Mexican patients and found to be acceptable and similar to other validation data.[45]

Strengths and weaknesses: It is a brief questionnaire, easy to implement. It has been specifically designed for PD patients. A recent independent validation confirmed that this scale was consistent, valid and precise. In a preliminary study comparing the use of SCOPA-AUT in MSA versus PD, sensitivity for screening orthostatic symptoms turned out to be low. The number of questions on orthostatic symptoms is limited, and this scale did not detect some symptoms related to OH.[46]

Conclusion

The SCOPA-AUT is a reliable, validated, and easily self-administered questionnaire for assessing frequency and burden of autonomic dysfunction in PD patients. Other groups than the developers have used it in studies in PD patients. It can be classified as "Recommended" for the assessment of presence and severity of OH-related symptoms, with the limitations previously mentioned.

COMPASS (COMPOSITE AUTONOMIC SYMPTOM SCALE) (ORTHOSTATIC SUBSECTION)[22]

Description

Developed in 1999 by Suarez and colleagues, the COMPASS comprises 73 questions assessing nine domains of autonomic dysfunction, including nine items for orthostatic symptoms. The authors aimed to develop a new, specific instrument to measure autonomic symptoms and test its validity. They first used a questionnaire called the Autonomic Symptom Profile, which had 169 items, including demographic questions. From this set of questions, 73 items emerged as the most important and frequently asked questions about autonomic symptoms. These 73 questions assess the following nine domains of autonomic symptoms: orthostatic (9 items); secretomotor, including sudomotor symptoms (8 items); male sexual dysfunction (8 items); urinary (3 items); gastrointestinal, including gastroparesis, diarrhea, and constipation (14 items); pupillomotor, including visual symptoms (7 items); vasomotor (11 items); reflex syncope (5 items); and sleep function (8 items). Seventy-three questions were grouped into key scorable areas of the autonomic nervous system to form the Composite Autonomic Symptom Scale (COMPASS). Each area was scored based on presence, severity, distribution, frequency, and progression of symptoms.

Key evaluation issues

USE IN PD AND USE BY MULTIPLE AUTHORS

The orthostatic section of the COMPASS has been used to study the efficacy of anti-hypotensive treatments (non-pharmacological, fludrocortisone and domperidone) in 17 patients with PD.[47] It has been used by multiple authors in other disorders[48,49] but not in PD, possibly because of its complexity and length.

CLINIMETRIC PROPERTIES

Content validity: Suarez et al. designed the evaluation tool after seeing patients with the disorders, having questionnaire design experience, engaging in discussions with clinicians about the disorders, reviewing other evaluation tools, and interviewing patients. The questionnaire underwent many revisions before it was studied in its current version.

Construct validity: Criterion validity was established by correlating the COMPASS scores with the scores of the CASS. The total CASS score is used, and the domain-specific COMPASS scores are used. Correlation coefficients are calculated and all COMPASS domains correlated with the CASS score, except the sleep-disorder domain. The total COMPASS score correlated well with the CASS score, although only 17 of 73 items measured OH and sweating disorders.

Time to administer/burden: The questionnaire is administered in less than 30 minutes.

Strengths and weaknesses: High accuracy in the definition of autonomic symptoms. Correlation with CASS, which is an objective-based measure of adrenergic and CV regulation (a scoring system for autonomic test results developed and validated by the same center).

Limitations: Complex questionnaire; the 73 items are time-consuming.

Conclusion

This questionnaire explores a wide range of autonomic dysfunctions and includes nine items for orthostatic symptoms. The COMPASS has shown a good correlation with autonomic tests results (CASS). It meets the designation of "Recommended" for the assessment of presence and severity of OH-related symptoms. This questionnaire has not been specifically validated in PD patients and has to be evaluated more thoroughly in this population.

NON-MOTOR SYMPTOMS QUESTIONNAIRE FOR PARKINSON'S DISEASE (NMS QUEST)

Description

The NMS Quest is a 30-item self-completed questionnaire, comprising the following autonomic domains: CV (2 questions: "Feeling light-headed, dizzy or weak on standing from sitting or lying"; "Falling"), gastrointestinal,[8] urinary,[2] sexual,[2] sleep/fatigue,[5] sudomotor,[1] and miscellaneous,[10] scoring as "yes" or "no." This questionnaire is the first validated instrument of this type designed for PD patients; it was evaluated in multiple centers internationally. There is no total score, and it is not a graded or rating instrument. This is a screening tool to show the presence of NMS and initiate further evaluation. Before the creation of this assessment tool, there was no single instrument that could provide a comprehensive assessment of the range of NMS in PD.

Key evaluation issues

USE IN PD AND USE BY MULTIPLE AUTHORS

The investigators who developed this scale used it in several studies.[22,23,50–52] Chaudhuri et al.[52] recently used it to determine the proportion of patients not declaring NMS to healthcare professional out of 242 PD patients. They showed, interestingly, that NMS are frequently undeclared at routine hospital consultations. Dizziness, which may be related to OH, was one of the most often undeclared symptoms, together with delusions, daytime sleepiness, and intense and vivid dreams.

Some groups beyond the group that developed the scale have also used this questionnaire. A Mexican group used it together with the NMSS to study the prevalence of NM symptoms in 100 Mexican PD patients.[53] They found that the prevalence of NM symptoms did not differ from other countries, and that mood, cognitive, and perceptual symptoms appeared to be more severe in this population.

CLINIMETRIC PROPERTIES

It is the first validated instrument of this type for PD patients and was evaluated in multiple centers internationally. This scale has been recently translated into German.[54] It has also been translated into Spanish, and its metric properties

have been checked in 100 consecutive Mexican patients.[45]

There is no total score, and it is not a graded or rating instrument. This is a screening tool to show the presence of NMS and initiate further evaluation. Before the creation of this assessment tool, there was no single instrument that could provide a comprehensive assessment of the range of NMS in PD.

Content validity: A multidisciplinary group of experts including patient representatives developed the questionnaire.

Construct validity: There was a significant correlation between the total NMS score (not designed to have a total score, but adding the positive "yes" responses in each person created one) in PD patients with Hoehn and Yahr stage (p = 0.0006). This also correlates with disease duration and disease progression.

Time to administer/burden: Five to seven minutes. The scoring is easily achieved; there is no total score to assess severity or burden.

Strengths and weaknesses: This scale is easy to complete.

Limitations: It is not a rating scale.

Conclusion

It is the first validated tool for screening for the presence of NMS in PD. It comprises autonomic domains including two questions possibly related to OH. This is not a rating scale, but it may be a good tool for screening orthostatic symptoms. The validation studies included patients and controls recruited worldwide; its use beyond the validation studies is increasing. Few key validation statistics have been performed on this instrument. The NMS meets the designation of "Recommended" as a screening tool.

NON-MOTOR SYMPTOMS SCALE (NMSS) (PHYSICIANS COMPLETE)[24,44,45]

Description

The NMSS was developed to provide a method to quantify NMS as evaluated in the previous NMS Quest. The NMS Scale is divided into nine major domains containing 30 questions, including two

CV items ("Does the patient experience light-headedness, dizziness, weakness on standing from sitting or lying position?"; "Does the patient fall because of fainting or blacking out?"). The NMSS reflects the questions flagged in the NMS Quest and is intended to be a practical tool for health professionals. Item scoring is obtained multiplying the severity score (ranging from 0 = *none* to 3 = *severe*) and the frequency score (from 1 = *rarely* to 4 = *very frequent*). The scale can, therefore, capture symptoms that are severe but relatively infrequent and those less severe but persistent.

Key evaluation issues

USE IN PD AND USE BY MULTIPLE AUTHORS

This scale was evaluated in multiple centers internationally.[24,55] A growing number of groups are using this scale worldwide. Honig et al.[56] used it to show the beneficial effects of infusion of levodopa/carbidopa gel compared to oral medications on NMS in 22 patients with advanced PD. In a small study, by using this scale, Kim et al.[57] showed that untreated de novo PD patients (n = 23) have more non-motor problems than controls (n = 23), and these non-motor symptoms are not ameliorated by three months of dopaminergic medication (n = 16).

As previously mentioned, Rodriguez-Violante et al.[52] used the NMS Quest and the NMS Scale to assess NMS in 100 Mexican PD patients. Its metric properties have been validated together with the NMS Quest and the SCOPA AUT in a Mexican population.[45]

This scale has been translated into German[54] and Chinese.[58] In this latter study, performed in 126 patients, the authors considered this scale to be a comprehensive, useful measure for NMS evaluation in Chinese PD patients. They compared these results with those measured with other already validated scales; however, these scales were only dealing with sleep, cognition, and mood, but none of them was dealing with autonomic symptoms.

Li et al.[59] showed in 86 Chinese patients that NMS were independently and negatively associated with quality of life. Sleep/fatigue, mood, gastrointestinal, urinary, and miscellaneous symptoms had a key impact on the health-related quality of life.

CLINIMETRIC PROPERTIES

Content validity: Patients and clinicians were involved in the creation of this instrument. A thorough literature review took place, a patient response survey was utilized and experts in the field were involved.

Comprehension and ease of readability: The validation study suggests that the questionnaire can be used in a clinical setting and can be translated for non–English speaking patients (already translated into Spanish, German, and Chinese).

Internal consistency was explored using Cronbach's alpha-coefficient and item homogeneity. Most domains showed very strong internal consistency. Sleep/fatigue and GI domains showed weak item homogeneity, but overall, the questionnaire was internally consistent.

Construct validity was evaluated by assessing both convergent validity (correlation with other measures assessing the same or similar constructs), as well as discriminative validity (the ability of the scale to differentiate between groups). A priori hypotheses were made concerning the correlations that the researchers expected to find between the NMS and domains of the UPDRS, duration of disease, and Hoehn and Yahr stage.

Floor/ceiling affects: The overall effects were 0.42%, well below the 15% limit. Overall, the scale exhibited strong acceptability.

Test-retest reliability: This was analyzed using the intra-class correlation coefficient. Reliability was shown to be satisfactory, except for the CV items and domain. The reason for the low cardiovascular ICC is unknown. The test-retest population was small; so this is an area for further examination.

MCID was examined and estimated by the means of the standard error of measurement (SEM) and the standard deviation. In the domains where the ICC was high, the SEM was less than one-half a standard deviation, which is a minimally important difference.

Time to administer/burden: This questionnaire is relatively easy to score (multiply the severity score [0–3] by the frequency score [1–4]). It takes 10 to 15 minutes to administer.

Factor analysis: An exploratory factor analysis (EFA) was carried out using the principal-component-factor method with orthogonal and oblique rotations. This EFA identified nine domains, and they corresponded approximately to the *a priori* defined domains.

Strengths and weaknesses: This is a questionnaire to quantify NMS, which may be used for evaluation of therapeutic effects, and is relatively easy to score. The scale can capture symptoms that are severe but relatively infrequent and those less severe but persistent.

Limitations: In the validation phase, the test-retest reliability was satisfactory except for the CV items and domain.

Conclusion

The NMSS (physicians complete) has been developed to quantify NMS as evaluated in the previous NMS Quest. It comprises only two questions related to OH. The NMSS fits the three criteria and merits the designation of "Recommended" for the assessment of presence and severity of OH-related symptoms.

UPDRS AND MDS-UPDRS PART I

Description

The UPDRS has been the most widely used scale for the clinical study of PD for many years. Because of some weaknesses, such as the absence of screening questions on several important non-motor aspects of PD, the Movement Disorder Society sponsored the development of a revised version of the UPDRS (MDS-UPDRS). The MDS-UPDRS retains the UPDRS structure of four parts with a total summed score, but the parts have been modified to provide a section that integrates non-motor elements of PD[60]: I, Non-motor Experiences of Daily Living; II, Motor Experiences of Daily Living; III, Motor Examination; and IV, Motor Complications. All items have five response options with uniform anchors of 0 = *normal*, 1 = *slight*, 2 = *mild*, 3 = *moderate*, and 4 = *severe*. Several questions in

Part I and all of Part II are written as a patient/caregiver questionnaire, so that the total rater time should remain approximately 30 minutes.[60] Detailed instructions for testing and data acquisition accompany the MDS-UPDRS in order to increase uniform usage.[61] The combined clinimetric tests have shown the validity of the MDS-UPDRS for rating PD.[25]

Key evaluation issues

USE IN PD AND USE BY MULTIPLE AUTHORS

The UPDRS has been used in numerous studies to assess motor and non-motor symptoms (including OH) in PD patients. However, in the original UPDRS, only one item is directly related to OH; light-headedness is assessed as *present* or *absent* in item 42 of the original UPDRS Part IV (related to treatment complications). In a few studies, results regarding OH are reported; for example, Zibetti et al.,[62] who used the UPDRS to evaluate motor and non-motor symptoms in PD patients undergoing bilateral deep brain stimulation, mentioned no effect on symptomatic OH. Because it does not provide any indication of quantification, it is really only a screening tool. The UPDRS is a multidimensional, reliable, and valid scale, translated into several languages. However, item 42 has not been clinimetrically analyzed as a single item.

In the new version of the UPDRS, MDS-UPDRS, Light-headedness on Standing is assessed in one item (0–4-point rating system) of Part I (non-motor experiences of daily living),[25] but there is still only one item in the scale that assesses orthostatic symptoms. The item "Fatigue," which may be related to OH, has been added in Part I (non-motor symptoms). Fatigue and lightheadedness on standing belong to the same factor.

Because of the single item related to orthostatic dizziness, the MDS-UPDRS and the original UPDRS can be used as screening tools to detect OH symptoms, with some limitations, since they are probably not sensitive enough to detect all cases of OH.

Strengths and weaknesses: The whole scale has been used widely.

Limitations: Only one item is directly related to OH.

Conclusion

The original UPDRS merits the designation of "Suggested" for screening. It meets criteria 1 and 2, but not 3 (the single item [Y/N] related to orthostatic dizziness has not been tested clinimetrically as isolated item). This item does not address severity.

The MDS-UPDRS merits the designation of "Listed" both for severity assessment and for screening the presence or absence OH symptoms. It meets criterion 1 but has not been used by other groups yet; the single question related to orthostatic dizziness has not been tested clinimetrically as isolated item.

FREIBURG QUESTIONNAIRE[26]

Description

Developed in 2004 by a German center in Freiburg, the questionnaire considers symptoms of autonomic failure in PD and their impact on daily life. In five short questions and three to six sub-items each, the main domains of autonomic failure are represented: orthostatic symptoms, bladder function, GI symptoms, male erectile dysfunction, sudomotor dysfunction. One question with three sub-items deals with OH.

Key evaluation issues

USE IN PD AND USE BY MULTIPLE AUTHORS

The questionnaire has been tested in 141 PD patients. In PD patients, the prevalence of autonomic symptoms was significantly higher compared with the age-matched control group. Of the 141 PD patients, 56% reported two or more symptoms of autonomic dysfunction. However, this short questionnaire has not been used by other groups beyond the developers.

CLINIMETRIC PROPERTIES

This is a five multi-part-item questionnaire. It has been translated from German into English, and the English version has not been validated.

Content validity: This tool discriminated well between PD patients and controls and supported the view that involvement of the autonomic nervous system is a characteristic of PD.

Time to administer/burden: It is fast and easily administered.

Strengths and weaknesses

The scale is easily administered, but limited data for evaluation are available.

Conclusion

This short questionnaire, easy to implement, and was developed for PD patients. As it was not used in other studies and was not validated, it is classified as "Listed." Further studies and validation are needed.

AUTONOMIC DYSFUNCTION IN PARKINSON'S DISEASE[27]

Description

This questionnaire was designed for a study. The purpose of this study was to examine autonomic dysfunction in a comprehensive manner by performing a global survey of autonomic symptoms in PD patients and in a control group without extra-pyramidal dysfunction. This questionnaire includes two CV items (orthostatic dizziness, syncope), six GI, seven urinary, three sexual dysfunction, 11 sudomotor function; the severity of symptoms was graded on a 0–4 scale.

Key evaluation issues

USE IN PD AND USE BY MULTIPLE AUTHORS

This questionnaire was used in 44 PD patients compared to 24 controls for the purpose of the study. The questionnaire specifically designed for this study has not been used beyond the developers.

CLINIMETRIC PROPERTIES

The study reporting the use of the instrument is a cross-sectional study, not a validation study.

Time to administer/burden: The total score for all items in the domain of interest is achieved by summing the individual item scores for each domain. The aggregate symptom score is the sum of the dysfunction in all systems. Time to administer was not discussed.

Methodological aspects: The study reporting the use of this instrument is a cross-sectional study comparing PD patients to controls. One aspect of the study compared the aggregate symptom scores between PD and non-PD patients to the scores of the symptom categories of autonomic dysfunction. The Wilcoxon rank-sum test was used. Another aspect of the study was to look at the presence or absence of symptoms in patients and controls. The findings confirm that autonomic dysfunction occurs in PD patients more often and more severely. Autonomic dysfunction did not correlate with disease severity, and that was not predicted. There were limitations to this study; one limitation being that the sample size was small, resulting in possible type II errors, another being no validation and no assessment of test-retest reliability. This is an important limitation.

Strengths and weaknesses

Limited data for evaluation are available.

Conclusion

This questionnaire has been developed for assessing autonomic symptoms specifically in PD, including two questions on the presence and severity of OH. This questionnaire has not been used in other studies. This scale only meets criterion 1 and is therefore "Listed."

ORTHOSTATIC GRADING SCALE (OGS)[29]

Description

The objective of the authors was to develop a brief self-report scale to rate the severity of orthostatic intolerance. They evaluated the relationship between the severity of orthostatic intolerance due to orthostatic hypotension as perceived by patients (symptoms) and the laboratory-measured autonomic deficits (composite autonomic severity score [CASS]).

The OGS is a short self-report questionnaire comprising five items, each on a scale from 1 to 4. The questions address frequency and severity of orthostatic symptoms, the relationship of symptoms to orthostatic stressors, and the impact of the symptoms on activities of daily living and standing time. Adding the scores for all items gives the total score for the instrument.

Key evaluation issues

USE IN PD AND USE BY MULTIPLE AUTHORS

145 patients were investigated in the validation study, including some PD patients. Among the five items on the questionnaire, the level of interference with activities of daily living showed the strongest correlation with the CASS sub-scores. This information emphasized the impact that OH has on patients' activities of daily living. However, the authors pointed out the possible limitations in PD patients, which may have postural instability that may render it difficult to isolate the effect of OH.[29] To our knowledge, this questionnaire has not been used in other studies in PD patients.

CLINIMETRIC PROPERTIES

Content validity: This questionnaire has been designed on the basis of questions asked by clinicians and researchers specializing in autonomic disorders during initial consultations with patients with definite OH and then tested with patients with suspected OH. There was no patient involvement in the creation of this instrument.

Internal consistency was explored using Cronbach's alpha-coefficient. The internal consistency was strong ($\alpha = 0.91$).

Time to administer/burden: Each item is rated on a 0–4-point scale. Adding the scores for all items gives the total score for the instrument. Time to administer is not specifically discussed, but the questionnaire is very brief.

Convergent/construct validity: This instrument was evaluated using the CASS score. Each scale item correlated significantly with the laboratory-based CASS scores. This shows good evidence for construct validity.

Factor analysis: This revealed a factor structure of one factor that accounted for 74% of the variance, and all factor loadings were greater than 0.78.

Strengths and weaknesses: Short and may be self-completed by the patient; correlation with CASS (developed and validated by the same center).

Limitations: This questionnaire has not yet been used specifically in PD patients.

Conclusion

This is a reliable tool designed for assessing presence and severity of orthostatic symptoms. This questionnaire needs further validation in PD patients. Some aspects have not been evaluated yet (floor/ceiling effects, MCID). The OGS fits criteria 1 and 3 and merits the designation of "Suggested."

L-THREO DOPS EVALUATION SCALE[30,31]

Some questionnaires have been used in clinical trials on treatment of OH. Multi-center studies have been conducted to assess effects of L-threo DOPS in MSA, pure autonomic failure, and PD [30,31,63–65]. L-threo-dihydroxyphenylserine (L-threo-DOPS) is an orally administered noradrenaline (NA) precursor that is metabolized to NA by L-aromatic amino acid decarboxylase. DOPS improved OH in patients with familial amyloid polyneuropathy, congenital deficiency of dopamine beta hydroxylase, pure autonomic failure, and multiple system atrophy.[65] It has also been tested against OH in some PD patients.[30,31,65] In these last studies, patients completed a "Clinical Symptoms Checklist" at different times. Each symptom was rated on

a 10-point scale: light-headedness, dizziness, feeling of weakness, fatigue, tiredness, blurred vision, maximal standing time, and maximal unassisted walking distance.

Conclusion

No clinimetric assessment of this scale is available in the literature. To our knowledge, this scale has not yet been used in other studies. This scale only meets criterion 1 for presence and severity of OH and therefore is "Listed."

ADDITIONAL QUESTIONNAIRES

The following questionnaires were specifically developed for a clinical study. They have not been validated or used beyond the original study they were developed for.

HOBSON SCALE[28]

This scale has been used in a study designed to estimate the prevalence of bladder and autonomic symptoms in a community-based sample of PD patients. Only one item is related to OH ("Feel dizzy on standing?"). Other items are listed as follows: nine bladder, four social functioning, one GI, one sudomotor, two sexual, five miscellaneous.

This scale only meets criterion 1 for presence and severity of OH and therefore is "Listed."

SENARD ET AL., 1997[6]

The questionnaire comprises eight subjective items on orthostatic symptoms (light-headedness, dizziness, postural instability, vertigo, blurred vision, fainting, asthenia, decreased hearing). It has been used to investigate the prevalence of OH and the nature of postural events related to a fall in BP in PD patients. It does not include a score for frequency and/or severity. This scale only meets criterion 1 for presence of OH and therefore is "Listed." Table 16-2 summarizes the main characteristics of the scales/questionnaires reviewed in this chapter.

Table 16-2. Scales Characteristics

"CHARACTERISTICS" SCALES	TYPE OF SCALE	SPECIFICALLY DESIGNED FOR PD PATIENTS	NUMBER OF ITEMS RELATED TOOH/ TOTAL NUMBER OF ITEMS	PATIENT VS. PHYSICIAN COMPLETED	ESTIMATED TIME TO ADMINISTER THE SCALE/ QUESTIONNAIRE
SCOPA AUT[20]	Autonomic symptoms scale	Yes	3/25	Self completed	10 min
COMPASS[21]	Autonomic symptoms scale	No	9/73	Physician completed	Less than 30 min
NMS Quest[22,23]	Non-motor symptoms questionnaire	Yes	2/30	Self completed	5–7 min
NMS Scale[24]	Non-motor symptoms scale	Yes	2/30	Physician completed	10–15 min
UPDRS	Global PD rating scales (motor and non-motor aspects)	Yes	1/55 (Part IV—Treatment complications)	Physician completed	30 min
MDS-UPDRS[25]			1/65 (Part I—Non-motor experiences)	Patient/caregiver completed for some items including this one	30 min (10 min for part I)
Freiburg Questionnaire[26]	Autonomic symptoms scale	Yes	1/5 questions with 3 sub-items	Self completed	Not mentioned but fast and easily administered
Autonomic Dysfunction in PD[27]	Autonomic symptoms scale	Yes	2/29	Physician completed	Not mentioned
Hobson et al. Scale[28]	Autonomic symptoms scale	Yes Designed for one study on autonomic symptoms in PD	1/23	Self completed	Not mentioned
Orthostatic Grading Scale[29]*	Focused on OH—including semi-quantitative maximal standing time assessment**	No	5/5	Self completed	Not mentioned but very brief
Senard et al.[6]	List of symptoms related to OH	Yes Designed for one clinical study on OH prevalence in PD	8/8	Physician completed	Not designed for clinical use
Matthias et al. (L-Threo DOPS)[30,31]	Focused on OH—including maximal standing time assessment**	No But most patients have Parkinsonian syndrome	10/10	Self completed	Not mentioned

* In the OGS, symptoms are not listed (see text). This group used the COMPASS[21] as a scale to assess autonomic symptoms. **The maximal standing time is a global criterion used in quantitative scales such as the OGS and scales designed to assess drug efficiency.

CLINICAL PERSPECTIVES

The assessment of OH varies across scales as their content varies considerably, and most include questions on OH as part of a larger scale on autonomic dysfunction or NM symptoms (see Table 16-2). Symptoms that may predict OH on standing are elicited in most of the scales (see Table 16-1). Other symptoms of OH such as postural headache, coathanger ache, and backache are under-recognized. Some scales (such as the OGS and those used in clinical trials) use the maximal standing time and emphasize the impact that OH has on patients' activities of daily living. In addition, some PD patients may have neurological symptoms such as postural instability that confound assessment of OH symptoms. Provoking and aggravating factors may help to relate such symptoms to OH; e.g., worse symptoms in the morning; aggravation by prolonged recumbency, heat, or a heavy meal; and improvement by sitting or supine position. Only the scales focusing on OH, such as the COMPASS orthostatic subsection or the OGS, clearly take these factors into account.

Based on clinimetric studies, there are few well-validated questionnaires on symptoms of OH that can be administered in the PD population. Some scales are used to screen for OH-related

Table 16-3. Overview of the Scales (with Scoring of Severity and/or Frequency) According to the Criteria

SCALES	USE IN PD	USE IN PD BEYOND ORIGINAL DEVELOPERS	SUCCESSFUL CLINIMETRIC TESTING IN PD	CLASSIFICATION
SCOPA-AUT[20]	X	X	X	Recommended (with some limitations)
COMPASS[21]	X limited number of patients with Parkinsonism	X one study (17 patients)	X strong but needs more validation	Recommended (with some limitations)
NMSS (physician complete)[24]	X	X	X	Recommended
MDS-UPDRS item on OH	X		not clinimetrically analyzed as a single item	Listed
Freiburg Questionnaire[26]	X			Listed
Autonomic Dysfunction in PD[27]	X			Listed
Orthostatic Grading Scale[29]	X (some PD patients in the population)		X needs more validation	Suggested
Hobson et al. Scale[28]	X			Listed
Mathias et al. (L-Threo-DOPS)[30, 31]	X			Listed

Table 16-4. Overview of the Scales (Screening Tools) According to the Criteria

SCALES	USE IN PD	USE IN PD BEYOND ORIGINAL DEVELOPERS	SUCCESSFUL CLINIMETRIC TESTING IN PD	CLASSIFICATION
NMS Quest[22,23]	X	X	X	Recommended
UPDRS item on lightheadedness	X	X limited use for OH screening	not clinimetrically analyzed as a single item (Y/N)	Suggested (with limitations)
Senard et al.[6]	X			Listed

symptoms and provide information on their severity and/or frequency (see Table 16-3).

Other scales can be considered as screening tools since they screen for OH symptoms but without scoring their severity and/or frequency (see Table 16-4).

All discussed questionnaires need to be tested further in both longitudinal and cross-sectional studies in PD patients, even the ones classified as "Recommended" or "Suggested." However, it does however not seem feasible for a single ideal scale to serve equally both epidemiological and interventional studies. Different scales can be applied for different purposes. In addition to a global scale designed to assess autonomic symptoms, there is a need to validate a simple scale specifically designed to screen for, or to assess the severity of, symptoms related to OH in PD. The OGS, the COMPASS orthostatic subsection, or some scales used in clinical trials designed to assess the effects of anti-hypotensive drugs may serve as a basis for such a severity scale. Complex and extensive scales such as COMPASS may be more useful in clinical research studies.

RECOMMENDED SCALES for Severity Rating
SCOPA-AUT
COMPosite Autonomic Symptom Scale (COMPASS)
Novel Non-Motor Symptoms Scale (NMSS)
RECOMMENDED SCALES for Screening
NMS Quest

References

1. The Consensus Committee of the American Autonomic Society and the American Academy of Neurology. Consensus statement on the definition of orthostatic hypotension, pure autonomic failure, and multiple system atrophy. *Neurology.* 1996;46:1470.
2. Kaufmann H. Consensus statement on the definition of orthostatic hypotension, pure autonomic failure and multiple system atrophy. *Clin Auton Res.* 1996;6:125–126.
3. Low PA. Prevalence of orthostatic hypotension. *Clin Auton Res.* 2008;18(suppl 1):8–13.
4. Rose KM, Eigenbrodt ML, Biga RL, et al. Orthostatic hypotension predicts mortality in middle-aged adults: the Atherosclerosis Risk in Communities (ARIC) Study. *Circulation.* 2006;114:630–636.
5. Verwoert GC, Mattace-Raso FU, Hofman A, et al. Orthostatic hypotension and risk of cardiovascular disease in elderly people: the Rotterdam study. *J Am Geriatr Soc.* 2008;56:1816–1820.
6. Senard JM, Raï S, Lapeyre-Mestre M, et al. Prevalence of orthostatic hypotension in Parkinson's disease. *J Neurol Neurosurg Psychiatry.* 1997;63:584–589.
7. Goldstein DS. Dysautonomia in Parkinson's disease: neurocardiological abnormalities. *Lancet Neurol.* 2003;2(11):669–676. Review. Erratum in: *Lancet Neurol.* 2004; 3:68.
8. Allcock LM, Ullyart K, Kenny RA, Burn DJ. Frequency of orthostatic hypotension in a community based cohort of patients with Parkinson's disease. *J Neurol Neurosurg Psychiatry.* 2004;75:1470–1471.
9. Pathak A, Senard JM. Pharmacology of orthostatic hypotension in Parkinson's disease: from pathophysiology to management. *Expert Rev Cardiovasc Ther.* 2004;2:393–403.

10. Pathak A, Senard JM. Blood pressure disorders during Parkinson's disease: epidemiology, pathophysiology and management. *Expert Rev Neurother.* 2006;6:1173–1180.

11. Kujawa K, Leurgans S, Raman R, Blasucci L, Goetz CG. Acute orthostatic hypotension when starting dopamine agonists in Parkinson's disease. *Arch Neurol.* 2000;57:1461–1463.

12. Senard JM, Brefel-Courbon C, Rascol O, Montastruc JL. Orthostatic hypotension in patients with Parkinson's disease: pathophysiology and management. *Drugs Aging.* 2001;18:495–505.

13. Goldstein DS, Eldadah BA, Holmes C, et al. Neurocirculatory abnormalities in Parkinson disease with orthostatic hypotension: independence from levodopa treatment. *Hypertension.* 2005;46:1333–1339.

14. Fujishiro H, Frigerio R, Burnett M, et al. Cardiac sympathetic denervation correlates with clinical and pathologic stages of Parkinson's disease. *Mov Disord.* 2008;23:1085–1092.

15. Novak V, Novak P, Spies JM, Low PA. Autoregulation of cerebral blood flow in orthostatic hypotension. *Stroke.* 1998;29:104–111.

16. Evatt ML, Chaudhuri KR, Chou KL, et al. Dysautonomia rating scales in Parkinson's disease: sialorrhea, dysphagia, and constipation. Critique and recommendations to Movement Disorders Task Force on Rating Scales for Parkinson's Disease. *Mov Disord.* 2009;24(5):635–646.

17. Lahrmann H, Cortelli P, Hilz M, Mathias CJ, Struhal W, Tassinari M. EFNS guidelines on the diagnosis and management of orthostatic hypotension. *Eur J Neurol.* 2006;13:930–936.

18. Gilman S, Wenning GK, Low PA, et al. Second consensus statement on the diagnosis of multiple system atrophy. *Neurology.* 2008;71:670–676.

19. Vinik AI, Ziegler D. Diabetic cardiovascular autonomic neuropathy. *Circulation.* 2007;115:387–397.

20. Visser M, Marinus J, Stiggelbout AM, Van Hilten JJ. Assessment of autonomic dysfunction in Parkinson's disease: the SCOPA-AUT. *Mov Disord.* 2004;19:1306–1312.

21. Suarez GA, Opfer-Gehrking TL, Offord KP, Atkinson EJ, O'Brien PC, Low PA. The Autonomic Symptom Profile: a new instrument to assess autonomic symptoms. *Neurology.* 1999;52(3):523–528.

22. Chaudhuri KR, Martinez-Martin P, Schapira AH, et al. International multicenter pilot study of the first comprehensive self-completed nonmotor symptoms questionnaire for Parkinson's disease: the NMSQuest study. *Mov Disord.* 2006;21:916–923.

23. Martinez-Martin P, Schapira AH, Stocchi F, et al. Prevalence of nonmotor symptoms in Parkinson's disease in an international setting; study using nonmotor symptoms questionnaire in 545 patients. *Mov Disord.* 2007;22:1623–1629.

24. Chaudhuri KR, Martinez-Martin P, Brown RG, et al. The metric properties of a novel non-motor symptoms scale for Parkinson's disease: results from an international pilot study. *Mov Disord.* 2007;22:1901–1911.

25. Goetz CG, Tilley BC, Shaftman SR, et al; for the Movement Disorder Society UPDRS Revision Task Force. Movement Disorder Society-sponsored revision of the Unified Parkinson's Disease Rating Scale (MDS-UPDRS): scale presentation and clinimetric testing results. *Mov Disord.* 2008;23:2129–2170.

26. Magerkurth C, Schnitzer R, Braune S. Symptoms of autonomic failure in Parkinson's disease: prevalence and impact on daily life. *Clin Auton Res.* 2005;15:76–82.

27. Siddiqui MF, Rast S, Lynn MJ, Auchus AP, Pfeiffer RF. Autonomic dysfunction in Parkinson's disease: a comprehensive symptom survey. *Parkinsonism Relat Disord.* 2002;8:277–284.

28. Hobson P, Islam W, Roberts S, Adhiyman V, Meara J. The risk of bladder and autonomic dysfunction in a community cohort of Parkinson's disease patients and normal controls. *Parkinsonism Relat Disord.* 2003;10:67–71.

29. Schrezenmaier C, Gehrking JA, Hines SM, Low PA, Benrud-Larson LM, Sandroni P. Evaluation of orthostatic hypotension: relationship of a new self-report instrument to laboratory-based measures. *Mayo Clin Proc.* 2005;80:330–334.

30. Mathias CJ, Senard JM, Braune S, et al. L-threo-dihydroxyphenylserine (L-threo-DOPS; droxidopa) in the management of neurogenic orthostatic hypotension: a multi-national, multi-center, dose-ranging study in multiple system atrophy and pure autonomic failure. *Clin Auton Res.* 2001;11:235–242.

31. Mathias CJ. L-dihydroxyphenylserine (Droxidopa) in the treatment of orthostatic hypotension: the European experience. *Clin Auton Res.* 2008;18(suppl 1):25–29.

32. Low PA, Gilden JL, Freeman R, Sheng KN, McElligott MA. Efficacy of midodrine vs placebo in neurogenic orthostatic hypotension. A randomized, double-blind multicenter study. Midodrine Study Group. *JAMA*. 1997;277:1046–1051.

33. Wright RA, Kaufmann HC, Perera R, et al. A double-blind, dose-response study of midodrine in neurogenic orthostatic hypotension. *Neurology*. 1998;51:120–124.

34. Wenning GK, Tison F, Seppi K, et al. Multiple System Atrophy Study Group. Development and validation of the Unified Multiple System Atrophy Rating Scale (UMSARS). *Mov Disord*. 2004;19:1391–402.

35. Low PA. Composite autonomic scoring scale for laboratory quantification of generalized autonomic failure. *Mayo Clin Proc*. 1993;68:748–752.

36. Low PA, Opfer-Gehrking TL, McPhee BR, et al. Prospective evaluation of clinical characteristics of orthostatic hypotension. *Mayo Clin Proc*. 1995;70:617–622.

37. Verbaan D, Marinus J, Visser M, van Rooden SM, Stiggelbout AM, van Hilten JJ. Patient-reported autonomic symptoms in Parkinson disease. *Neurology*. 2007;69:333–341.

38. Papapetropoulos S, Argyriou AA, Chroni E. No correlation between the clinical severity of autonomic symptoms (SCOPA-AUT) and electrophysiological test abnormalities in advanced Parkinson's disease. *Mov Disord*. 2006;21:430–431.

39. Idiaquez J, Benarroch EE, Rosales H, Milla P, Ríos L. Autonomic and cognitive dysfunction in Parkinson's disease. *Clin Auton Res*. 2007;17:93–98.

40. Martinez-Martin P, Arroyo S, Rojo-Abuin JM, Rodriguez-Blazquez C, Frades B, de Pedro Cuesta J. Longitudinal Parkinson's Disease Patient Study (Estudio longitudinal de pacientes con enfermedad de Parkinson-ELEP) Group. Burden, perceived health status, and mood among caregivers of Parkinson's disease patients. *Mov Disord*. 2008;23:1673–1680.

41. Oh ES, Lee JH, Seo JG, Sohn EH, Lee AY. Autonomic and cognitive functions in Parkinson's disease (PD). *Arch Gerontol Geriatr*. 2011;52:84–88.

42. Rodriguez-Blazquez C, Forjaz MJ, Frades-Payo B, de Pedro-Cuesta J, Martinez-Martin P. Longitudinal Parkinson's Disease Patient Study, estudio longitudinal de pacientes con enfermedad de Parkinson Group. Independent validation of the scales for outcomes in Parkinson's disease–autonomic (SCOPA-AUT). *Eur J Neurol*. 2010;17:194–201.

43. Forjaz MJ, Ayala A, Rodriguez-Blazquez C, Frades-Payo B, Martinez-Martin P. Longitudinal Parkinson's Disease Patient Study, estudio longitudinal de pacientes con enfermedad de Parkinson-ELEP Group. Assessing autonomic symptoms of Parkinson's disease with the SCOPA-AUT: a new perspective from Rasch analysis. *Eur J Neurol*. 2010;17:273–279.

44. Carod-Artal FJ, Ribeiro Lda S, Kummer W, Martinez-Martin P. Psychometric properties of the SCOPA-AUT Brazilian Portuguese version. *Mov Disord*. 2010;25:205–212.

45. Cervantes-Arriaga A, Rodríguez-Violante M, Villar-Velarde A, López-Gómez M, Corona T. Metric properties of clinimetric indexes for non-motor dysfunction of Parkinson's disease in Mexican population. *Rev Invest Clin*. 2010;62:8–14. (Article in Spanish).

46. Damon-Perrière N, Foubert-Samier N, Cochen De Cock V, Gerdelat-Mas A, Debs R, Pavy-Le Traon A, Rascol O, Tison F, Meissner W. Assessment of the Scopa-Aut questionnaire in multiple system atrophy: Relation to UMSARS scores and progression over time. *Parkinsonism & Related Disorders*, in press.

47. Schoffer KL, Henderson RD, O'Maley K, O'Sullivan JD. Nonpharmacological treatment, fludrocortisone, and domperidone for orthostatic hypotension in Parkinson's disease. *Mov Disord*. 2007;22:1543–1549.

48. Newton JL, Okonkwo O, Sutcliffe K, Seth A, Shin J, Jones DE. Symptoms of autonomic dysfunction in chronic fatigue syndrome. *QJM*. 2007;100:519–526.

49. Cai FZ, Lester S, Lu T, et al. Mild autonomic dysfunction in primary Sjögren's syndrome: a controlled study. *Arthritis Res Ther*. 2008;10:31.

50. Chaudhuri KR, Martinez-Martin P. Quantitation of non-motor symptoms in Parkinson's disease. *Eur J Neurol*. 2008;15 (suppl 2):2–7.

51. Chaudhuri KR, Naidu Y. Early Parkinson's disease and non-motor issues. *J Neurol*. 2008;255(suppl5):33–38.

52. Chaudhuri KR, Prieto-Jurcynska C, Naidu Y, et al. The nondeclaration of nonmotor symptoms of Parkinson's disease to health care professionals: an international study using the nonmotor symptoms questionnaire. *Mov Disord*. 2010;25(6):697–701.

53. Rodríguez-Violante M, Cervantes-Arriaga A, Villar-Velarde A, Corona T. Prevalence of non-

motor dysfunction among Parkinson's disease patients from a tertiary referral center in Mexico City. *Clin Neurol Neurosurg.* 2010;112:883–885.

54. Storch A, Odin P, Trender-Gerhard I, et al. Non-motor Symptoms Questionnaire and Scale for Parkinson's disease. Cross-cultural adaptation into the German language. *Nervenarzt.* 2010;81(8):980–985 (Article in German).

5. Martinez-Martin P, Rodriguez-Blazquez C, Abe K, et al. International study on the psychometric attributes of the non-motor symptoms scale in Parkinson disease. *Neurology.* 2009;73(19):1584–1591.

56 Honig H, Antonini A, Martinez-Martin P, et al. Intrajejunal levodopa infusion in Parkinson's disease: a pilot multicenter study of effects on nonmotor symptoms and quality of life. *Mov Disord.* 2009;24(10):1468–1474.

57. Kim HJ, Park SY, Cho YJ, et al. Nonmotor symptoms in de novo Parkinson disease before and after dopaminergic treatment. *J Neurol Sci.* 2009;287(1–2):200–204.

58. Wang G, Hong Z, Cheng Q, et al. Validation of the Chinese non-motor symptoms scale for Parkinson's disease: results from a Chinese pilot study. *Clin Neurol Neurosurg.* 2009;111(6): 523–526.

59. Li H, Zhang M, Chen L, et al. Nonmotor symptoms are independently associated with impaired health-related quality of life in Chinese patients with Parkinson's disease. *Mov Disord.* 2010;25(16):2740–2746.

60. Movement Disorder Society Task Force on Rating Scales for Parkinson's Disease. The Unified Parkinson's Disease Rating Scale (UPDRS): status and recommendations. *Mov Disord.* 2003;18(7):738–750.

61. Goetz CG, Fahn S, Martinez-Martin P, et al. Movement Disorder Society-sponsored revision of the Unified Parkinson's Disease Rating Scale (MDS-UPDRS): process, format, and clinimetric testing plan. *Mov Disord.* 2007;22(1):41–47.

62. Zibetti M, Torre E, Cinquepalmi A, et al. Motor and nonmotor symptom follow-up in parkinsonian patients after deep brain stimulation of the subthalamic nucleus. *Eur Neurol.* 2007;58(4):218–223.

63. Kaufmann H. Could treatment with DOPS do for autonomic failure what DOPA did for Parkinson's disease? *Neurology.* 1996;47:1370–1371.

64. Sobue I, Senda Y, Hirayama K, et al. Clinical pharmacological evaluation of L-threo-3-4-dihydroxyphenylserine (L-DOPS) in Shy-Drager's syndrome and its related diseases. A nation-wide double-blind comparative study. *Jpn J Clin Exp Med.* 1987;141:353–378.

65 Kaufmann H. L-dihydroxyphenylserine (Droxidopa): a new therapy for neurogenic orthostatic hypotension: the US experience. *Clin Auton Res.* 2008;18(suppl 1):19–24.

17

FATIGUE RATING SCALES IN PARKINSON'S DISEASE

Guido Alves

Summary

Fatigue is a frequent and potentially disabling non-motor problem in patients with Parkinson's disease. Fatigue may occur in all stages of PD, including the pre-motor phase. A number of studies on the epidemiology of fatigue in PD have been conducted, but rather few on its neurobiology and treatment. A task force commissioned by the Movement Disorder Society recently assessed psychometric and clinical properties of clinical fatigue rating scales and provided critique and recommendations for their use to screen or measure severity of fatigue in PD. Based on the MDS report on fatigue rating scales and systematic review of more recent literature, this chapter provides an overview of scale properties of clinical fatigue rating scales that have been applied in PD. Scales were rated as "Recommended," "Suggested," or "Listed" with respect to their usefulness to screen for or measure severity of fatigue, according to criteria used by the MDS task force for fatigue rating scales. A scale was "recommended" if it (1) has been used in PD, (2) has been used in clinical studies by others than the developers, and (3) has been shown to be valid, reliable and sensitive to change in PD. A scale was "suggested" when it did not meet all the criteria of a "recommended" scale, usually the criterion of documented sensitivity to change in PD. Scales were "listed" if they had been used in PD studies but had little or no psychometric data to assess. The Fatigue Severity Scale and the Parkinson Fatigue Scale were "recommended" for both screening and severity rating. The Fatigue Assessment Inventory was "suggested" for both screening and severity. The Functional Assessment of Chronic Illness Therapy-Fatigue was "recommended" for screening and "suggested" for severity. The Multidimensional Fatigue Inventory was "suggested" for screening and "recommended" for severity. The Fatigue Impact Scale for Daily Use was "listed" for screening and "suggested" for severity. The Fatigue Severity Inventory, the Chalder Fatigue Questionnaire, and the Visual Analogue and Global Impression Scales were all "listed" for both screening and severity. Several of the "suggested" scales show good clinimetric properties in non PD-populations and have the potential to achieve "recommended" status if successfully tested in PD. In particular, formal validation of responsiveness is warranted for all scales. No new scales are needed until the available scales are fully tested clinimetrically.

INTRODUCTION

Fatigue is a frequent complaint in a wide range of medical, psychiatric, and neurological conditions, including Parkinson's disease.[1] In PD, fatigue may antedate the motor onset[2] and is common in early, yet-untreated patients.[3] The prevalence of fatigue tends to increase with disease progression,[2,4] affecting 60% or more of patients with more advanced disease.[1,4-6] The etiology of fatigue in PD is little explored and hence poorly understood, although some progress has been made in recent years.[3,7] There is no established treatment for fatigue in PD.[8-12] Effective therapies, however, are urgently needed, given the negative impact of fatigue on daily functioning, work ability,[13] and quality of life.[6,14-16] Still, fatigue is under-recognized in the clinical setting, even by specialists.[17-19]

Both in clinical practice and research there is a need for clinical fatigue measures that are appropriate for the use in PD and sufficiently comprehensive, valid, reliable, and responsive. The Movement Disorders Society commissioned a task force to evaluate existing clinical rating scales addressing symptoms of fatigue in PD. Based on the report[20] of the MDS task force on fatigue rating scales and systematic review of more recent literature, this chapter provides a critique of clinical and psychometric properties of fatigue measures in PD, as well as recommendations for their use to screen or measure severity of fatigue in PD.

METHODS

This chapter is largely based on a task force report to the MDS. The definitions of "Recommended," "Suggested" and "Listed" and the following methods here are consistent with those used by the MDS Task Force on fatigue rating scales in PD. To be "recommended," a scale had to have been applied to PD populations with adequate clinimetric properties in PD.[20]

In addition to the literature research conducted by the members of the MDS Task Force on fatigue rating scales,[20] which included publications up until October of 2008, PubMed was searched for relevant papers published between November, 2008, and May, 2011. The search terms were "PD," "Parkinsonism," "Parkinson disease," and "fatigue." For each scale identified, another search was conducted for the term "PD" ("Parkinsonism" or "Parkinson disease") and the name of the scale. The search was limited to published or "in press" peer-reviewed papers or published abstracts. In addition, the review limited the term's use for severity ratings to those scales shown to be sensitive to change.

Only scales devoted to the assessment of fatigue and those that have been used in PD were considered. Scales that include fatigue items but assess clinical symptoms more broadly, such as health-status measures, health-related quality of life scales, the non-motor symptoms scale (NMSS),[21] or the MDS-UPDRS,[22] were not evaluated.

RESULTS

Identified scales

In the MDS Task Force report,[20] seven fatigue rating scales had been identified that have undergone some validation and have been used in PD: the Fatigue Severity Scale (FSS), Fatigue Assessment Inventory (FAI), Functional Assessment of Chronic Illness Therapy–Fatigue (FACIT-F) scale, Multidimensional Fatigue Inventory (MFI), Parkinson Fatigue Scale (PFS), Fatigue Severity Inventory (FSI), and the Fatigue Impact Scale for Daily Use (D-FIS). Search of more recent literature identified another scale, the Chalder Fatigue Questionnaire (CFQ), which had been used (but not validated) in one PD study. Visual analogue scales (VASs) and clinical global impression scales (CGIS), including the Rhoten Fatigue Scale (RFS), are also addressed as they have been used in PD. However, these scales were used primarily to provide confirmatory support for the other identified scales, but their psychometric properties have not been studied in PD.

The scale characteristics are provided in Table 17-1. Each scale was given a separate rating for screening and for measuring severity of fatigue, as summarized in Table 17-2.

Table 17-1. Characteristics of Clinical Fatigue Measures Used in PD

SCALE NAME	DEFINITION OF FATIGUE PROVIDED	SCORE RANGE	DIMENSIONS	NO. OF ITEMS INCLUDED	TIME FRAME (WEEKS) COVERED	NO. OF POINTS FOR SEVERITY RATING	CUTOFF PROPOSED	TIME (MINUTES) TO ADMINISTER
FSS	No	1–7	Unidimensional	9	2	7	Yes	5
FAI	Yes	1–7	Multidimensional	29	2	7	Yes	10–30
FACIT-F	No	0–52	Unidimensional	13	1	5	Yes	5
MFI	No	4–20*	Multidimensional	20	"Lately"	5	No	10–20
PFS	No	Variable	Unidimensional	16	2	2 or 5	Yes	15
D-FIS	Yes	0–32	Unidimensional	8	Today	5	No	5
FSI	No	Not stated	Multidimensional	33	Not stated	7	No	20–30
CFQ	Yes	Variable	Two-dimensional	11	4	2 or 4	Yes	5
VAS	No standard	Variable	-	1	Variable	Continuous	No	1
CGI	No standard	Variable	-	1	Variable	Variable	No	1

*Score range for each dimension.

Table 17-2. Rating of Fatigue Measures in PD According to Criteria Used by the MDS Task Force for Fatigue Rating Scales in Parkinson's Disease

	APPLIED IN PD	USED BY MULTIPLE GROUPS	SATISFACTORY CLINIMETRIC ASSESSMENT IN PD			ENDORSEMENT FOR SEVERITY RATING	ENDORSEMENT FOR SCREENING
			RELIABILITY	VALIDITY	RESPONSIVENESS		
SCALE NAME							
FSS	√	√	√	√	√c	Recommended	Recommended
FAI	√	√			√c	Suggested	Suggested
FACIT-F	√	√	√	√		Suggested	Recommended
MFI	√	√	√	√a	√c	Recommended	Suggested
PFS	√	√	√	√	√c	Recommended	Recommended
D-FIS	√	√	√	√b		Suggested	Listed
FSI	√					Listed	Listed
CFQ	√					Listed	Listed
VAS	√					Listed	Listed
CGI	√					Listed	Listed

a Lack of data to support discriminant validity.
b No cutoff established.
c Clinical data to support responsiveness.

Confounds associated with the application of fatigue rating scales

INCONSISTENT DEFINITIONS

As explained in the task force report on which this chapter is based,[20] in the absence of a biological marker or gold standard for defining fatigue, the lack of a consistent definition for fatigue represents the greatest challenge to its measurement. The presence of subtypes of fatigue is another source of scale variation that influences psychometric performance. "Peripheral fatigue" refers to actual muscle fatigue induced by repetitive contractions[23,24] and can be measured objectively as decreased force generation or the inability to sustain repetitive movements. Although "central fatigue," the perception of feeling fatigued, is the usual focus of subjective complaints of fatigue, patients do not necessarily distinguish muscular fatigue that occurs with exercise from their subjective perceptions of fatigue.[25] Central fatigue is generally described as an abnormal degree of persistent tiredness, weakness, or exhaustion that is mental, physical, or both, in the absence of motor or physical impairment outside the central nervous system.[23,24] Physical fatigue (PF) involves a sense of physical exhaustion and lack of energy to perform physical tasks despite the ability and motivation to perform them. Mental fatigue (MF) refers to the cognitive effects experienced during and after prolonged periods of demanding cognitive activities and tasks that require sustained concentration and mental endurance. Assessments of cognitive and motor processing over a given time interval provide objective measurements of the mental and physical components of central fatigue. However, the overlap between MF and PF symptoms may not be clear on rating scales; not all scales distinguish the two types of fatigue. Sleep may be a confounding factor as well.

Only three of the eight reviewed scales provide an explicit definition of fatigue for the respondent. These were the D-FIS, FAI, and CFQ. Although there are objective measures of neuromuscular fatigue, the experience of fatigue as a symptom is subjective, and all of the rating scales are, appropriately, self-rated. However,

as the constructs of fatigue are variably defined by the developer of each scale, the various scales may attach different weights to different aspects of fatigue depending upon the scale developer's conceptualization of fatigue, which features of fatigue are addressed by the scale items, and the respondent's own interpretation of the questions.[24] Because there are controversies around the definition of fatigue, provision of a definition preceding the scale generally represents an advantage; it makes explicit what concepts are embedded in the definition of fatigue for that scale and the constructs inherent to the development of the scale. Such knowledge facilitates selection of the most adequate instrument for a given purpose.

The subjective nature of fatigue also affects the ability of fatigue rating scales to provide valid measures of variations in fatigue severity. Some scales measure the presence or absence of fatigue-related symptoms on a spectrum without creating a threshold for a determination of yes—"fatigued" or no—"not fatigued." Other scales may be used to classify patients as suffering from fatigue. Availability of a metric that defines minimal, mild, moderate, and severe fatigue provides a basis for clinical interventions and outcomes assessments.

However, without "external markers" for fatigue, the limits and thresholds for perceptions such as fatigue are difficult to determine. The same theoretical degree of fatigue will not be perceived with the same intensity by different subjects, and its manifestation will be differentially modulated by personal factors.

OVERLAP OF FATIGUE WITH NEUROPSYCHIATRIC DISTURBANCES

The interpretation of fatigue assessments is significantly confounded by the association of fatigue with other non-motor symptoms frequently associated with PD, such as depression, anxiety, cognitive dysfunction, apathy, and sleep disturbances. Fatigue is one of the diagnostic criteria for the DSM-IV diagnoses of a major depressive episode as well as generalized anxiety disorder,[26] and it is often included as one of the items in mood symptom rating scales. Sleep and cognitive difficulties are also diagnostic criteria for depressive and anxiety disorders. In patients with PD, fatigue is associated with higher rates of depressive symptoms, but it also occurs in non-depressed patients.[4,27] In some regression analyses, the presence of fatigue was predicted only by depressive symptoms, whereas in other studies, a variety of symptoms, including depression, anxiety, pain, axial symptoms, reduced motivation (RM), daytime sleepiness, and motor impairment were predictive.[2,4] As treatments for fatigue may be different than those used to treat depression or anxiety, it is important that rating scales are sensitive to the detection of fatigue in patients without mood symptoms. Longitudinal analyses that include DSM-IV diagnoses, mood symptom ratings, and fatigue rating scales provide a basis for determining whether the scales are sensitive to changes in fatigue over time relative to the experience of mood symptoms.

Symptoms of fatigue and cognitive dysfunction may also overlap in PD, with potential influence on the validity of self-report fatigue rating scales. Cognitive impairment in PD, especially the presence of dementia, may preclude valid completion of self-report scales, and patients with significant cognitive dysfunction are therefore usually excluded from validation studies. Cognitive changes in PD, even early in its course, may include attentional difficulties that overlap with the phenomenon of MF, manifesting as difficulties with sustained attention or with initiation of activities.[25] Several studies show that fatigue is associated with greater cognitive dysfunction in PD.[4,28] Even though fatigue also occurs in patients with PD with no or limited cognitive dysfunction, presence of MF may be least evident to those most affected by cognitive dysfunction and may be difficult to distinguish from apathy. Patients may also be unable to distinguish fatigue symptoms from sleepiness on self-report scales.

UNIDIMENSIONAL VERSUS MULTIDIMENSIONAL SCALES

Scales may be aimed at measuring a single (unidimensional) or diverse (multidimensional) attributes of the construct being measured. Unidimensionality is a characteristic inherent to a physical measure (e.g., distance or volume), but the constructs in health-related areas are often complex, so that it may be easier to capture a set of aspects connected to them by means of multidimensional evaluations. However, although scales that assess different manifestations of a feature (e.g., PF and MF) are multidimensional, each *domain* (subscale) needs to be unidimensional. This is a fundamental assumption in traditional as well as modern psychometric theory[29] that may or may not be met at both the subscale and the total scale levels, depending on conceptualization and operationalization of the construct. Frequently, multidimensional scales intend to represent the construct's value by means of a global score obtained from the sum of their components' scores, but such strategy has scientific problems.[30,31] For example, individual item scores are usually ordinal rather than continuous. In addition, response options from different items are considered equivalent, and the contribution of the items to the final score is assumed to be homogeneous, which is not always accurate. Solutions for this dilemma are not easy because the alternatives are not free of problems.[32] In this situation, it is recommended that: (1) development and analysis of rating scales be carried out with strict compliance to the highest and most updated quality standards; (2) outcomes must always be interpreted with caution; and (3) new theories and models must be developed and explored.

THE FATIGUE SEVERITY SCALE
Scale description
STRUCTURE

The FSS is a self-rated unidimensional generic nine-item fatigue rating scale.[33] The FSS emphasizes functional impact of fatigue and contains items on physical and mental fatigue and social aspects, although these are not divided into explicit domains. Items are brief and easily understandable statements related to fatigue that are rated on a seven-grade Likert scale. Only the respective ends of the scale are defined (*completely disagree* = 1 to *completely agree* = 7). The total FSS score represents the mean score of each of the nine items, yielding a score range between 1 and 7. Higher scores indicate a higher level of fatigue. Although not explicitly recommended in the original study,[33] a cutoff of 4 and a time frame covering the past two weeks are used by the developers (personal communication) and most other groups.[34] However, other cutoff values have been used and suggested to be more appropriate.[35] The FSS provides no definition of fatigue.[33]

HANDLING COMORBIDITIES

Potential overlap with PD symptoms (physical limitations due to PD [3 items] and apathy [1 item]) is present in at least 4 items (44%).

ADDITIONAL POINTS

The FSS has been translated into numerous languages. The scale is copyrighted but freely available from its developers.

Key evaluation issues

USE IN PD AND APPLICATIONS ACROSS THE DISEASE SPECTRUM

The clinimetric properties of the FSS have been assessed in various diseases[34,36-52] and the general population.[35] In PD, the FSS has been used as outcome measure in numerous studies. The scale has been validated in PD by independent groups[36,52] in non-demented patients without clinically significant neuropsychiatric comorbidities.[36,52] No restrictions are mentioned regarding disease stage.[36,52]

USE BY MULTIPLE AUTHORS

The FSS is the most frequently used fatigue-specific scale in chronic diseases[53] and has been tested clinimetrically by multiple authors.

CLINIMETRIC ISSUES

Studies in non-PD populations usually demonstrate high rates (>95%) of data being fully computable.[37,54] Floor and ceiling effects are generally low.[37,46] Score distribution is normal.[37,55]

Reliability: Internal consistency is high (Cronbach's alpha > 80).[33,38,43,44,46,48-51,56] Inter-item correlations range from 0.35 to 0.91 in diseased people, with somewhat lower values found in the general population.[35,37,51,56] Corrected item-total correlations and intra-class correlation coefficients exceed the minimal standard values.[35,37,39,43,48-51,56]

Validity: The FSS discriminates significantly between diseased and non-diseased subjects.[39,47,49,51] Construct validity of the FSS is further supported by usually moderate to strong correlations with visual analogue scales and various fatigue rating scales.[34,45,47,48,50,51,56-59] Expected correlations have also been observed with scales measuring partly related constructs including depression,[33,56,60,61] daytime sleepiness,[51,62] sleep quality, and quality of life.[19,37,43,49,63,64] Factor analysis demonstrates unidimensionality of the FSS in various patient groups,[43,44,50] although misfit of single items has been reported.[40,48]

Responsiveness: Results on the FSS's sensitivity to change compared to other fatigue measures in non-PD disorders are inconsistent.[33,59,65-67] The *MCID* for the FSS was estimated to be 0.6 (95% CI 0.3-0.9) in systemic lupus erythematosus.[68] In rheumatoid arthritis, a 10% to 15% change in FSS was suggested to be clinically meaningful.[41]

Psychometric properties in PD generally resemble those in non-PD populations. In a PD sample comprising non-demented patients with HY stages ranging from I to V, missing item responses were 0.8% and data were fully computable in 95.8% of subjects.[52] Floor and ceiling effects were minimal (2.5%).[52] These data support the appropriateness of the FSS in PD.

Reliability: The FSS demonstrates excellent reliability with a Cronbach's alpha value of 0.94 found in two independent studies, and a split half reliability of 0.86 and 0.91.[36,52] Observed inter-item correlations in PD range from 0.27 to 0.78.[36]

Validity: The FSS discriminates PD from healthy controls [36,69] and severe coxarthrosis,[69] and correctly, but to a lesser extent than the FACIT-F, discriminates between PD patients classified as non-fatigued and fatigued as measured by the Energy subscale of the Nottingham Health Profile (NHP-EN).[4,52] Construct validity of the FSS in PD is further supported by moderate to strong correlations with other fatigue measures, such as the FACIT-F (r = −0.77),[52] the NHP-EN (r = 0.62),[52] the Parkinson Fatigue Scale (PFS) (r = 0.84),[36] and a one-question fatigue rating (r = 0.80).[36] Low to moderate correlations were found between FSS scores and quality of life measures (PDQ-39: r = 0.22–0.47; MOS-SF-36: r = 0.37),[14,70] the HY stage (r = 0.38), and the UPDRS total score (r = 0.41).[14] Low correlations were observed between the FSS and the HAM-D (r = 0.19).[3] Correlations were also found in PD between the FSS and reduced physical activity and function, and functional capacity.[71] No correlations were found with striatal dopamine transporter density.[3] While Rasch analysis identified FSS-item 1 as not meeting unidimensionality criteria, exploratory factor analysis resulted in one factor, supporting the unidimensionality of the FSS in PD.[52] Potential DIF by age was found for items 1 and 8 using t-tests, but this difference did not remain significant after Bonferroni correction for multiple comparisons.[52]

Responsiveness: Two clinical trials suggest the FSS to be sensitive to change with time and treatment in PD.[3,10] In the ELLDOPA trial, the mean FSS score increased by 0.75 points (19%) during 42 weeks in the placebo group, while the increase in FSS score was 0.30 to 0.36 (7%–8%) in those receiving levodopa.[3] In a six-week double-blind placebo-controlled trial of methylphenidate in PD, FSS scores improved by 14.8% in those receiving active treatment vs. 4.2% improvement in patients on placebo.[10] Cohen's effect size for the reduction in FSS score was 0.79, compared to 0.62 for the reduction in MFI score.[10] The MCID has not been assessed in PD.

Strengths and weaknesses

Strengths of the FSS include the good psychometric properties in non-PD and PD populations (including discrimination between fatigued and non-fatigued patients), and its

brevity and ease of administration. In addition, the FSS has been translated into and validated in various languages. Limitations include the lack of definition of the underlying variable it intends to measure. In addition, the extent to which the scale items overlap with self-rated mood symptoms in PD has not been explored. Finally, although sensitivity to change has been demonstrated in two clinical trials, responsiveness in terms of MCID remains to be determined in PD.

Final assessment

The FSS fulfils the criteria of a "Recommended" scale, both for screening and severity rating of fatigue in PD.

THE FATIGUE ASSESSMENT INVENTORY

Scale description

STRUCTURE

The Fatigue Assessment Instrument (FAI) is an expanded version of the FSS.[34] This self-administered multidimensional fatigue rating scale was developed to allow the assessment of fatigue symptomatology across various medical conditions. The 29 items including in the FAI are statements related to fatigue which are rated on a seven-grade Likert scale. As in the FSS, only the respective ends of the scale are defined (*completely disagree* = 1 to *completely agree* = 7). The FAI comprises four subscales measuring global severity (11 items, of which 8 are from the FSS), situation-specificity (6 items), consequences (3 items), and responsiveness to rest/sleep (2 items) of fatigue, and additional seven items that are not part of these subscales. Subscales and the total FAI scores are calculated by averaging the included item responses, providing a score range from 1 to 7. Higher FAI scores indicate more severe fatigue. Although not explicitly recommended in the original paper, a cutoff of 4 is frequently used. The explored time frame is "the past two weeks."[34] The FAI provides instructions to the user and an explicit definition of fatigue.[34]

HANDLING COMORBIDITIES

There is potential overlap with other PD-related symptoms in at least 13 out of 29 (45%) items (5 items for physical limitations due to PD, and 2 items each for sleep/rest, cognitive impairment, apathy, and depression).

ADDITIONAL POINTS

The scale is copyrighted but freely available from its developers.

Key evaluation issues

USE IN PD AND APPLICATIONS ACROSS THE DISEASE SPECTRUM

A slightly modified version of the FAI (see below) has been used in three studies in PD, conducted by two independent groups. These studies comprised PD patients in various Hoehn and Yahr stages.[11,28,72,73]

USE BY MULTIPLE AUTHORS

The psychometric properties of the FAI were originally validated in a sample of patients with a variety of diagnoses including MS, SLE, Lyme disease, chronic fatigue syndrome, and dysthymia.[34] Since, the FAI has been applied in various other conditions.[11,28,46,72–81]

CLINIMETRIC ISSUES

In non-PD disorders, the FAI possesses acceptable data quality, with low floor and ceiling effects,[46] although missing item responses of up to 17% have been reported.[54]

Reliability: Internal consistency of the FAI subscales is good to excellent, with Cronbach's alpha ranging from 0.70 (consequences of fatigue) to 0.93 (fatigue severity).[34,79,81] Inter-factor correlations are low to moderate.[34] Test-retest correlations in patients with MS were found to be low for the "responsiveness to rest/sleep" subscale (r = 0.29) and moderate for the three other subscales (r = 0.51–0.69).[34] High intra-observer reliability (0.81) was demonstrated in patients with epilepsy.[82]

Validity: The FAI is able to distinguish between several different diagnoses as well as diseased and non-diseased patients, although some studies found no differences between healthy controls and patient groups in one or more subscales.[34,54,74,77,79] As expected, high correlations between the FAI fatigue severity subscale and the FSS have been reported (r = 0.98), indicating appropriate convergent validity for this subscale.[34] Convergent correlations with other measures of fatigue[34,81,83] and divergent correlations with measures of energy[34] are usually found to be moderate.

Responsiveness: Sensitivity to change with time and treatment has been demonstrated for the total FAI and the FAI fatigue severity subscale in clinical trials and observational longitudinal studies.[74,84,85] However, the MCID of the FAI subscales and total FAI has not been determined.

In PD, a slightly modified version of the FAI (one additional item: "During the past week, I have slept very well") has been applied and partly validated.[11,28,72,73] Analysis of the acceptability of the FAI in PD has not been performed. Face validity appears acceptable, although the appropriateness of some situation-specific items for PD is uncertain.

Reliability: Principal components analysis of the modified FAI resulted in nine factors. Cronbach's alpha for these nine factors ranged from 0.27 to 1,[72] but Cronbach's alpha for the FAI subscales were not provided, and other analysis of reliability were not performed.

Validity: FAI total scores discriminate significantly between PD patients and controls.[11,28] Convergent validity with other fatigue scales has not been studied in PD. Low to moderate negative correlations (r ≤ –0.68) with a visual analogue energy scale and positive correlations with depression scores (r < 0.62) have been found.[11,28,72] No correlation was found between the FAI total score and clinical measures of motor and disease severity in PD.[28] One study found significant differences in FAI total score between PD patients with normal vs. reduced perfusion in the frontal lobe as measured by SPECT.[28] In a five-week open clinical trial, total FAI scores significantly decreased in PD patients on pergolide mesilate (5.1 to 4.4) but not in those receiving bromocriptine (4.8 to 4.7), supporting its *responsiveness* to change with treatment.[11] The MCID has not been determined in PD.

Strengths and weaknesses

Strengths include that the FAI is a comprehensive instrument that covers various aspects of fatigue and allows comparison between different disease groups. An explicit definition of fatigue and clear instructions are provided. Items are brief and easily understandable. Weaknesses of the FAI include the lack of data to support its validity (including discriminant) and reliability in PD. Although the FAI shows generally acceptable psychometric properties in non-PD disorders, test-retest reliability is only moderate in non-PD populations. Clinical data support its responsiveness but the MCID has not been assessed. Because of its overall length, the FAI appears less suitable for screening purposes and large-scale studies.

Final Assessment

The (modified) FAI fulfills criteria for a "suggested" fatigue scale in PD for both diagnostic screening and severity of fatigue, as it has not been validated sufficiently in PD.

FUNCTIONAL ASSESSMENT OF CHRONIC ILLNESS THERAPY– FATIGUE SCALE

Scale description

STRUCTURE

The Functional Assessment of Chronic Illness Therapy-Fatigue (FACIT-F) scale was developed from interviews with oncology patients and clinical experts to assess anemia-associated fatigue.[86] It is a patient-reported rating scale consisting of 13 items (statements) with five ordered response categories (*not at all—a little bit—somewhat—quite a bit—very much*) regarding the respondents' situation during the past week.[86,87] It yields a summed total score ranging

between 0 and 52 (52 = less fatigue). Item contents cover the experience (e.g., feelings of tiredness, listlessness, energy) as well as the impact (e.g., trouble doing things, need to sleep, social limitations) of fatigue. Different cutoff scores have been suggested. In patients with cancer, a score of 34 was proposed as a cutoff for cancer-related fatigue.[88] Based on general population and clinical trial data, others have suggested a FACIT-F score of 30 as a cutoff for significant fatigue.[87] This corresponds to fatigue scores associated with troublesome levels of activity limitations.[89] The FACIT-F does not provide a definition of fatigue.

HANDLING COMORBIDITIES

There is potential overlap with other PD-related symptoms (sleep, motor disability) in at least four of 13 (31%) items.

ADDITIONAL POINTS

Although typically used as a traditional paper-and-pencil rating scale, the FACIT-F can be administered via a range of modes (e.g., interview and touch-screen computers).[90] General population norms are available for the United States.[91] The FACIT-F is part of the larger FACIT measurement system[96] and is copyrighted but freely available from its developers (www.facit.org). A manual and scoring algorithm is also available (www.facit.org). The FACIT-F is available in 48 official language versions (facit.org) that have been produced according to rigorous standardized methodology.[93,94]

Key evaluation issues

USE IN PD AND APPLICATIONS ACROSS THE DISEASE SPECTRUM

In PD, the FACIT-F was validated and used as outcome measure in two studies, conducted by the same group and in the same cohort.[2,52] Patients included in these studies were in various disease stages (Hoehn and Yahr stages I to V) but free from significant cognitive impairment and depression.[2,52]

USE BY MULTIPLE AUTHORS

The FACIT-F is one of the most widely used fatigue scales today[95] and has been validated in a range of patient groups, such as rheumatoid arthritis, PD, various forms of cancer, and in the general population.[52,91,96,97]

CLINIMETRIC ISSUES

Studies in non-PD populations conducted by its developers as well as by independent investigators have found the FACIT-F to yield good data quality and *reliability* (coefficient α, 0.86–0.95; test-retest, 0.89–0.90) with a standard error of measurement (SEM) of about 2.3 to 4.3.[86–88,91,97–99] Internal *validity* of the scale has been found adequate with mean inter-item correlations of 0.51, corrected item-total correlations >0.4, and identification of a single dimension in factor analysis.[88,91,99] Construct validity has been supported by expected (−0.68 to −0.88) correlations with other fatigue-related scales.[88,97,99] Divergent validity has been supported by an inverse correlation (0.61) with the POMS vigor scale. Further supporting its validity is its ability to discriminate between people with various hemoglobin and performance levels.[86,88,98,99] Comparisons with other fatigue scales have found the FACIT-F equally or more able to distinguish between such subgroups, and it has been found to represent a broader range of fatigue severity levels than, e.g., the Vitality (VT) scale of the SF-36 and the MAF.[97,99] One study found some DIF between cancer patients and the general population for three FACIT-F items.[100] However, it is unclear whether this influenced the total score. The FACIT-F has been used as an outcome measure in many clinical trials.[97,98,101,102] These studies have supported its *responsiveness*, showing effect sizes in the magnitude of about 0.5 to >0.8. These data have enabled guidance to be developed to aid interpretation of FACIT-F scores and planning of interventional trials.[87] Studies have identified a MCID and change score of about 3 to 4, corresponding to about 1 SEM, 0.5 standard deviation, and an effect size >0.2.[87,97,98,103] However, the MCID appears to be larger among people in palliative cancer care.[102]

In PD, the measurement properties of the FACIT-F resemble those in non-PD populations.[52] The scale has been easy to use with good data quality (<1% missing item responses). *Reliability* has been good (test-retest reliability, 0.85; coefficient alpha, 0.90–0.92), with a SEM of 3.13. Floor and ceiling effects were low (1.7% and 0%, respectively). Construct *validity* was supported by expected correlations with scores on the FSS and the Nottingham Health Profile–energy scale (NHPEN) (−0.77 and −0.70). In a different study,[104] FACIT-F scores correlated strongly (−0.89) with scores on the Parkinson Fatigue Scale. Correlations have also been observed between FACIT-F and MMSE ($r_s = -0.19$) Epworth Sleepiness Scale ($r_s = 0.30$), HADS depression ($r_s = 0.55$) and anxiety ($r_s = 0.54$) scores, pain ($r_s = 0.34$), disease duration ($r_s = 0.23$), UPDRS motor score ($r_s = 0.31$), and Hoehn and Yahr stage.[2] FACIT-F scores discriminated between fatigued and non-fatigued PD patients.[52] The relative efficacy of the FACIT-F and the FSS suggested that the former was about 50% more efficient in detecting differences than the latter. Explorative factor analysis and Rasch analysis provided support for the unidimensionality of the scale. Rasch analysis also suggested that the response categories work as expected and that there is no DIF between genders or older and younger respondents.[52] That is, items work the same way and have the same meaning across these subgroups. There is no evidence regarding the *responsiveness* or MCID of FACIT-F scores in PD. However, the MCID found in non-PD studies is in general agreement with the SEM found in PD.[52] The resemblance between its SEM and MCID in non-PD populations[91,97,98,103] could therefore suggest that an MCID of about 4 FACIT-F points may apply also to PD.[105] Empirical data are, however, needed to confirm or reject this.

Strengths and weaknesses

Strengths: The FACIT-F is brief and has very good psychometric properties, including evidence for good reliability, and internal and external validity in PD. It compares well to other fatigue scales in both PD and non-PD populations. Interpretation guidelines that relate changes and differences in scores to tangible clinical criteria are available in non-PD populations. It is available in a large range of languages, and all translations have been produced in association with the developers of the scale using rigorous methodology.

Weaknesses: There is no clearly stated definition of the underlying variable that it intends to measure. Replication studies are needed to more firmly establish its measurement properties in PD, including evaluations of responsiveness and MCID, which currently are lacking, although available observations indicate better measurement precision than the FSS, thus suggesting it should be responsive.

Final Assessment

The FACIT-F fulfills criteria for a recommended scale for screening and suggested scale for severity rating (as it has not been shown to be sensitive to change in PD).

THE MULTIDIMENSIONAL FATIGUE INVENTORY

Scale description

STRUCTURE

The MFI is a 20-item self-report measure with five dimensions: general fatigue (GF), PF, MF, RM, and reduced activity.[106] Each dimension contains four items, with two items formulated in a positive and two formulated in a negative direction. There are five response options. Items indicative of fatigue must be recoded before adding up, after which higher scores indicate a higher degree of fatigue. Scores range from 4 to 20 for subscales. If one score is required, the GF scale is recommended.[106] The addressed time frame is "lately." The MFI does not provide a definition of fatigue.

HANDLING COMORBIDITIES

Seven of the 16 items (44%) address physical aspects (e.g., "physically I feel only able to do a

little") and may be influenced by physical limitations due to motor impairment. Some further items my also be affected by mood, as well as motivational and cognitive aspects.

ADDITIONAL POINTS

The scale is available in 15 languages. Population-based norm values for healthy populations are available.[107] The scale can be used free of charge for academic use on the condition that the original publication is properly referenced.

Key evaluation issues

USE IN PD AND APPLICATION ACROSS THE DISEASE SPECTRUM

The MFI has been used by independent groups in 16 PD studies. These assessed patients in various disease stages (Hoehn and Yahr stages I to V).

USE BY MULTIPLE AUTHORS

The MFI has been used in over 150 studies and has been validated by independent groups, both in PD and non-PD diseases.

CLINIMETRIC ISSUES

In non-PD populations, the acceptability of the MFI is generally good,[106,108,109] and the scale does not suffer from floor or ceiling effects.[110] The five dimensions of the MFI were postulated in advance and subsequently tested using confirmatory factor analysis. The fit indices in the original publication were good, and retesting by the developers in a different sample confirmed the factor structure.[106,111] Other studies, however, sometimes found different factor solutions.[108,109,112–114] In support of its *reliability*, Cronbach's alpha for the five scales in clinical populations ranged from 0.76 to 0.93 in the original publication.[106] In most independent studies, satisfactory results were also obtained, with values usually well above 0.7 for subscales and above 0.9 for the total score,[108,109] although values <0.70 have occasionally been reported.[112,113,115] The test-retest reliability of the MFI was tested in various patient groups and generally was good, with intra-class correlation coefficients and test-retest correlations ranging from 0.50 to 0.85.[108,112,114,116,117] *Validity* has been extensively evaluated in non-PD populations. All scales discriminated significantly between diseased and non-diseased and between fatigued and non-fatigued subjects.[106,110] Correlations of MFI subscales with other fatigue scales were generally moderate to high.[106,107,112,113,115,118–121] Correlations with scales measuring partly related constructs generally ranged from 0.40 to 0.60 for mood scales and from 0.45 to 0.67 for quality-of-life scales.[107,116] Correlations with hemoglobin values in different patient groups ranged from −0.05 to −0.34.[110,122] *Responsiveness* of the MFI in non-PD populations has been demonstrated, with Cohen's effect sizes of the subscales in different patient groups ranging from 0.16 to 1.55.[110,114,116] A significant decrease in MFI score was found in patients indicating an improvement of more than 2 cm on a VAS-f over a one-month period.[108] The *MCID* for MFI, only provided for the total score (range 20–100), was estimated to be 11.5 (95% CI 8.0–15.0) in systemic lupus erythematosus.[68]

In PD, independent studies[5,123] demonstrate *reliability* of the MFI (Cronbach's alpha = 0.84[5] and intra-class correlation coefficients between 0.70 and 0.87[123]), although test-retest reliability has not been assessed. The *validity* of the MFI has been demonstrated in several studies. PD patients exhibited higher scores in all subscales compared to various control groups.[25,124,125] Convergent validity with other fatigue scales has been established with the FSI, POMS fatigue scale, VAS-energy, VAS-fatigue (VAS-f), D-FIS, and Global Perception of Fatigue.[16,25] Significant correlations have been observed with the PDQ-8 and PDQ-39[15,16] and several depression scales,[5,15,16,25,125,126] but less so with anxiety measures.[5]

Responsiveness of the MFI in PD was assessed in only one randomized controlled trial where the MFI total scale decreased significantly, showing a Cohen's effect size of 0.63, which was somewhat smaller than the 0.79 that was found for the FSS.[10] The MCID of the MFI has not been assessed in PD.

Strengths and weaknesses

Strengths: The MFI is a relatively short but comprehensive scale with good psychometric properties. Validity and reliability have been demonstrated in both PD and non-PD populations. The scale has been shown to be sensitive to change outside of PD and in one study in PD. The MFI includes a subscale to measure MF. Weaknesses: The proposed factor structure has not always been confirmed in independent studies. The covered time frame ("lately") is vague. The MFI does not define fatigue, and there is no information on the MCID.

Final assessment

The MFI fulfils the criteria for a suggested scale for screening (as discrimination between fatigued and non-fatigued PD patients has not been demonstrated) and a recommended scale for severity rating.

PARKINSON FATIGUE SCALE

Scale description

STRUCTURE

The PFS is a 16-item patient-rated scale that was developed to assess a single construct reflecting the physical aspects of fatigue in patients with PD and to measure both the presence of fatigue and its impact on daily function.[127] The scale was developed for use in clinical practice and in research as a screen or to assess fatigue severity in PD. Seven items tap the presence or absence of the subjective experience of fatigue, with an emphasis on the physical effects of fatigue. Nine items address the impact of fatigue on daily functioning and activities, including socialization and work, but not exercise specifically. Neither severity nor frequency of fatigue symptoms is specifically measured. Ratings are based on feelings and experiences over the prior two weeks. The item response options for each PFS item range from 1 (*strongly disagree*) to 5 (*strongly agree*). There are three scoring options. A total PFS score, the average item score across all 16 items, ranges from 1 to 5. A binary scoring method yields scores from 0 to 16, with positive scores for each item generated by agree and strongly agree responses. A third option, calculates total PFS score (range 16–80) based on the sum of scores for the 16 individual items. Based on general population and clinical data, a score of 3.3 (ordinal scoring method, 1–5 range) or 8 (binary scoring method, 0–16 range) have been suggested as cutoff for significant fatigue.[127,128] The scale does not provide a definition of fatigue.

HANDLING COMORBIDITIES

Although the scale was designed to exclude cognitive and emotional features of fatigue, several items assessing the impact of fatigue may reflect mood states or effects on motivation, or may be affected by sleepiness and cognitive impairment.

ADDITIONAL POINTS

The scale, in English, can be obtained free of charge from its developer for academic use. It was formally translated into Swedish[104] and Brazilian-Portuguese[128] as part of separate studies.

Key evaluation issues

USE IN PD AND APPLICATION ACROSS THE DISEASE SPECTRUM

The PFS has been applied by independent groups in several observational studies and clinical trials (see below).

USE BY MULTIPLE AUTHORS

Original testing of the scale was in patients with Parkinsonism identified through PD support groups, of whom the majority were expected to have idiopathic PD. Three additional studies assessed the psychometric properties of the PFS, one in a PD sample relative to healthy controls[36] and the two others in Swedish[104] and Brazilian[128] PD patients using translated versions of the instrument. In addition, a number of more recent clinical and clinicobiological studies used

the PFS to measure fatigue in PD.[7,129–131] The PFS has also been used as outcome measure in several clinical drug trials and other interventional studies.[132–135] Except for healthy controls, the scale has not been used in non-PD patient samples.

CLINIMETRIC ISSUES

Psychometric assessment of the PFS yielded no significant floor or ceiling effects and good data quality and *reliability* (Cronbach's alpha = 0.93–0.98; test-retest = 0.82 using the total score and 0.82 for the binary scoring method).[104,127,128] Internal *validity* of the scale was adequate to high. Split-half analysis showed correlations of 0.93 to 0.95 and internal consistencies of 0.90 to 0.97.[36,127] Inter-item correlations ranged from 0.44 to 0.87.[36] Corrected item-total correlations ranged from 0.37 to 0.79 for the ordinal scoring method and 0.27 to 0.75 for the binary scoring method.[128] Confirmatory factor analyses replicated the single factor for the 16-item scale.[127] For individual PFS-16 items, test-retest reliability (Spearman R) ranged from 0.52 to 0.72 (mean 0.63 + 0.06) for actual scores. Using the binary scoring method, concordance rate (percentage of subjects rating the same on both occasions) was high (71.9%–89.7%, mean 80.7% ± 5.2), and there was a moderate degree of agreement between subsequent administrations (Cohen's coefficient kappa range 0.41 to 0.70 (mean [0.55 ± 0.08]). Construct *validity* is supported by correlation with the FSS[34] (Pearson r = 0.84), the RFS[140] (r = 0.68 to 0.78), and FACIT-F.[36,52,87,127] Correlations (Spearman R) have been demonstrated for measures of depression (0.60 to 0.62), anxiety (0.55), sleepiness (PDSS −0.49, ESS 0.40), and cognition (MMSE −0.256, FAB −0.363).[128,129] Significant correlations (0.667) have been observed between the PFS and the PDQ-39.[129] The PFS discriminates people with Parkinsonism with and without fatigue and PD patients from healthy controls and the presence of clinically significant fatigue in people with Parkinsonism.[36,129] PD patients with high PFS scores displayed reduced serotonergic function in the basal ganglia and limbic structure compared to patients with low PFS scores.[7] *Responsiveness* to change with time and treatment is supported by several recent studies,[132–135,137] including a large clinical trial[132] in PD that observed significantly greater progression in PFS scores (ordinal scoring method, personal communication) in the placebo group compared to those receiving active treatment (Rasagaline). The *MCID* of the PFS has not been assessed.

Strengths and weaknesses

Strengths: The PFS is a brief and easily completed scale developed specifically for use in patients with PD. The scale has good psychometric properties and compares well to generic fatigue scales used in PD samples. The scale is easily scored, particularly when the binary approach is used. Weaknesses: The coexistence of different scoring methods is not ideal, and whether one of these is superior to the others has to be clarified. Further studies are also needed to formally validate its responsiveness and to explore the potential overlap with other PD-related features. Although the PFS was designed to address physical aspects of fatigue, the observed correlations with mood, sleepiness, and cognitive measures (and the high correlations with fatigue scales that include mental aspects of fatigue) suggest that the PFS does not provide a measure of fatigue that is independent from these features. The PFS does not define fatigue.

Final assessment

The PFS fulfills criteria for a recommended scale for screening and severity rating.

FATIGUE SEVERITY INVENTORY

Scale description

STRUCTURE

The FSI is a 33-item questionnaire[25] modified from the FAI,[34] originally designed for measuring fatigue severity in patients with multiple sclerosis and systemic lupus erythematosus, adapted for PD. Items are statements related to fatigue perceptions scored from 1 (*completely disagree*) to 7 (*completely agree*). Eight items are specifically related to PD. In the original study, the scale was used as having two parts: (1) general, for use on PD patients and control subjects; (2) specific, for use only on PD patients. It is a patient-based assessment and contains items related to physical, mental, and social aspects, although not grouped in explicit domains. A proportion of items may overlap the symptoms and complications of PD. It does not include a definition of fatigue.

HANDLING COMORBIDITIES

About 50% of items included in the FSI may be affected by other PD-related symptoms, including motor disability, sleepiness, depressive symptoms, and cognitive impairment.

ADDITIONAL POINTS

None.

Key evaluation issues

USE IN PD AND APPLICATION ACROSS THE DISEASE SPECTRUM

The FSI has been used in one study.[25] This study restricted inclusion to patients with Hoehn and Yahr stages I to III.[25]

USE BY MULTIPLE AUTHORS

None.

CLINIMETRIC ISSUES

Analysis of acceptability and *reliability* were not performed.[25] Face validity seems acceptable, although some statements may appear contradictory or may be confounded with PD manifestations. The convergent *validity* with the MFI was "statistically significant (p < 0.001)," but the coefficient value was not given. Correlations with other measures (Hoehn and Yahr staging, depression, energy) were weak to moderate.

No more information about the attributes of this scale is available.

Strengths and weaknesses

Strengths: The FSI covers diverse aspects related to fatigue, including factors influencing this symptom and the impact of the fatigue on daily functioning, work, and social activities. The 1 to 7 scoring per item could furnish a sensitive measure, but this attribute has not been explored. Weaknesses: The FSI has not been formally validated, and most of its psychometric properties are unknown.

Final assessment

The FSI is "Listed" as an instrument for screening and measuring fatigue severity in PD as it has not been used by multiple authors and its psychometric properties are unknown in PD.

THE FATIGUE IMPACT SCALE FOR DAILY USE

Scale description

STRUCTURE

The D-FIS,[138] an adaptation of the Fatigue Impact Scale (FIS),[139] was specifically designed for daily administration to measure severity (impact) of fatigue on daily life. The D-FIS is a self-administered rating scale composed of eight items that were selected from the FIS pool of items using Rasch analysis. Each item scores with five options of response from 0 (*no problem*) to 4 (*extreme problem*). The total score is obtained from the sum of each item's ordinal score and, therefore, runs from 0 to 32. The higher the score, the greater the impact of fatigue. There is no established cutoff. The eight items of the D-FIS cover mental (4 items), physical (3 items), and psychosocial (1 item) aspects of fatigue. Statements and response options are clear and concise. It provides a definition of fatigue for the users. The explored time frame is "today." The use in chronic conditions, such as PD, may be appropriate for monitoring effects of medication

(e.g., clinical trials with anti-fatigue drugs, side effects of treatments) and comorbidity.

HANDLING COMORBIDITIES

Overlap with PD symptoms (psychomotor retardation, slowness or clarity of thinking, attention, and apathy) may be present in at least six of eight items (75%)

ADDITIONAL POINTS

None.

Key evaluation issues

USE IN PD AND APPLICATIONS ACROSS THE DISEASE SPECTRUM

The psychometric properties of the D-FIS in PD were studied in one study of patients in Hoehn and Yahr stages of 1 to 4, in the "on" state.[16]

USE BY MULTIPLE AUTHORS

The D-FIS was initially tested in patients with a flu-like illness, a condition allowing changes in the fatigue state in a brief time span.[138] Two additional studies assessed the psychometric properties of the D-FIS in PD and multiple sclerosis,[16,120] and further one study used the scale in patients with celiac disease.[140]

PSYCHOMETRIC PROPERTIES

In non-PD populations, the D-FIS possesses excellent data quality, with 95.6% to 98.9% of data fully computable.[120,138] No significant floor (1.5%) or ceiling (1.5%) effects were found, and other parameters of acceptability were satisfactory.[120,138] The D-FIS was found to be *reliable*, with Cronbach's alpha = 0.91, item-total correlation between 0.62 and 0.84, intra-class correlation coefficient = 0.81, item homogeneity = 0.55, and a standard error of measurement of 3.18. Construct *validity* is supported by moderate to strong correlations (r_s = 0.46 to 0.60) with other fatigue measures.[120] Strong correlations were found between D-FIS scores and health-related quality of life measures.[120,140] D-FIS scores were found to be significantly lower in treated than untreated patients with celiac disease.[140] Divergent validity has not been assessed. In terms of *responsiveness*, significant changes of D-FIS scores over time were observed in patients with flu-like illness.[138] The *MCID* has not been studied in non-PD populations.

In PD, floor (4.2%) and ceiling (1.1%) effects were low.[16] D-FIS *reliability* was satisfactory, with Cronbach's alpha = 0.93, item homogeneity coefficient = 0.63, item-total correlation ranging from 0.68 to 0.82, and a standard error of measurement of 2.15.[16] High correlations were found with global self-assessments (VAS and global perception of FSS [r_S = 0.55–0.62]), indicative of appropriate convergent *validity*.[16] Factor analysis identified a single factor explaining 69.5% of the variance.[16] D-FIS scores were significantly different between PD patients grouped by severity of fatigue levels (discriminative validity).[16] Criterion validity and *responsiveness*, including *MCID*, have not been assessed in PD.

Strengths and weaknesses

Strengths: The D-FIS is a brief and comprehensive scale with satisfactory psychometric attributes, potentially useful for application in PD when daily assessment of fatigue is needed or convenient. It includes a definition of fatigue. In contrast to other scales, it emphasizes the impact of fatigue rather than the perceived severity of fatigue symptoms. Weaknesses: There have been few validation studies in PD, a setting in which overlapping of fatigue with some disease manifestations may be problematic. Responsiveness has not been determined in PD, albeit the precision level predicts an acceptable sensitivity to change.

Final assessment

D-FIS is a "Listed" scale for screening for fatigue (no cutoff value established) and "Suggested"

measure for daily assessment of fatigue severity in PD as it has not been used to assess changes in fatigue in this disease.

THE CHALDER FATIGUE QUESTIONNAIRE

Scale description

STRUCTURE

The CFQ[141] is a 11-item self-rated scale that was developed to assess fatigue in general practice settings. The eleven items were selected from a larger scale containing 14 items using principal component analyses (PCA) and item discriminative properties based on ROC analysis. PCA resulted in two components, one comprising seven items that relate to physical symptoms and the other four items related to mental symptoms of fatigue. Items are brief and easily understandable statements which are rated on a 4-point Likert scale assessing the frequency of fatigue (*less than usual—no more than usual—more than usual—much more than usual*). There are two scoring options. Using the Likert scoring system, a item is scored from 0 to 3. The total score is the sum of scores for the 11 individual items, and ranges from 0 to 33. Alternatively, a binary scoring method has been used, with positive scores for each item generated by *more than usual* and *much more than usual*, yielding a score range from 0 to 11. Based on general population and clinical data, a score of 4 (binary method) has been suggested as cutoff for significant fatigue.[142] The time frame is "the past month". The CFQ provides a definition of fatigue and scoring instructions.

HANDLING COMORBIDITIES

Nine of the 11 items (82%) may be affected by other PD-related symptoms, including motor disability, sleepiness, and cognitive symptoms.

ADDITIONAL POINTS

The scale, originally in English, has been translated into numerous other languages. General population norms are available.[143]

Key evaluation issues

USE IN PD AND APPLICATION ACROSS THE DISEASE SPECTRUM

In PD, the use of the CFQ is restricted to one hospital-based study[144] that included PD patients who were mentally (MMSE score > 22) and physically (not specified) able to complete assessments lasting for at least two hours.

USE BY MULTIPLE AUTHORS

In non-PD populations, the CFQ has been used and validated by independent authors and in a variety of settings (epidemiological and interventional studies, general population, primary and secondary care) and patient groups, including chronic fatigue syndrome, cancer, and post-polio syndrome.[141-143,145]

CLINIMETRIC ISSUES

In non PD-populations, clinimetric assessment of the CFQ yielded no significant floor or ceiling effects and good data quality and *reliability*. In the original publication, Cronbach's alpha was 0.89 for the total (11-item) scale, 0.85 for the PF subscale, and 0.82 for the MF subscale.[141] Independent studies have confirmed these findings (Cronbach's alpha for total score 0.86–0.98), although alpha values < 0.70 have been reported for the MF subscale.[143,146,147] The two-factor structure found in the original study[141] was replicated in independent samples by the developers and others.[142,146,147] Other studies, however, sometimes found different factor solutions.[148,149] Test-retest reliability of a slightly modified version was excellent, with ICC for the total scale and both subscales >0.95.[148]
Validity: The CFQ discriminated significantly between diseased and non-diseased and between fatigued and non-fatigued subjects.[141,142,147,150] Convergent validity is supported by moderate to strong correlations with other fatigue measures.[145,151] CFQ scores have been shown to correlate with scales measuring partly related constructs, including depressive symptoms[152] (0.53–0.55), and impaired sleep quality $(r = 0.54)$[146] and physical functioning $(r = -0.38)$.[152]

Moderate to strong inverse correlations have been observed with quality of life $(r = -0.66)$[152] and general health status (-0.62) measures.[153]

Interventional studies support the *responsiveness* of the CFQ.[154] In patients with systemic lupus erythematosus,[68] the *MCID* for the CFQ (ordinal scoring, 0–33 range) was estimated to be 2.3 (95% CI 1.0–3.7).

In PD, only one study has used the CFQ.[144] CFQ scores were higher in PD patients than in the normal population. The magnitude of differences in the total CFQ score and both subscores were low to moderate (Cohen's d = 0.33–0.65).[144] Linear regression analysis showed that female gender, UPDRS score, symptoms of anxiety and depression, and sleep disturbances predicted CFQ scores.[144] Clinimetric analyses were not performed, so the *validity*, *reliability*, and *responsiveness* of the scale in PD are unknown.

Strengths and weaknesses

Strengths: The CFQ is a brief and easily completed scale that assesses physical and mental aspects of fatigue. The scale has good clinimetric properties in non-PD populations. It provides a definition of fatigue and scoring instructions. Weaknesses: The majority of items may be affected by other PD-related symptoms, including motor disability, sleepiness, and cognitive symptoms. The scale has not been formally validated in PD or related disorders.

Final assessment

The CFQ fulfills criteria for a "Listed" scale for screening and severity rating as there are no data on its clinimetric properties in PD.

VISUAL ANALOGUE SCALES

Scale description

STRUCTURE

A VAS can be used to measure any subjective phenomenon. Subjects are asked to put a mark on a straight line to estimate where they believe their perception of the sensation being measured belongs. The lines may be of any length, but most commonly are 10 cm. Studies of VAS have shown that: length less than 10 cm is more subject to error variance[155]; horizontal lines are associated with a more uniform distribution of scores than vertical[156]; descriptions should be at each end and not below or above[157]; and right-angle endpoints, rather than arrows or other markers, are "critical."[157,158]

Key evaluation issues

USE IN PD AND APPLICATIONS ACROSS THE DISEASE SPECTRUM

VAS have been used to assess fatigue in independent PD cohorts.[16,72,73]

USE BY MULTIPLE AUTHORS

Yes.

CLINIMETRIC ISSUES

VAS have been applied to help validate other fatigue scales in PD.[16,72,73] The first publication using the VAS in fatigue[72] found a statistically significant correlation (P < 0.01) between the VAS and six of the nine principal components identified in a principal components analysis of the same subjects completing the FAI.[72] The mean score of the subjects on the VAS was 53.74 (sigma 25.89) versus controls of 73.59 (sigma 21.91), P < 0.001. Convergent validity with other fatigue scales (D-FIS, MFI, VAS) was further demonstrated in another study.[16] Two studies measured fatigue as a secondary outcome variable using VAS,[16,159] but no data other than the mean scores were published. There are no data on *reliability* and *responsiveness*.

Strengths and weaknesses

Strengths: VAS are easy to use and generally easy for the subject to understand. The scales can be used to measure virtually any self perception with a simple change in labels on the ends of the scale. Weaknesses: VAS for assessment of fatigue in PD has not been sufficiently validated.

In addition, VAS (test-retest) reliability might be affected by motor or visual-spatial deficits.

Final assessment

VAS scales are classed as "Listed" instruments for the assessment of fatigue in PD as there are no sufficient data on their clinimetric properties in PD.

CLINICAL GLOBAL IMPRESSION SCALE

Scale description

STRUCTURE

The CGIS, has, in some form, probably been used from time immemorial, for studies of all types. It is a scale that embraces all aspects of the condition under investigation and attaches a number to rate severity. Probably the most commonly used form in psychiatric publications is a clinician-rated seven-point scale[160] codified to assess severity of mental illness in which 0 = not assessed; 1 = normal; 2 = borderline mentally ill; 3 = mildly ill; 4 = moderately ill; 5 = markedly ill; 6 = severely ill; 7 = among the most extremely ill. The choice of seven options (0 not really being a rating) reflects analyses showing that seven options are "ideal."[161–163]

Key evaluation issues

USE IN PD AND APPLICATION ACROSS THE DISEASE SPECTRUM

Several studies have used the CGIS, with scoring possibilities of 5, 7, and 11 choices, in PD fatigue studies. One long-term study[4,27] used the CGIS for a screen for fatigue but not for measurement. The 5-point scale was used in two PD studies.[16,164] The Rhoten Scale,[136] used primarily in cancer, is another CGIS that was applied in a single publication in PD to help validate the PFS.[127]

USE BY MULTIPLE AUTHORS

Yes.

CLINIMETRIC ISSUES

One PD study[16] obtained data on convergent *validity* with the D-FIS ($r_s = 0.55$) and fatigue scales, depression, and PD measures. However, other psychometric data on validity, *reliability*, or *responsiveness* are not reported in PD.

Strengths and weaknesses

Strengths: The CGIS is easy to use and has been widely used in many medical and psychiatric disorders. Patients are familiar with the scale format in the ordinary context of their lives in rating likes and dislikes. Weaknesses: There are few data on its value in fatigue and consensus is lacking regarding the number of choices that should be included in a CGIS.

Final assessment

The CGIS is classed as a "Listed" scale for the assessment of fatigue in PD as there are no sufficient data on its psychometric properties in PD.

CONCLUSIONS AND RECOMMENDATIONS

Three scales meet criteria for the designation of "Recommended" as defined by the MDS for rating severity of fatigue. These scales are the FSS, MFI, and PFS. The latter scale was "upgraded" from the "Suggested" status provided by the previous MDS Task Force[20] because more recent clinical data demonstrate the responsiveness of the PFS in PD. Three scales meet criteria for the designation of "Recommended" for screening purposes, and these are the FSS, the FACIT-F, and the PFS.

A "Recommended" status was given to scales with satisfactory clinimetric attributes, including responsiveness, *in PD*. This definition of the "Recommended" status is more restrictive as compared to previously published MDS scale reviews, in which a "Recommended" status could be achieved if evidence from non-PD populations demonstrated a scale to be clinimetrically sound. The lack of a "Recommended" status for a scale assessed here may be due to lack

of published data in PD rather than a clinimetric problem with the scale. Several "Suggested" fatigue scales have shown good clinimetric properties in non-PD populations and have the potential to achieve "Recommended" status if successfully tested in PD.

Notably, a "Recommended" status does not mean that a scale is "perfect" and that further clinimetric evaluation is unnecessary. None of the recommended scales provides a definition of the construct it intends to measure. This would, however, be valuable, given the existence of different subtypes and the lack of a commonly accepted definition of fatigue. Although the focus in PD is on central fatigue, the subjective perception of being fatigued, this might not be obvious to the patient. In addition, it might be extremely difficult or impossible to distinguish the fatigue one experiences from PD from fatigue related to concurrent depression, anxiety, cognitive dysfunction, apathy, medication, or other medical or psychiatric conditions. This might hamper appropriate treatment and clinical care, as well as studies into the neurobiology of fatigue in PD. The assessment of fatigue therefore requires a broader approach with systematic evaluation of overlapping symptoms.

There is no doubt that fatigue is a very common and often debilitating feature in patients with PD. Therefore, there is a major need for studies on the pathophysiology and the treatment of fatigue. Such research depends on clinical instruments that are valid, reliable, and sensitive to change. The following issues in the area of fatigue rating scales require further exploration:

1. Studies on the sensitivity to change and minimal clinically important differences of the various fatigue scales.

2. Studies on the sensitivity and specificity of fatigue rating scales for detecting clinically significant fatigue in patients with PD as well as the ability of the scales to provide distinct measures of fatigue irrespective of concurrent depressive, anxiety, or cognitive symptoms.

3. Studies on MF versus PF, to determine whether rating scales are more sensitive to PF versus MF.

4. To determine possible differences in the structure of fatigue in PD patients compared to other neuropsychiatric disorders.

5. To determine if there are quantitative measures or biomarkers that reflect fatigue presence or severity.

RECOMMENDED SCALES for Screening
Fatigue Severity Scale
Parkinson Fatigue Scale
Functional Assessment of Chronic Illness Therapy-Fatigue
RECOMMENDED SCALES for Severity Rating
Fatigue Severity Scale
Parkinson Fatigue Scale
Multidimensional Fatigue Inventory

References

1. Friedman JH, Brown RG, Comella C, et al. Fatigue in Parkinson's disease: a review. *Mov Disord.* 2007;22:297–308.
2. Hagell P, Brundin L. Towards an understanding of fatigue in Parkinson disease. *J Neurol Neurosurg Psychiatry.* 2009;80:489–492.
3. Schifitto G, Friedman JH, Oakes D, et al. Fatigue in levodopa-naive subjects with Parkinson disease. *Neurology.* 2008;71:481–485.
4. Alves G, Wentzel-Larsen T, Larsen JP. Is fatigue an independent and persistent symptom in patients with Parkinson disease? *Neurology.* 2004;63:1908–1911.
5. Havlikova E, Rosenberger J, Nagyova I, et al. Clinical and psychosocial factors associated with fatigue in patients with Parkinson's disease. *Parkinsonism Relat Disord.* 2008;14:187–192.
6. Martinez-Martin P, Rodriguez-Blazquez C, Kurtis MM, Chaudhuri KR. The impact of non-motor symptoms on health-related quality of life of patients with Parkinson's disease. *Mov Disord.* 2011;26:399–406.
7. Pavese N, Metta V, Bose SK, et al. Fatigue in Parkinson's disease is linked to striatal and limbic serotonergic dysfunction. *Brain.* 2010;133:3434–3443.
8. Lou JS, Dimitrova DM, Park BS, et al. Using modafinil to treat fatigue in Parkinson disease: a double-blind, placebo-controlled pilot study. *Clin Neuropharmacol.* 2009;32:305–310.
9. Tyne HL, Taylor J, Baker GA, Steiger MJ. Modafinil for Parkinson's disease fatigue. *J Neurol.* 2011;257:452–456.
10. Mendonca DA, Menezes K, Jog MS. Methylphenidate improves fatigue scores in Parkinson disease: a randomized controlled trial. *Mov Disord.* 2007;22:2070–2076.
11. Abe K, Takanashi M, Yanagihara T, Sakoda S. Pergolide mesilate may improve fatigue in patients with Parkinson's disease. *Behav Neurol.* 2001;13:117–121.
12. Oved D, Ziv I, Treves TA, et al. Effect of dopamine agonists on fatigue and somnolence in Parkinson's disease. *Mov Disord.* 2006;21:1257–1261.
13. Zesiewicz TA, Patel-Larson A, Hauser RA, Sullivan KL. Social Security Disability Insurance (SSDI) in Parkinson's disease. *Disabil Rehabil.* 2007;29:1934–1936.
14. Herlofson K, Larsen JP. The influence of fatigue on health-related quality of life in patients with Parkinson's disease. *Acta Neurol Scand.* 2003;107:1–6.
15. Havlikova E, Rosenberger J, Nagyova I, et al. Impact of fatigue on quality of life in patients with Parkinson's disease. *Eur J Neurol.* 2008;15:475–480.
16. Martinez-Martin P, Catalan MJ, Benito-Leon J, et al. Impact of fatigue in Parkinson's disease: the Fatigue Impact Scale for Daily Use (D-FIS). *Qual Life Res.* 2006;15:597–606.
17. Shulman LM, Taback RL, Rabinstein AA, Weiner WJ. Non-recognition of depression and other non-motor symptoms in Parkinson's disease. *Parkinsonism Relat Disord.* 2002;8:193–197.
18. Sullivan KL, Ward CL, Hauser RA, Zesiewicz TA. Prevalence and treatment of non-motor symptoms in Parkinson's disease. *Parkinsonism Relat Disord.* 2007;13:545.
19. Gallagher DA, Lees AJ, Schrag A. What are the most important non-motor symptoms in patients with Parkinson's disease and are we missing them? *Mov Disord.* 2010;25:2493–2500.
20. Friedman JH, Alves G, Hagell P, et al. Fatigue rating scales critique and recommendations by the Movement Disorders Society Task Force on rating scales for Parkinson's disease. *Mov Disord.* 2010;25:805–822.
21. Chaudhuri KR, Martinez-Martin P, Brown RG, et al. The metric properties of a novel non-motor symptoms scale for Parkinson's disease: results

from an international pilot study. *Mov Disord.* 2007;22:1901–1911.

22. Goetz CG, Tilley BC, Shaftman SR, et al. Movement Disorder Society-sponsored revision of the Unified Parkinson's Disease Rating Scale (MDS-UPDRS): scale presentation and clinimetric testing results. *Mov Disord.* 2008;23:2129–2170.

23. Chaudhuri A, Behan PO. Fatigue and basal ganglia. *J Neurol Sci.* 2000;179:34–42.

24. Chaudhuri A, Behan PO. Fatigue in neurological disorders. *Lancet.* 2004;363: 978–988.

25. Lou JS, Kearns G, Oken B, et al. Exacerbated physical fatigue and mental fatigue in Parkinson's disease. *Mov Disord.* 2001;16: 190–196.

26. American Psychiatric Association. *Diagnostic and Statistical Manual of Mental Disorders.* 4th ed. Text revision (DSM-IV-TR). Washington, DC: American Psychiatric Association; 2000.

27. Karlsen K, Larsen JP, Tandberg E, Jorgensen K. Fatigue in patients with Parkinson's disease. *Mov Disord.* 1999;14:237–241.

28. Abe K, Takanashi M, Yanagihara T. Fatigue in patients with Parkinson's disease. *Behav Neurol.* 2000;12:103–106.

29. Nunnally JC, Bernstein IH. *Psychometric Theory.* 3rd ed. New York: McGraw-Hill Inc; 1994.

30. Hobart J. Rating scales for neurologists. *J Neurol Neurosurg Psychiatry.* 2003;74 (suppl 4):iv22–iv26.

31. Hobart JC, Cano SJ, Zajicek JP, Thompson AJ. Rating scales as outcome measures for clinical trials in neurology: problems, solutions, and recommendations. *Lancet Neurol.* 2007;6: 1094–1105.

32. Martinez-Martin P, Rodriguez-Blazquez C, Frades-Payo B. Specific patient-reported outcome measures for Parkinson's disease: analysis and applications. *Expert Rev Pharmacoecon Outcomes Res.* 2008;8:401–418.

33. Krupp LB, LaRocca NG, Muir-Nash J, Steinberg AD. The fatigue severity scale. Application to patients with multiple sclerosis and systemic lupus erythematosus. *Arch Neurol.* 1989;46:1121–1123.

34. Schwartz JE, Jandorf L, Krupp LB. The measurement of fatigue: a new instrument. *J Psychosom Res.* 1993;37:753–762.

35. Lerdal A, Wahl A, Rustoen T, et al. Fatigue in the general population: a translation and test of the psychometric properties of the Norwegian version of the fatigue severity scale. *Scand J Public Health.* 2005;33:123–130.

36. Grace J, Mendelsohn A, Friedman JH. A comparison of fatigue measures in Parkinson's disease. *Parkinsonism Relat Disord.* 2007;13:443–445.

37. Mattsson M, Moller B, Lundberg I, et al. Reliability and validity of the Fatigue Severity Scale in Swedish for patients with systemic lupus erythematosus. *Scand J Rheumatol.* 2008;37:269–277.

38. Flachenecker P, Muller G, Konig H, et al. [Fatigue in multiple sclerosis. Development and validation of the Wurzburger Fatigue Inventory for MS]. *Nervenarzt.* 2006;77:165–166, 168–170, 172–164.

39. Armutlu K, Korkmaz NC, Keser I, et al. The validity and reliability of the Fatigue Severity Scale in Turkish multiple sclerosis patients. *Int J Rehabil Res.* 2007;30:81–85.

40. Mills RJ, Young CA, Nicholas RS, et al. Rasch analysis of the Fatigue Severity Scale in multiple sclerosis. *Mult Scler.* 2009;15:81–87.

41. Pouchot J, Kherani RB, Brant R, et al. Determination of the minimal clinically important difference for seven fatigue measures in rheumatoid arthritis. *J Clin Epidemiol.* 2008;61:705–713.

42. Taylor RR, Jason LA, Torres A. Fatigue rating scales: an empirical comparison. *Psychol Med.* 2000;30:849–856.

43. Kleinman L, Zodet MW, Hakim Z, et al. Psychometric evaluation of the fatigue severity scale for use in chronic hepatitis C. *Qual Life Res.* 2000;9:499–508.

44. Winstead-Fry P. Psychometric assessment of four fatigue scales with a sample of rural cancer patients. *Psychol Med.* 1998;6:111–122.

45. LaChapelle DL, Finlayson MA. An evaluation of subjective and objective measures of fatigue in patients with brain injury and healthy controls. *Brain Inj.* 1998;12:649–659.

46. Dijkers MP, Bushnik T. Assessing fatigue after traumatic brain injury: an evaluation of the Barroso Fatigue Scale. *J Head Trauma Rehabil.* 2008;23:3–16.

47. Vasconcelos OM Jr, Prokhorenko OA, Kelley KF, et al. A comparison of fatigue scales in postpoliomyelitis syndrome. *Arch Phys Med Rehabil.* 2006;87:1213–1217.

48. Horemans HL, Nollet F, Beelen A, Lankhorst GJ. A comparison of 4 questionnaires to measure fatigue in postpoliomyelitis syndrome. *Arch Phys Med Rehabil.* 2004;85:392–398.

49. Merkies IS, Schmitz PI, Samijn JP, et al. Fatigue in immune-mediated polyneuropathies. European Inflammatory Neuropathy Cause

and Treatment (INCAT) Group. *Neurology.* 1999;53:1648–1654.

50. Laberge L, Gagnon C, Jean S, Mathieu J. Fatigue and daytime sleepiness rating scales in myotonic dystrophy: a study of reliability. *J Neurol Neurosurg Psychiatry.* 2005;76: 1403–1405.

51. Valko PO, Bassetti CL, Bloch KE, et al. Validation of the fatigue severity scale in a Swiss cohort. *Sleep.* 2008;31:1601–1607.

52. Hagell P, Hoglund A, Reimer J, et al. Measuring fatigue in Parkinson's disease: a psychometric study of two brief generic fatigue questionnaires. *J Pain Symptom Manage.* 2006;32:420–432.

53. Hjollund NH, Andersen JH, Bech P. Assessment of fatigue in chronic disease: a bibliographic study of fatigue measurement scales. *Health Qual Life Outcomes.* 2007;5:12.

54. Chipchase SY, Lincoln NB, Radford KA. Measuring fatigue in people with multiple sclerosis. *Disabil Rehabil.* 2003;25:778–784.

55. Lerdal A, Celius EG, Krupp L, Dahl AA. A prospective study of patterns of fatigue in multiple sclerosis. *Eur J Neurol.* 2007;14: 1338–1343.

56. Gencay-Can A, Can SS. Validation of the Turkish version of the fatigue severity scale in patients with fibromyalgia. *Rheumatol Int.* 2012;32:27–31.

57. Kos D, Kerckhofs E, Carrea I, et al. Evaluation of the Modified Fatigue Impact Scale in four different European countries. *Mult Scler.* 2005;11:76–80.

58. Marrie RA, Cutter G, Tyry T, et al. Validation of the NARCOMS registry: fatigue assessment. *Mult Scler.* 2005;11:583–584.

59. Kos D, Kerckhofs E, Nagels G, et al. Assessing fatigue in multiple sclerosis: Dutch modified fatigue impact scale. *Acta Neurol Belg.* 2003;103:185–191.

60. Measurement of fatigue in systemic lupus erythematosus: a systematic review. *Arthritis Rheum.* 2007;57:1348–1357.

61. Krupp LB, LaRocca NG, Muir J, Steinberg AD. A study of fatigue in systemic lupus erythematosus. *J Rheumatol.* 1990;17:1450–1452.

62. Hossain JL, Reinish LW, Kayumov L, et al. Underlying sleep pathology may cause chronic high fatigue in shift-workers. *J Sleep Res.* 2003;12:223–230.

63. Tench CM, McCurdie I, White PD, D'Cruz DP. The prevalence and associations of fatigue in systemic lupus erythematosus. *Rheumatology (Oxford).* 2000;39:1249–1254.

64. Merkelbach S, Sittinger H, Koenig J. Is there a differential impact of fatigue and physical disability on quality of life in multiple sclerosis? *J Nerv Ment Dis.* 2002;190:388–393.

65. Krupp LB, Coyle PK, Doscher C, et al. Fatigue therapy in multiple sclerosis: results of a double-blind, randomized, parallel trial of amantadine, pemoline, and placebo. *Neurology.* 1995;45:1956–1961.

66. Wingerchuk DM, Benarroch EE, O'Brien PC, et al. A randomized controlled crossover trial of aspirin for fatigue in multiple sclerosis. *Neurology.* 2005;64:1267–1269.

67. Rammohan KW, Rosenberg JH, Lynn DJ, et al. Efficacy and safety of modafinil (Provigil) for the treatment of fatigue in multiple sclerosis: a two center phase 2 study. *J Neurol Neurosurg Psychiatry.* 2002;72:179–183.

68. Goligher EC, Pouchot J, Brant R, et al. Minimal clinically important difference for 7 measures of fatigue in patients with systemic lupus erythematosus. *J Rheumatol.* 2008;35:635–642.

69. Herlofson K, Larsen JP. Measuring fatigue in patients with Parkinson's disease—the Fatigue Severity Scale. *Eur J Neurol.* 2002;9:595–600.

70. McKinlay A, Grace RC, Dalrymple-Alford JC, et al. A profile of neuropsychiatric problems and their relationship to quality of life for Parkinson's disease patients without dementia. *Parkinsonism Relat Disord.* 2008;14:37–42.

71. Garber CE, Friedman JH. Effects of fatigue on physical activity and function in patients with Parkinson's disease. *Neurology.* 2003;60: 1119–1124.

72. Friedman J, Friedman H. Fatigue in Parkinson's disease. *Neurology.* 1993;43:2016–2018.

73. Friedman JH, Friedman H. Fatigue in Parkinson's disease: a nine-year follow-up. *Mov Disord.* 2001;16:1120–1122.

74. Ramirez C, Piemonte ME, Callegaro D, Da Silva HC. Fatigue in amyotrophic lateral sclerosis: frequency and associated factors. *Amyotroph Lateral Scler.* 2008;9:75–80.

75. O'Dell MW, Meighen M, Riggs RV. Correlates of fatigue in HIV infection prior to AIDS: a pilot study. *Disabil Rehabil.* 1996;18:249–254.

76. Perry MB, Suwannarat P, Furst GP, et al. Musculoskeletal findings and disability in alkaptonuria. *J Rheumatol.* 2006;33: 2280–2285.

77. Girgrah N, Reid G, MacKenzie S, Wong F. Cirrhotic cardiomyopathy: does it contribute to chronic fatigue and decreased health-related quality of life in cirrhosis? *Can J Gastroenterol.* 2003;17:545–551.

78. Obhrai J, Hall Y, Anand BS. Assessment of fatigue and psychological disturbances in patients with hepatitis C virus infection. *J Clin Gastroenterol.* 2001;32:413–417.

79. de Leeuw R, Studts JL, Carlson CR. Fatigue and fatigue-related symptoms in an orofacial pain population. *Oral Surg Oral Med Oral Pathol Oral Radiol Endod.* 2005;99:168–174.

80. Gramigna S, Schluep M, Staub F, et al. [Fatigue in neurological disease: different patterns in stroke and multiple sclerosis]. *Rev Neurol (Paris).* 2007;163:341–348.

81. Kapella MC, Larson JL, Patel MK, et al. Subjective fatigue, influencing variables, and consequences in chronic obstructive pulmonary disease. *Nurs Res.* 2006;55:10–17.

82. Hernandez-Ronquillo L, Moien-Afshari F, Knox K, et al. How to measure fatigue in epilepsy? The validation of three scales for clinical use. *Epilepsy Res.* 2011;95:119–129.

83. Yang CM, Wu CH. The situational fatigue scale: a different approach to measuring fatigue. *Qual Life Res.* 2005;14:1357–1362.

84. Mohr DC, Hart SL, Goldberg A. Effects of treatment for depression on fatigue in multiple sclerosis. *Psychosom Med.* 2003;65:542–547.

85. Krupp LB, Hyman LG, Grimson R, et al. Study and treatment of post Lyme disease (STOP-LD): a randomized double masked clinical trial. *Neurology.* 2003;60:1923–1930.

86. Yellen SB, Cella DF, Webster K, et al. Measuring fatigue and other anemia-related symptoms with the Functional Assessment of Cancer Therapy (FACT) measurement system. *J Pain Symptom Manage.* 1997;13:63–74.

87. Cella D. *The Functional Assessment of Chronic Illness Therapy-Fatigue (FACT-F) Scale: Summary of Development and Validation.* Evanston, IL: Center on Outcomes, Research and Education (CORE), Evanston Northwestern Healthcare and Northwestern University; 2003.

88. Van Belle S, Paridaens R, Evers G, et al. Comparison of proposed diagnostic criteria with FACT-F and VAS for cancer-related fatigue: proposal for use as a screening tool. *Support Care Cancer.* 2005;13:246–254.

89. Mallinson T, Cella D, Cashy J, Holzner B. Giving meaning to measure: linking self-reported fatigue and function to performance of everyday activities. *J Pain Symptom Manage.* 2006;31:229–241.

90. Hahn EA, Cella D. Health outcomes assessment in vulnerable populations: measurement challenges and recommendations. *Arch Phys Med Rehabil.* 2003;84:S35–S42.

91. Cella D, Zagari MJ, Vandoros C, et al. Epoetin alfa treatment results in clinically significant improvements in quality of life in anemic cancer patients when referenced to the general population. *J Clin Oncol.* 2003;21:366–373.

92. Cella D, Nowinski CJ. Measuring quality of life in chronic illness: the functional assessment of chronic illness therapy measurement system. *Arch Phys Med Rehabil.* 2002;83:S10–S17.

93. Bonomi AE, Cella DF, Hahn EA, et al. Multilingual translation of the Functional Assessment of Cancer Therapy (FACT) quality of life measurement system. *Qual Life Res.* 1996;5:309–320.

94. Eremenco SL, Cella D, Arnold BJ. A comprehensive method for the translation and cross-cultural validation of health status questionnaires. *Eval Health Prof.* 2005;28:212–232.

95. Minton O, Stone P. A systematic review of the scales used for the measurement of cancer-related fatigue (CRF). *Ann Oncol.* 2009;20:17–25.

96. Cella D, Lai JS, Chang CH, et al. Fatigue in cancer patients compared with fatigue in the general United States population. *Cancer.* 2002;94:528–538.

97. Cella D, Yount S, Sorensen M, et al. Validation of the Functional Assessment of Chronic Illness Therapy Fatigue Scale relative to other instrumentation in patients with rheumatoid arthritis. *J Rheumatol.* 2005;32:811–819.

98. Cella D, Eton DT, Lai JS, et al. Combining anchor and distribution-based methods to derive minimal clinically important differences on the Functional Assessment of Cancer Therapy (FACT) anemia and fatigue scales. *J Pain Symptom Manage.* 2002;24:547–561.

99. Hwang SS, Chang VT, Kasimis BS. A comparison of three fatigue measures in veterans with cancer. *Cancer Invest.* 2003;21:363–373.

100. Lai JS, Cella D, Chang CH, et al. Item banking to improve, shorten and computerize self-reported fatigue: an illustration of steps to create a core item bank from the FACIT-Fatigue Scale. *Qual Life Res.* 2003;12:485–501.

101. Osterborg A, Brandberg Y, Molostova V, et al. Randomized, double-blind, placebo-controlled trial of recombinant human erythropoietin, epoetin Beta, in hematologic malignancies. *J Clin Oncol.* 2002;20:2486–2494.

102. Reddy S, Bruera E, Pace E, et al. Clinically important improvement in the intensity of fatigue in patients with advanced cancer. *J Palliat Med.* 2007;10:1068–1075.

103. Patrick DL, Gagnon DD, Zagari MJ, et al. Assessing the clinical significance of health-related quality of life (HrQOL) improvements in anaemic cancer patients receiving epoetin alfa. *Eur J Cancer.* 2003;39:335–345.

104. Hagell P, Rosblom T, Pålhagen S. Initial validation of the Swedish version of the 16-item Parkinson Fatigue Scale (PFS-16). *Qual Life Res.* 2008;17(suppl):A43.

105. Wyrwich KW, Bullinger M, Aaronson N, et al. Estimating clinically significant differences in quality of life outcomes. *Qual Life Res.* 2005;14:285–295.

106. Smets EM, Garssen B, Bonke B, De Haes JC. The Multidimensional Fatigue Inventory (MFI) psychometric qualities of an instrument to assess fatigue. *J Psychosom Res.* 1995;39:315–325.

107. Schwarz R, Krauss O, Hinz A. Fatigue in the general population. *Onkologie.* 2003;26: 140–144.

108. Gentile S, Delaroziere JC, Favre F, et al. Validation of the French multidimensional fatigue inventory (MFI 20). *Eur J Cancer Care (Engl).* 2003;12:58–64.

109. Lin JM, Brimmer DJ, Maloney EM, et al. Further validation of the Multidimensional Fatigue Inventory in a US adult population sample. *Popul Health Metr.* 2009;7:18.

110. Jansen AJ, Essink-Bot ML, Duvekot JJ, van Rhenen DJ. Psychometric evaluation of health-related quality of life measures in women after different types of delivery. *J Psychosom Res.* 2007;63:275–281.

111. Smets EM, Garssen B, Cull A, de Haes JC. Application of the multidimensional fatigue inventory (MFI-20) in cancer patients receiving radiotherapy. *Br J Cancer.* 1996;73:241–245.

112. Fillion L, Gelinas C, Simard S, et al. Validation evidence for the French Canadian adaptation of the Multidimensional Fatigue Inventory as a measure of cancer-related fatigue. *Cancer Nurs.* 2003;26:143–154.

113. Goodchild CE, Treharne GJ, Booth DA, et al. Measuring fatigue among women with Sjogren's syndrome or rheumatoid arthritis: a comparison of the Profile of Fatigue (ProF) and the Multidimensional Fatigue Inventory (MFI). *Musculoskeletal Care.* 2008;6:31–48.

114. Meek PM, Nail LM, Barsevick A, et al. Psychometric testing of fatigue instruments for use with cancer patients. *Nurs Res.* 2000;49:181–190.

115. Schneider RA. Reliability and validity of the Multidimensional Fatigue Inventory (MFI-20) and the Rhoten Fatigue Scale among rural cancer outpatients. *Cancer Nurs.* 1998;21: 370–373.

116. van Tubergen A, Coenen J, Landewe R, et al. Assessment of fatigue in patients with ankylosing spondylitis: a psychometric analysis. *Arthritis Rheum.* 2002;47:8–16.

117. d'Elia HF, Rehnberg E, Kvist G, et al. Fatigue and blood pressure in primary Sjogren's syndrome. *Scand J Rheumatol.* 2008;37: 284–292.

118. Hagelin CL, Wengstrom Y, Runesdotter S, Furst CJ. The psychometric properties of the Swedish Multidimensional Fatigue Inventory MFI-20 in four different populations. *Acta Oncol.* 2007;46:97–104.

119. Dagnelie PC, Pijls-Johannesma MC, Pijpe A, et al. Psychometric properties of the revised Piper Fatigue Scale in Dutch cancer patients were satisfactory. *J Clin Epidemiol.* 2006;59:642–649.

120. Benito-Leon J, Martinez-Martin P, Frades B, et al. Impact of fatigue in multiple sclerosis: the Fatigue Impact Scale for Daily Use (D-FIS). *Mult Scler.* 2007;13:645–651.

121. Ericsson A, Mannerkorpi K. Assessment of fatigue in patients with fibromyalgia and chronic widespread pain. Reliability and validity of the Swedish version of the MFI-20. *Disabil Rehabil.* 2007;29:1665–1670.

122. Jansen AJ, Essink-Bot ML, Beckers EA, et al. Quality of life measurement in patients with transfusion-dependent myelodysplastic syndromes. *Br J Haematol.* 2003;121:270–274.

123. Elbers R, van Wegen EE, Rochester L, et al. Is impact of fatigue an independent factor associated with physical activity in patients with idiopathic Parkinson's disease? *Mov Disord.* 2009;24:1512–1518.

124. Rochester L, Jones D, Hetherington V, et al. Gait and gait-related activities and fatigue in Parkinson's disease: what is the relationship? *Disabil Rehabil.* 2006;28:1365–1371.

125. Zenzola A, Masi G, De Mari M, et al. Fatigue in Parkinson's disease. *Neurol Sci.* 2003;24:225–226.

126. Havlikova E, van Dijk JP, Rosenberger J, et al. Fatigue in Parkinson's disease is not related to

excessive sleepiness or quality of sleep. *J Neurol Sci.* 2008;270:107–113.

127. Brown RG, Dittner A, Findley L, Wessely SC. The Parkinson fatigue scale. *Parkinsonism Relat Disord.* 2005;11:49–55.

128. Kummer A, Scalzo P, Cardoso F, Teixeira AL. Evaluation of fatigue in Parkinson's disease using the Brazilian version of Parkinson's Fatigue Scale. *Acta Neurol Scand.* 2011;123:130–136.

129. Okuma Y, Kamei S, Morita A, et al. Fatigue in Japanese patients with Parkinson's disease: a study using Parkinson fatigue scale. *Mov Disord.* 2009;24:1977–1983.

130. Nakamura T, Hirayama M, Hara T, et al. Does cardiovascular autonomic dysfunction contribute to fatigue in Parkinson's disease? *Mov Disord.* 2011;26:1869–1874.

131. Kummer A, Cardoso F, Teixeira AL. Loss of libido in Parkinson's disease. *J Sex Med.* 2009;6:1024–1031.

132. Rascol O, Fitzer-Attas CJ, Hauser R, et al. A double-blind, delayed-start trial of rasagiline in Parkinson's disease (the ADAGIO study): prespecified and post-hoc analyses of the need for additional therapies, changes in UPDRS scores, and non-motor outcomes. *Lancet Neurol.* 2011;10:415–423.

133. Kieburtz K. Twice-daily, low-dose pramipexole in early Parkinson's disease: a randomized, placebo-controlled trial. *Mov Disord.* 2011;26:37–44.

134. Makoutonina M, Iansek R, Simpson P. Optimizing care of residents with Parkinsonism in supervised facilities. *Parkinsonism Relat Disord.* 2010;16:351–355.

135. Iansek R, Danoudis M. A single-blind cross over study investigating the efficacy of standard and controlled release levodopa in combination with entacapone in the treatment of end-of-dose effect in people with Parkinson's disease. *Parkinsonism Relat Disord.* 2011;17:533–536.

136. Rhoten D. Fatigue and the postsurgical patient. In: Norris C, ed. *Concept Classification in Nursing.* Rockville, MD: Aspen Systems Corporation; 1982:277–300.

137. Iansek R. Key points in the management of Parkinson's disease. *Aust Fam Physician.* 1999;28:897–901.

138. Fisk JD, Doble SE. Construction and validation of a fatigue impact scale for daily administration (D-FIS). *Qual Life Res.* 2002;11:263–272.

139. Fisk JD, Ritvo PG, Ross L, et al. Measuring the functional impact of fatigue: initial validation of the fatigue impact scale. *Clin Infect Dis.* 1994;18(suppl 1):S79–S83.

140. Jorda FC, Lopez Vivancos J. Fatigue as a determinant of health in patients with celiac disease. *J Clin Gastroenterol.* 2010;44:423–427.

141. Chalder T, Berelowitz G, Pawlikowska T, et al. Development of a fatigue scale. *J Psychosom Res.* 1993;37:147–153.

142. Cella M, Chalder T. Measuring fatigue in clinical and community settings. *J Psychosom Res.* 2010;69:17–22.

143. Loge JH, Ekeberg O, Kaasa S. Fatigue in the general Norwegian population: normative data and associations. *J Psychosom Res.* 1998;45:53–65.

144. Beiske AG, Loge JH, Hjermstad MJ, Svensson E. Fatigue in Parkinson's disease: prevalence and associated factors. *Mov Disord.* 2010;25:2456–2460.

145. Strohschein FJ, Kelly CG, Clarke AG, et al. Applicability, validity, and reliability of the Piper Fatigue Scale in postpolio patients. *Am J Phys Med Rehabil.* 2003;82:122–129.

146. Patterson PD, Suffoletto BP, Kupas DF, et al. Sleep quality and fatigue among prehospital providers. *Prehosp Emerg Care.* 2010;14:187–193.

147. Cho HJ, Costa E, Menezes PR, et al. Cross-cultural validation of the Chalder Fatigue Questionnaire in Brazilian primary care. *J Psychosom Res.* 2007;62:301–304.

148. Ferentinos P, Kontaxakis V, Havaki-Kontaxaki B, et al. The Fatigue Questionnaire: standardization in patients with major depression. *Psychiatry Res.* 2010;177:114–119.

149. Morriss RK, Wearden AJ, Mullis R. Exploring the validity of the Chalder Fatigue scale in chronic fatigue syndrome. *J Psychosom Res.* 1998;45:411–417.

150. Kaasa S, Loge JH, Knobel H, et al. Fatigue. Measures and relation to pain. *Acta Anaesthesiol Scand.* 1999;43:939–947.

151. Knobel H, Loge JH, Brenne E, et al. The validity of EORTC QLQ-C30 fatigue scale in advanced cancer patients and cancer survivors. *Palliat Med.* 2003;17:664–672.

152. Wagner GJ, Rabkin JG, Rabkin R. Testosterone as a treatment for fatigue in HIV+ men. *Gen Hosp Psychiatry.* 1998;20:209–213.

153. Pawlikowska T, Chalder T, Hirsch SR, et al. Population based study of fatigue and

psychological distress. *BMJ*. 1994;308: 763–766.

154. White PD, Goldsmith KA, Johnson AL, et al. Comparison of adaptive pacing therapy, cognitive behaviour therapy, graded exercise therapy, and specialist medical care for chronic fatigue syndrome (PACE): a randomised trial. *Lancet*. 2011;377:823–836.

155. Revill SI, Robinson JO, Rosen M, Hogg MI. The reliability of a linear analogue for evaluating pain. *Anaesthesia*. 1976;31:1191–1198.

156. Scott J, Huskisson EC. Graphic representation of pain. *Pain*. 1976;2:175–184.

157. Huskisson EC. Visual analogue scales. In: Melzack R, ed. *Pain Measurement and Assessment*. New York: Raven Press; 1983:33–40.

158. Wewers ME, Lowe NK. A critical review of visual analogue scales in the measurement of clinical phenomena. *Res Nurs Health*. 1990;13:227–236.

159. Nutt JG, Carter JH, Carlson NE. Effects of methylphenidate on response to oral levodopa: a double-blind clinical trial. *Arch Neurol*. 2007;64:319–323.

160. Guy W. *Clinical Global Impression. ECDEU Assessment Manual for Psychopharmacology— revised*. Rockville, MD: National Institute of Mental Health; 1976.

161. Kadouri A, Corruble E, Falissard B. The improved Clinical Global Impression Scale (iCGI): development and validation in depression. *BMC Psychiatry*. 2007;7:7.

162. Cox EP. The optimal number of response alternatives for a scale: a review. *J Mark Res*. 1980;17:407–422.

163. Miller GA. The magical number seven plus or minus two: some limits on our capacity for processing information. *Psychol Rev*. 1956;63:81–97.

164. van Hilten JJ, Hoogland G, van der Velde EA, et al. Diurnal effects of motor activity and fatigue in Parkinson's disease. *J Neurol Neurosurg Psychiatry*. 1993;56: 874–877.

18

PSYCHOSIS RATING SCALES IN PARKINSON'S DISEASE

Hubert H. Fernandez

Summary

Psychotic symptoms are a frequent occurrence in Parkinson's disease, affecting up to 50% of patients. This chapter is mainly based on the published review of PD psychosis rating scales by the Movement Disorders Society Task Force on Rating Scales.[1] It also incorporates part of the supplementary materials produced by the task force that was published online on the *Movement Disorders* journal website. The critiques apply only to published, peer-reviewed psychosis rating scales used in PD psychosis studies. Thirteen psychosis scales and question-naires are reviewed in this chapter. Overall, none of the reviewed scales adequately captured the entire phenomenology of PD psychosis. While the task force has labeled some scales as "Recommended" or "Suggested" based on the fulfilling predefined criteria, none of the cur-rent scales contains all the basic content, mechanistic, and psychometric properties needed to capture PD psychotic phenomena and to measure clinical response over time. Different scales may be better for some settings versus others. Since one scale may not be able to serve all needs, a scale used to measure clinical response and change over time (such as the Clinical Global Impression Scale [CGIS]) may need to be combined with another scale better at cataloguing specific features (such as the Neuropsychiatric Inventory [NPI] or Schedule for Assessment of Positive Symptoms [SAPS]). Therefore, at present, for clinical trials on PD psychosis assessing new treatments, the following are the recommended scales: NPI (for the cognitively impaired PD population or when a caregiver is required), SAPS, Positive and Negative Syndrome Scale (PANSS), or Brief Psychiatric Rating Scale (BPRS) (for the cognitively intact PD population or when the patient is the sole informant). The CGIS is suggested as a secondary scale to meas-ure change and response to treatment over time.

INTRODUCTION

Psychotic symptoms are a frequent occurrence in Parkinson's disease (PD), affecting up to 50% of patients.[1-3] Studies on psychosis have mostly focused on visual hallucinations, the commonest type of psychotic symptom in PD.[4-7] However, hallucinations can occur in all sensory domains, and delusions of various types are also relatively common.[5,8-10]

Over the course of PD, psychotic symp-toms, once present, tend to be persistent and progressive.[11-13] The impact of psychosis is substantial in that it is associated with dementia, depression, earlier mortality, greater caregiver strain, and nursing-home placement.[13-17]

The first challenge encountered in trying to critique scales used for PD psychosis is that, until recently, there have been no standardized criteria specifically designed to diagnose PD-related psychosis.[1] *The Diagnostic and Statistical Manual of Mental Disorders, Fourth Edition* (DSM-IV-R)[18] and the Structured Clinical Interview for DSM-IV-TR Axis I disorders (SCID)[19] has been used, but they rely on general categories like "psychotic disorder due to a general medical condition" or "substance-induced psychotic disorder."

A National Institutes of Health–sponsored workshop recently reviewed the PD psychosis literature to provide criteria that distinguished PD psychosis from other causes of psychosis.[20] Based on these data, provisional criteria for PD psychosis in the style of the DSM-IV-R were proposed (see Table 18-1). The criteria are inclusive and contain descriptions of the full range of characteristic symptoms, chronology of onset, duration of symptoms, exclusionary diagnoses, and associated features, such as dementia. They describe a distinctive constellation of clinical features that are not shared by other psychotic syndromes. These criteria require validation and perhaps refinement, but form a useful starting point for studies on PD psychosis.

To critique the psychosis scales used in PD studies for the MDS Rating Scales Task Force review (Fernandez et al.), PubMed searches (from 1950 to September, 2005) were conducted using Parkinson's disease AND psychosis/hallucinations/delusions in combination with each

Table 18-1. Proposed Diagnostic Criteria for PD-Associated Psychosis

A. Characteristic Symptoms

Presence of at least one of the following symptoms (specify which of the symptoms fulfill the criteria):

Illusions

False sense of presence

Hallucinations

Delusions

B. Primary Diagnosis

    U.K. brain bank criteria for PD

C. Chronology of the onset of symptoms of psychosis

    The symptoms in Criterion A occur after the onset of PD

D. Duration

    The symptom(s) in Criterion A are recurrent or continuous for one month

E. Exclusion of other causes

    The symptoms in Criterion A are not better accounted for by another cause of Parkinsonism such as dementia with Lewy bodies, psychiatric disorders such as Schizophrenia, Schizoaffective Disorder, Delusional Disorder, or Mood Disorder with Psychotic Features, or a general medical condition including delirium

F. Associated Features (specify if associated)

    With/without insight

    With/without dementia

    With/without treatment for PD (specify drug, surgical, other)

of the following terms: *clinical course, functional outcome, clinical features, antipsychotic drugs, neuroleptics, diagnosis, diagnostic criteria, rating scales,* and *clinical trials.* The resulting articles were then screened before distribution to the task force members to determine that they dealt specifically with PD and that they were original contributions. While several other psychosis scales exist, this critique was limited to the scales used in published, peer-reviewed PD psychosis studies.[1] The primary reference for the psychosis scale along with all articles in which the scales were used in patients with PD were then carefully reviewed. Each scale's strengths, weaknesses, and psychometric properties[21–23] were then determined and summarized. Specific recommendations concerning the recommended use of each scale in PD were made according to the following definitions similarly used in other Movement Disorders Society (MDS) Task Force on Rating Scales initiatives.[24–26]
1. **Recommended:** a scale that has been applied to PD populations; there are data on its use in clinical studies beyond the group that developed the scale; and it has been studied clinimetrically and considered valid, reliable, and sensitive to the given behavior being assessed. Ideally this latter criterion is met for PD psychosis specifically, but can be met if strong clinimetric results are available for hallucinations and psychosis in other contexts. 2. **Suggested:** the scale has been applied to PD populations, but only one of the other criteria is fulfilled. 3. **Listed:** the scale has been applied to PD populations, but neither of the other criteria is fulfilled. This chapter is an adaptation of a peer-reviewed manuscript published previously (Fernandez et al.), with one additional scale, the University of Miami Parkinson's Disease Hallucinations Questionnaire,[26] which was described after the task force published its review, included.

SCALES

Table 18-2 summarizes characteristics of each scale, and Table 18-3 shows how each scale fulfilled the criteria for use recommendations as a scale to assess PD psychosis.

Psychosis scales specific for Parkinson's disease

PARKINSON PSYCHOSIS RATING SCALE (PPRS)

Scale description This scale is designed to "rate the content, quality, severity, and frequency of six domains (of psychotic phenomenology in PD), and their functional impact based on family report,"[27] The six domains are: visual hallucinations, illusions/misidentification, paranoid ideation, sleep disturbance, confusion, and sexual preoccupation.

The original publication was based on 29 generally elderly and demented PD patients with psychosis. The six items are scored on a 4-point scale (1 = *absent* to 4 = *severe symptoms*), anchor points are provided, with total scoring guidelines: *mild* = 8–12; *moderate* = 13–18, *severe* = 19–24. An additional item with the same scoring system rates the overall functional impact of psychosis based on family report.

In the original report, little information is given regarding administration. It appears to be based on an interview by an experienced clinician. The authors describe the scale as "easily administered," but the time required for administration was not given.

Key evaluation issues The scale has been used in the PD psychosis population. However, it has not been utilized by others beyond the author's group.

Validity and reliability evaluation is limited to the original report on the scale.[27] Given the small sample size ($n = 29$), those data must be viewed as preliminary. Furthermore, responsiveness of the PPRS to active or passive intervention in a longitudinal setting has not been fully tested. Inter-rater reliability for individual items and total score was good to very good (rho = 0.80–0.99) (though it is not specified why this type of correlation coefficient was employed). Internal consistency of items across three raters ranged from 0.31 to 0.80. Values for hallucination and paranoid ideation items are fair (0.64–0.75); others are quite weak. Test-retest reliability is described by the authors as

Table 18-2. Summary of the General Properties of Psychosis Scales and Inventories Reviewed in This Chapter

SCALE	TIME REQUIRED TO ADMINISTER THE SCALE (IN MINUTES)	ARE THE ITEMS ASKED IN A STRUCTURED MANNER? (Y/N)	SPECIAL TRAINING REQUIRED TO ADMINISTER THE SCALE? (Y/N)	HAS A VALIDATION STUDY BEEN REPORTED IN PD? (Y/N)	DOES THE SCALE LOOK INTO THE FULL SPECTRUM OF PD PSYCHOSIS? (Y/N)
Parkinson Psychosis Rating Scale	5–15	N	N	Y	N
Parkinson Psychosis Questionnaire	5–15	Y	N	Y	N
Rush Hallucination Inventory	>30	Y	N	N	N
Baylor Hallucination Questionnaire	5–15	Y	N	N	N
University of Miami Parkinson's Disease Hallucinations Questionnaire	5–15	Y	N	N	N
Neuropsychiatric Inventory	15–30	Y	Y	N	N
Behavioral Pathology in Alzheimer's Disease Rating Scale	15–30	Y	N	N	N
Brief Psychiatric Rating Scale	15–30	N	Y	N	N
Positive and Negative Syndrome Scale	>30	N	Y	N	N
Schedule for Assessment of Positive Symptoms	>30	Y	N	N	N
Nurses' Observation Scale for Inpatient Evaluation	5–15	Y	N	N	N
Clinical Global Impression Scale	<5	N	N	N	N
Unified Parkinson Disease Rating Scale Part I	<5	N	N	Y	N

Table 18-3. Summary of "Use Recommendations" of Psychosis Scales Used in PD

PSYCHOSIS SCALE	APPLIED IN PD	USED IN STUDIES BEYOND ORIGINAL PAPER	SATISFACTORY CLINIMETRIC ASSESSMENT	SCALE DESIGNATION*
Parkinson Psychosis Rating Scale	√		√	Suggested
Parkinson Psychosis Questionnaire	√		√	Suggested
Rush Hallucination Inventory	√			Listed
Baylor Hallucination Questionnaire	√			Listed
University of Miami Parkinson's Disease Hallucinations Questionnaire	√			Listed
Neuropsychiatric Inventory	√	√	√	Recommended
Behavioral Pathology in Alzheimer's Disease Rating Scale	√	√		Suggested
Brief Psychiatric Rating Scale	√	√	√	Recommended
Positive and Negative Syndrome Scale	√	√	√	Recommended
Schedule for Assessment of Positive Symptoms	√	√	√	Recommended
Nurses' Observation Scale for Inpatient Evaluation	√			Listed
Clinical Global Impression Scale	√	√		Suggested
Unified Parkinson Disease Rating Scale Part I	√			Listed

* **Recommended**—a scale that has been applied to PD populations; there are data on its use in clinical studies beyond the group that developed the scale; and, it has been studied clinimetrically and considered valid, reliable and sensitive to the given behavior being assessed; **Suggested**—the scale has been applied to PD populations, but only one of the other criteria is fulfilled; **Listed**—the scale has been applied to PD populations, but neither of the other criteria is fulfilled.

"high" for six weeks, but coefficients ranged from quite poor to fair (0.06–0.70). Concurrent validity examining correlation of scores with BPRS (presumably using total scores) was high (0.92); however, the relationship was weak with Nurses' Observation Scale for Inpatient Evaluation (NOSIE) psychotic dimension score (0.48). The instrument appears sensitive to treatment (i.e., on ondansetron).

Strengths and Weaknesses: Strengths: The PPRS was specifically designed to assess psychotic symptoms in patients with PD. It is short (6 items, plus a global assessment item) and allows measurement of change over time. The visual hallucinations item takes into account the frequency of hallucinatory events and insight, two important characteristics of hallucinations in PD.

Weaknesses: The PPRS fails to capture the heterogeneity of psychosis in PD, and the single items for hallucinations and delusions each provide a narrow range of scores for tracking clinical change. Furthermore, the symptoms that accompany psychosis include "confusion," "sexual preoccupancy," and "sleep disturbances," which are not specifically felt to be part of the specific syndrome of psychosis. With only three items devoted to psychosis and three other items devoted to the associated features, the final score risks being burdened with non-psychotic confounds. Finally, the anchors have multiple features collapsed together (i.e., "3 = frequent; absence of full insight; can be convinced," leaving no options for the frequent hallucinations with full insight retained).

Final Assessment The PPRS fulfills criteria as a **Suggested** scale for rating PD psychosis.

PARKINSON PSYCHOSIS QUESTIONNAIRE (PPQ)

Scale description The PPQ[28] was developed as a screening instrument for early recognition of psychosis in PD. The scale was reviewed by clinicians regarding its appropriateness and underwent further analysis of its internal validity by studying test results in 50 patients with Parkinsonism relative to results on the BPRS and the DSM-IV.[17]

The scale includes screening probes followed by detailed questions regarding the presence or absence of sleep disturbance, hallucinations/illusions, delusions, and orientation. Any positive answers within a domain trigger inquiries about frequency and severity. A subscore is the product of the frequency multiplied by the severity score for that symptom category. The total score is the sum of the subscores.

Key evaluation issues The scale has been used in the PD psychosis population. However, it has not been utilized beyond the original report.

There is limited psychometric evidence based on the original study of 50 PD patients.[28] The scale has not been tested extensively, and it has not been subject to evaluation in clinical trials or larger samples and its sensitivity to change has not been tested.

Internal consistency (of presumably the total scale) was moderate to good (alpha 0.68). Interrater reliability is unknown. Divergent validity with UPDRS Part III (rho = −0.13) and MMSE (rho = −0.27) is good. The scale has excellent agreement with SCID (100% sensitivity, 92% specificity). There is a significant, but unspecified, correlation with the BPRS. The use of additive vs. multiplicative scores is not justified adequately.

Strengths and weaknesses Strengths: The PPQ is one of a few scales developed specifically for PD and provides detailed anchors and guidelines for rating items. It provides a mechanism for cataloguing the presence or absence of most discrete psychotic phenomena. Unlike the PPRS, it scores both severity and frequency, and two of the four categories are devoted specifically to hallucinations/illusions and to delusions.

Weaknesses: The PPQ does not include all hallucinatory phenomena (such as olfactory, tactile, kinesthetic; sense of presence). Insight into hallucinations is not taken into consideration. Some forms of delusions, including somatic delusions, are not assessed, and there is no mechanism for cataloguing psychotic phenomena outside the specific questions. Delusions (5 items) are more detailed than hallucinations (4 items) although they are less common in PD psychosis. One item, *delusional ideas of control or influence on actions and thoughts,* is rare in PD. The sleep and orientation items reduce the specificity of the scale.

Final assessment The PPQ fulfills criteria as a "Suggested" scale for rating PD psychosis.

RUSH HALLUCINATION INVENTORY

Scale description This 53-item inventory allows four answers to most questions, but also includes informational questions (how long to fall asleep? what is bedtime?) and yes/no answers to others.[29] The questions with four answers allow for frequency and duration ratings. These questions are not given weights. Illusions and hallucinations as well as emotional coloration (fear) are considered, and visual, auditory, tactile, and olfactory domains are separately assessed.

The first set of questions addresses sleep disorders. There are 11 questions, including informational questions such as: quality of sleep, frequency questions on vivid dreams, nightmares, excessive daytime sedation, and use of sedative medications.

The second section is devoted to visual illusions and consists of seven questions, the first being a screening question, asking if illusions occur. If not, one skips to the next section. The third section pertains to auditory illusions, and has a maximum frequency of three times per week. The six further questions are the same as for the visual illusions. The fourth section is on hallucinations, with an initial focus on visual hallucinations. The initial screening question defines maximal frequency as three times per week. This section asks how long the hallucination persists, what time of day, environmental circumstances, and whether they are frightening. Similar questions are then asked about auditory hallucinations. Then, a section on presence hallucinations, phrased somewhat ambiguously, asks, "During the past month, have you had the experience of feeling something or someone out of nowhere... that is, have you had a sensation when nothing was there?" The last section asks about olfactory hallucinations.

Key evaluation issues The inventory has been used in PD hallucinators, but has not been used in other PD psychosis trials. The inventory has unknown psychometric properties. The correlation between the scale and MMSE (measuring cognitive state) and the UPDRS motor score at baseline is difficult to interpret. That is, is the Rush Hallucinations Inventory score simply a proxy for disease severity? Or, does it indicate, as one might expect, that persons with more marked motor problems and cognitive compromise are also more likely to have hallucinations?

Strengths and weaknesses Strengths: This scale specifically states that it covers "the past month." It comprehensively probes into the major and minor forms of hallucinations and includes detailed questioning about associated sleep disturbances. The questions take into account the frequency and duration of each type of hallucination.

Weaknesses: This inventory assumes that severity is based on frequency and negative emotional association. There is no overall rating for any section. Furthermore, although it is written as a questionnaire, there are no specific instructions. Delusions are not included in the inventory. None of the information is solicited from an observer. Content-wise, there is no mechanism for applying the scale to patients with dementia.

In the visual illusions section, there is no question on how clearly the vision is seen, how persistent it is, or anything about the content other than whether it is frightening. The most severe rating for visual illusion frequency is three times per week (which may not be unlikely for a normal person with impaired vision). There are questions of interest, such as what situations (day, night, dark, light) are most likely to stimulate visual illusions, but these are not useful for either treatment studies or diagnosis. There is no question on visual acuity. Similarly, in the auditory illusions section, no questions on hearing impairment are asked. Duration of the illusion is not ascertained, nor are any questions about content asked (e.g., are the sounds isolated, such as a bark or a name being called; or is it sustained music, conversations, clearly heard, heard at a distance, etc.). For olfactory hallucinations, there is no question about smell or taste impairment and no question on taste. The lack of description of the hallucinated content or whether there is an emotional reaction (other than fear) is another drawback.

Final assessment The Rush Hallucination Inventory fulfills criteria as a **Listed** scale for rating PD psychosis.

BAYLOR HALLUCINATIONS QUESTIONNAIRE

Scale description This six-item, 4-point scale questionnaire assesses only hallucinations[30]: (1)

visual hallucinations; (2) auditory hallucinations; (3) presence hallucinations; (4) insight: "can you tell that the hallucinations are not real?"; (5) "do you attempt to communicate with the hallucinations?"; and, (6) "how upset is your family by the hallucinations?" The answers to questions 1 to 3 are: 0 = *I don't have this problem*; 1 = *rare*; 2 = *occasionally* (about once a week); 3 = *frequently* (more than 3 times a week); 4 = *all the time* (more than once each day).

Key evaluation issues Similar to the Rush Hallucinations Inventory, this questionnaire has been used in PD patients with hallucinations, but it has not been utilized by other groups beyond that of the authors' first description.

The psychometric properties are unknown. The score reportedly correlates with global impression but the correlation coefficient was not reported.[30] The scale has been used in one small study only.[30]

Strengths and weaknesses Strengths: The strengths of this scale are its ease and rapidity of administration, characterization of the distress caused to the family, and delineation of symptom frequency. It focuses specifically on hallucinations in PD, and is anchored in frequency and insight, two clinically important dimensions of PD hallucinations.

Weaknesses: The frequency anchors are unclear, and the equivalence of "daily" and "all the time" is likely to be a problem for many patients and caregivers. The spectrum used to rate symptom frequency seems disproportionate. For example, patients or raters may not view hallucinations experienced more than once a day as occurring "all the time" if they are very fleeting. A person with frequent presence hallucinations may have them three of four times daily without being terribly bothered by them. Despite focusing on hallucinations only, not all hallucinations are included. It does not assess tactile hallucinations or other rare modalities such as olfactory hallucinations. Delusions are not taken into account. The last item concerning the reactions of "the family" is interesting but debatable, as reactions of the family may not reflect the severity of the patient's hallucinations.

Final assessment The Baylor Hallucinations Questionnaire fulfills criteria as a **Listed** scale for rating PD psychosis.

UNIVERSITY OF MIAMI PARKINSON'S DISEASE HALLUCINATIONS QUESTIONNAIRE (UM-PDHQ)

Scale description The UM-PDHQ is a 20-item clinician-administered questionnaire that is completed during a structured interview.[26] The 20 items were derived by its original authors through consultations with PD patients, caregivers, and a panel of experts including four movement disorders specialists, one geriatric psychiatrist, three neuropsychologists, one nurse specialist, and one neuro-opthalmologist. The questions are divided into two groups; a quantitative group that consists of six questions (modality, frequency, duration, insight, emotional burden) and a qualitative group that consists of 14 questions.

In the "quantitative section," the first item is a gating question to assess the presence or absence of hallucinations. If present, the questionnaire probes into whether these are visual, auditory, somatic, gustatory, or olfactory, or combinations thereof. It then asks how often and how long do these experiences last, whether insight is retained, and how distressing it is.

The "qualitative section" comprised of 14 items probes into comorbid eye conditions, current medications, and changes in treatment, whether the hallucinations occurred in the "on" or "off" state, what the patient does to make the hallucinations disappear, etc. It also probes into the quality of the hallucinations—whether or not they are formed, moving, normal size, transparent, solid, colored, etc.

Key evaluation issues Similar to the Rush Hallucinations Inventory and the Baylor Hallucinations Questionnaire, this questionnaire has been used in PD patients with hallucinations, but has not been utilized by other groups beyond that of its original composers.

In its original description, the scale has been used in a PD hallucinations survey of 70 consecutive PD patients, but not in a clinical trial.[26]

Therefore, its psychometric properties are unknown. However, the authors did find in their survey that using the UM-PDHQ, 31 patients (44.3%) were classified as hallucinators and 39 were classified as non-hallucinators, while the Unified Parkinson Disease (UPDRS) Part I identified 26 (37.1%) and failed to report hallucinations in five patients.

Strengths and weaknesses Strengths: The strengths of this scale are its ease of use and thorough quantification of the types of hallucinations. It probes all the less common types of hallucinations (such as somatic, olfactory, gustatory). The questionnaire goes to great lengths to characterize the hallucinations. It also assesses key characteristics that are important in this patient population, such as degree of distress, insight, frequency, and severity. Unique to the questionnaire are items that probe into comorbidities, medication, and recent therapeutic changes.

Weaknesses: It only assesses hallucinations, and not delusions. It is unclear if the questionnaire is able to capture illusions. There are no questions regarding "sense of presence" hallucinations. It does not clearly state the time frame of the assessment. The scoring ranges are not uniform in each item. And it does not separate the different types of hallucinations when scoring frequency, duration, insight, and degree of distress. There is only a single item that probes each of these elements. The authors, in their original publication, did conclude that "the UM-PDHQ in its current form does not provide an overall score of severity and is not a graded or rating instrument. Instead, it is a screening tool designed to draw attention to the presence of hallucinations and initiate further investigation."[26]

Final assessment The UM-PDHQ fulfills criteria as a **Listed** scale for rating PD psychosis.

Scales developed to assess psychosis in patients with dementia

NEUROPSYCHIATRIC INVENTORY (NPI)

Scale description The NPI is a 12-item scale developed primarily for the assessment of psychopathology in patients with dementia.[31] While the NPI has also been used in studies of neuropsychiatric disturbances with non-demented patients, its standard administration assumes that the subject has dementia and that the interview is conducted by a trained rater with a knowledgeable caregiver. There are now other validated and widely used versions: the Nursing Home NPI and the Questionnaire Version (NPIQ), but informant report remains the source of information about the patient.

The twelve items covered by the NPI are: delusions; hallucinations; agitation/aggression; depression/dysphoria; anxiety/elation/euphoria; apathy/indifference; disinhibition; irritability; aberrant motor behavior; nighttime behaviors; and appetite/eating behaviors. To facilitate detection of behavioral changes in these domains and minimize administration time, the NPI uses screening questions about symptoms and behaviors for each of the 12 items. More specific questions are asked only if the screening probe is positively endorsed. For each positive screening probe, the severity and frequency of the related symptoms are rated and a product of these two ratings is multiplied to obtain the score for each domain. A separate rating is attached to the "distress caused to the caregiver," or the "occupational disruption" at the nursing home.

The NPI is copyrighted.

Key evaluation issues The scale has been used by different groups in several PD psychosis studies. In Alzheimer's disease, the NPI showed good internal consistency (Cronbach's alpha 0.87–0.88). The *test-retest reliability* over two to three weeks for the 10 constituent scales and the total score of the NPI ranged from 0.51 to 0.97 for frequency of occurrence of symptoms and from 0.51 to 1.00 for ratings of the severity of symptoms. The inter-rater agreement was "90%–100%." Concurrent validity was established with Behave-AD: the Behave-AD score and NPI frequency score correlation was 0.66; while the correlation with the NPI severity rating of symptoms was 0.71. Correlations among corresponding (similar) subscales of the Behave-AD and NPI tended to be weaker: 0.54 to 0.78 for frequency of symptoms and 0.47 to 0.80

for severity of symptoms.[31] The NPI has been used in several studies related to PD psychosis. Whereas the NPI may be useful for tracking the incidence and presence of psychosis, some antipsychotic treatment studies suggest that the NPI may not be as sensitive to change in the PD population[32–34] as the Brief Psychiatric Rating Scale. This may be related to the multiplicative scoring metric, which results in non-continuous scores as symptom frequency and severity increase. In addition, there probably is a non-linear relationship between symptom severity (intensity) and frequency, and these constructs may have differential sensitivity to treatment. Clinimetric testing has been performed on the total score and not the specific subscores related to hallucinations and psychotic behaviors.

Strengths and weaknesses Strengths: The NPI has a number of strengths. Administration of this scale is relatively efficient, with screening probes that capture delusions and hallucinations as well as the range of most psychiatric symptoms in patients with PD. The structured interview questions potentially enable administration of the NPI by less clinically experienced professionals without reducing scale validity or reliability. Open-ended questions for each item also allow recording of behaviors not listed for a particular domain. Separating symptom frequency from symptom severity provides a means to track the frequency, incidence, prevalence, and the dynamics of various psychiatric phenomena over time. As such, the NPI allows the rater to capture mild but very frequent phenomena or moderate but less frequent phenomena. The scale also provides some questions to characterize specific psychotic phenomena. Ratings of other symptoms, e.g., agitation, and anxiety, allow characterization of additional psychiatric phenomena that may occur with psychosis and improve when the psychotic symptoms improve.

Weaknesses: While the NPI is applicable to a range of neuropsychiatric conditions, its development as an instrument to evaluate patients with dementia potentially limits its application in PD patients who are not demented. Accordingly, if the NPI is to be used in clinical studies of PD patients, the scale needs to be modified so that informant- and patient-derived information is obtained in a standardized fashion. The instrument inquires about most psychotic phenomena, but it does not provide a systematic way of capturing the presence or character of the "minor" forms of psychosis (i.e., illusions and passage and "sense of presence" hallucinations). The total score does not provide a specific index of psychosis, because other behaviors are included in the final outcome.

Final assessment The NPI fulfills criteria as a **Recommended** scale for rating PD psychosis, especially in the cognitively impaired population.

BEHAVIORAL PATHOLOGY IN ALZHEIMER'S DISEASE RATING SCALE (BEHAVE-AD)

Scale description The BEHAVE-AD[35] was designed to measure behavioral disturbances in dementia, especially those occurring in AD, by excluding symptoms that primarily result from cognitive and functional impairments. Hallucinations (5 items) and delusions (7 items) are assessed, and therefore the scale has been applied to PD psychosis. The BEHAVE-AD is a two-part scale. Part 1 (symptomatology) includes 25 items that measure behavioral disturbances classified in seven categories: paranoid and delusional ideation (7 items); hallucinations (5 items); activity disturbances (3 items); aggressiveness (3 items); diurnal rhythm disturbances (1 item); affective disturbance (2 items); and anxieties and phobias (4 items). Each symptom is scored on 4-point scale of severity, where 0 means "not present" and 3 means "present, generally with an emotional and physical component." Part 2 (global rating) is a 4-point global assessment of the overall magnitude of the behavioral symptoms in terms of disturbance to the caregiver and dangerousness to the patient. Ratings are based on caregiver reports of symptoms occurring in the preceding two weeks. The scale takes approximately 20 minutes or less to administer. A shorter, 12-item, observer-rated derived scale has been developed.[36]

Key evaluation issues While the scale as been used extensively in AD studies, it has only been used rarely in PD studies.

In AD, inter-rater agreement for total scores and for paranoia and delusions subscales were very high (greater than 0.90). Strong internal consistency and validity evaluations have been established for AD. Its internal consistency appears to be excellent for the scale overall (0.96 total).[37] Regarding validity, the items are grouped to "measure" seven areas; recent factor analysis with 151 AD patients supports five factors,[38] only one measuring psychosis. A study on its concurrent validity shows a 0.92 correlation between the BEHAVE-AD paranoid and delusional ideation category and the Dementia Signs and Symptoms Scale (DSS); 0.93 between BEHAVE-AD hallucinations and DSS. Paranoid and delusional ideation scores are sensitive to serotonergic and antipsychotic treatment.[37] In spite of these positive evaluations in AD, however, the scale has only rarely been used in PD psychosis.[38]

Strengths and weaknesses Strengths: In the setting of AD, this relatively brief scale is sensitive to therapeutic interventions, such as the use of antipsychotic drugs.[39] Its administration is operationalized to provide low variability. The emphasis of the scale is on delusions (7 items) and hallucinations (5 items). In particular, the detailed rating of delusions is well fitted to the PD population. It is a caregiver-based scale, which is an advantage in demented populations.

Weaknesses: The scale was specifically constructed for the assessment of behavioral disorders of AD, not in patients with PD, in which the profile of behavioral disorders is different. In particular, hallucinations are more frequent than delusions in PD and should receive heavier representation. Of the five items on hallucinations, only one item is on visual hallucinations. Equal weight is then placed on auditory, olfactory, haptic, and "other" hallucinations that are less prevalent in PD. "Minor" forms, such as illusions, passage hallucinations, and "sense of presence" are not taken into account. Retained or lost insight and frequency, both clinically considered as key features of PD hallucinations

and delusions, are not considered. The frequency of hallucinations and delusions is also not considered.

On the other hand, the scale includes "diurnal rhythm disturbances," which are common in PD, such as in response to anti-PD medications. They should, therefore, not be considered *a priori* as a psychiatric symptom. Basing symptom severity on the caregiver's response carries the risk of indirectly measuring other features such as "agitation impression" rather than the actual delusion or psychosis. Some items are confounded by motor, cognitive, and behavioral features of PD, such as the items on depression and anxiety. Since the scale is caregiver-based, non-observable intra-psychic symptoms may not directly measured.

Final assessment The BEHAVE-AD fulfills criteria as a **Suggested** scale for rating PD psychosis.

Scales developed to assess psychosis in schizophrenia

BRIEF PSYCHIATRIC RATING SCALE (BPRS)

Scale description The BPRS was designed to measure clinical changes in patients with schizophrenia.[40] Developers of the BPRS intended for it to be administered by experienced psychiatrists and psychologists, and that the 20- to 30-minute scale required staff training and monitoring to ensure adherence to item definitions. The BPRS includes 18 items, with one item devoted to hallucinatory behavior, one to suspiciousness, and one to unusual thought content. Ratings are to be based solely on clinician-observed symptom severity.

Each item is scored on a 7-point scale ranging from *not present* to *extremely severe*. The total BPRS score is the sum of the scores for each of the 18 items and can be used as a global measure of psychopathology.

Key evaluation issues This scale has been used repeatedly in PD psychosis studies. In fact, it is perhaps the most commonly utilized scale in this unique patient population.

In general, the BPRS-total score and the BPRS "psychosis subscore" appear to be sensitive to changes in overall psychopathology in placebo-controlled and open-label clinical studies on the treatment of psychosis in PD. Despite its extensive use in PD psychosis studies, however, the scale has yet to undergo formal psychometric evaluation in this population. It might be difficult to replicate the tight psychometric properties originally reported in schizophrenia—Hedlund and Vieweg[41] reported item inter-rater reliabilities (Pearson coefficients) of 0.63 to 0.83—unless significant effort is spent in training observers, especially on observational vs. patient-report items. One study reported needing more than 30 training sessions using seven psychiatrists to achieve intra-class correlation coefficients > 0.80.[42] Modified descriptive anchors may help improve reliability. Positive and negative symptom items have good internal consistency, with alpha > 0.81.[43]

Regarding internal consistency, a recent meta-analysis of 26 factor analytic studies[44] showed good support for the core 4-factor model (meaning that the instrument measures 4 domains relevant to psychosis); however, a 5-factor solution is also supported by meta-analysis: affect, positive symptoms, negative symptoms, resistance, and activation (the fifth best emerges in studies of schizophrenia). Most validity studies examined convergent validity: BPRS positive and negative symptom scores correlate well with same scales from PANSS (0.92 and 0.82). Construct validity in terms of sensitivity to change with treatment is supported in many studies. The BPRS may be less useful in patients with mild symptoms.[45]

Strengths and weaknesses Strengths: The BPRS has been used more often than any other symptom rating scale in clinical trials of antipsychotic agents in patients with PD.[11,32–34,46–59] It is relatively brief to administer. It is a good measure of overall psychopathology in a wide range of patient groups. This is relevant in studies of PD psychosis because patients frequently experience other psychiatric symptoms (e.g., depression and anxiety) or behaviors

(e.g., uncooperativeness) that cut across diagnostic categories and may be affected by antipsychotic treatment. In addition, empirically derived subscores, based on patients with schizophrenia, provide an index of the severity of related psychotic phenomena as well as independent symptom areas (e.g., mood phenomena). The BPRS contains items that enable characterization of different delusional phenomena that can occur in PD, such as bizarre delusions, somatic delusions (or concerns), and grandiosity. The 7-point scoring system allows a large gradation of measures including minor (i.e., "very mild") hallucinations when scoring.

Weaknesses: The scale does not provide adequate detailed characterization of the various psychotic phenomena that occur in PD. The scale does not permit differential scoring of the intensity and frequency of different types of hallucinatory phenomena (e.g., frequently formed visual hallucinations and rare auditory hallucinations). Anchors for the item on hallucinations exclude "vivid mental imagery," which could represent illusions in PD patients.

Raters for the BPRS need training. Some items, such as "physical tension," "mannerisms," "blunted affect" and "motor retardation" may be confounded by the motor aspects of PD, dementia, or apathy. It may also be unclear how to evaluate the items on "conceptual disorganization," "guilt feelings," "grandiosity," and "excitement" in patients with PD and psychosis. In cognitively impaired patients, the restricted use of patient-report during the interview and direct observation of the patient may limit the validity of the BPRS.

Final assessment The BPRS fulfills criteria as a **Recommended** scale for rating PD psychosis, especially in the cognitively intact population and as a means to track response to treatment or other interventions.

POSITIVE AND NEGATIVE SYNDROME SCALE (PANSS)

Scale description The Positive and Negative Syndrome Scale (PANSS) is a 30-item scale with seven *positive symptom* items, seven *negative symptom* items, and 16 *general psychopathology symptom* items. The scale is completed by the physician, on the basis of "verbal report and manifestations during the course of the interview as well as reports of behavior by primary care workers or family."[60] Each item is scored on a 7-point severity scale from 1 (*symptom absent, definition does not apply*) to 7 (*extreme*). The positive and negative symptom scales are often reported separately. The PANSS was based originally on the BPRS and on the Psychopathology Rating Schedule. It was designed to measure symptoms in schizophrenia and is commonly used in that setting in trials of antipsychotic agents.

Key evaluation issues The PANSS or its *positive symptom subscore* has been used in several studies of the treatment of drug-induced psychosis in PD.[12,61–64]

The positive symptom scale and the individual items for "hallucinations" and "delusions" have been sensitive to changes in therapeutic trials in PD.[12] In studies among persons with schizophrenia, inter-rater reliability is good with intra-class correlation coefficients of 0.80 or above.[65] For individual items, inter-rater correlations (with patients with schizophrenia) have ranged from 0.54 to 0.93[66] or 0.23 to 0.88.[67] Adequate inter-rater reliability can be achieved in three training sessions.[68] For the positive and negative scales, inter-rater reliability has been reported at 0.82 and 0.86.[67] Internal consistency is good with: Cronbach's alpha 0.73 to 0.87 for both subscales in all rating sessions.[69]

That PANSS shows correlation with BPRS (convergent validity) is not surprising, since the items were derived in part from the BPRS. Correlations between positive scale with SAPS and between negative scale with SANS are 0.77.[69] Though it has three original scales (positive symptoms, negative symptoms, general psychopathology), almost all factor analytic studies with schizophrenic and mood-disordered patients have shown this to be not supported. Instead, most studies support a five- to six-factor model.[70]

Strengths and weaknesses Strengths: Detailed definitions and specific criteria for all rating points are provided in the scale. The positive scale also includes behavioral phenomena (hostility, suspiciousness, excitement) that can accompany hallucinations or delusions. It provides a "minimal" rating and therefore permits rating the presence of minor forms of hallucinations in a standardized fashion.

The general psychopathology subscale includes other psychiatric phenomena that are frequently, though not invariably, present in PD patients with psychosis. And the scale has a sufficient number of items to permit conduction of factor analyses for psychosis in PD, to determine whether the syndrome of PD psychosis is associated with specific patterns of psychotic symptoms.

Weaknesses: The scale was specifically constructed for the assessment of the psychopathology of schizophrenia, not PD. The duration of administration is relatively long (recommended interview time is 30–40 minutes) and includes assessment of complex phenomena. The examiner should have experience in psychiatry, but its applicability in PD samples may be limited. The positive scale of the PANSS includes a single item devoted to hallucinatory behavior, and the operational criteria for severity scoring are based on the hallucinatory syndrome of schizophrenia (which are mostly "verbal and distressing"). Among the other items of the positive symptoms subscale of the PANSS, only the delusions one is well fitted to patients with PD, the other items (conceptual disorganization, excitement, grandiosity, suspiciousness/persecution fears, and hostility) are not well adapted to PD psychopathology. The negative symptoms subscale has many items that can overlap with the presence of dementia or apathy.

Final assessment The PANSS fulfills criteria as a **Recommended** scale for rating PD psychosis, especially for tracking treatment response. The scale can be used in cognitively intact or impaired populations as it relies not only on patient report and clinician observation during the interview but also on the reports of primary caregivers and family.

SCHEDULE FOR ASSESSMENT OF POSITIVE SYMPTOMS (SAPS)

Scale description The SAPS was developed to assess and provide qualitative information about specific features of hallucinations, delusions, behavioral changes associated with psychosis, and thought disorder.[71] The instructions state that the interview should be administered as part of a standardized interview with additional information obtained from nursing staff or others who have observed the patient. The scale is designed to include single items as well as global ratings for each symptom cluster. The rater is instructed to take detailed notes when the patient describes the symptoms. The scale was not developed as a tool for measuring change, although it has been used this way in treatment trials for PD psychosis. The hallucinations section includes seven items: one each on visual hallucinations, olfactory hallucinations, and somatic or tactile hallucinations; three items on auditory hallucinations, of which two rate certain "first rank" symptoms (such as "voices conversing" and "voices commenting," which should be rated independently of the more typical auditory hallucinations); and a global rating. The rater is instructed not to rate illusions or hallucinations that occur when the person is falling off to or waking up from sleep or in the context of an illness or medication exposure that might be associated with the occurrence of hallucinations. The individual hallucination items are rated on a continuum based on their frequency (*occasional* to *daily*, with the latter being most severe). However, the global hallucinations item scoring is based on both the frequency and the extent to which the hallucinations are disruptive. The delusions section has 13 items, including 12 individual items reflecting various types of delusions and one global delusions score. The types of delusions rated include persecutory, grandiose, jealousy, guilt, religious, somatic, and referential, as well as first-rank symptoms of being controlled, mind-reading, thought-broadcasting, thought-insertion, and thought-withdrawal.

These items are rated according to the patient's degree of conviction about the idea, the frequency with which the idea is considered, and whether it affects behavior. The global rating also takes into account bizarre delusions, but is otherwise rated in a fashion similar to the individual items. The next section rates "bizarre behavior" and includes four items plus a global score that reflects a range of phenomena, including abnormal dress, manneristic behavior that is socially inappropriate behavior, aggressive behavior, and repetitive stereotyped behaviors. The final section rates formal "thought disorder," which is characterized by a disruption in how ideas are linked to one another in the context of communication. This section includes eight items. There are no specific instructions for scoring the SAPS. Some studies in PD patients use the sum of all the items as well as the global scores. Others look only at global scores or just the hallucinations and delusions scores.

Key evaluation issues The scale has been used in PD psychosis clinical trials. Studies using the SAPS in clinical trials of PD psychosis (especially the subsection on delusions and hallucinations) show that it is sensitive to change in response to effective treatment.[34,56] However, SAPS has not been subject to careful psychometric analysis in PD.

Nonetheless, inter-rater reliability for the SAPS summary score in psychotic patients is good (0.84).[67] The intra-class coefficient (ICC) is 0.94.[72] For the global domain, intra-class correlations ranged from 0.50 to 0.91[67] Test-retest reliability is weak to moderate (0.54).[72,73] Internal consistency is weaker for the overall instrument (Cronbach's alpha 0.48) than for the four global domain scores (alpha ranging from 0.66 to 0.79).[74] Correlations with PANSS and BPRS are consistently high. For example, Norman et al.[67] found correlation 0.91 between PANSS positive and SAPS summary score. Nicholson et al. (1995) found BPRS positive symptoms (various definitions) correlated well with SAPS composite (0.89+). Single factor structure generally not supported.[75]

Strengths and weaknesses Strengths: The SAPS is easy to administer, with a structured interview and clear anchors provided as part of the scale. It assesses the range of various subtypes of hallucinations and delusions, and this may provide a tool for cataloguing the range of hallucinatory and delusional phenomena in PD.

The global severity rating for each subsection provides a useful measure of overall symptom severity. In particular, the global rating of hallucinations is a good question, as it rates severity by its impact, with *mild* (patient unsure if they are real), *moderate* (vivid and mildly bothersome), *marked* (vivid, frequent and "pervade his life") and *severe* (very vivid and extremely troubling). The global rating for delusions is similarly useful.

Weaknesses: Like other scales, the SAPS was developed for use in patients with schizophrenia, not PD, so the items do not rate the more common types of hallucinations or delusions in PD or capture the range of severity of those symptoms and vice versa (covering many symptoms that are uncommon in PD). The scale specifically excludes illusions. It does not provide a systematic way of capturing the presence or character of all psychotic phenomena, including other minor forms. The hallucination items are weighted towards auditory hallucinations. The presence of insight is not taken into account with scoring.

The scale was not intended for use in patients with dementia or cognitive impairment that limits awareness that symptoms are present. Furthermore, the anchors for scoring hallucinations are confusing to apply in PD and may not reflect the overall severity of the phenomena, because frequency and severity are dissociated in the scoring metric. For example, vivid visual hallucinations with insight that occur daily and do not disrupt behavior would score a "5" (*severe*) in this item, but it is unclear where they would be rated for the global item.

The behavioral section includes disparate items that are poorly defined and cover too-varied dimensions in a single rating. Phenomena in the thought disorder section overlap with features of aphasia, and it would be impossible to distinguish the etiology of the language disturbance in a patient with psychosis. An inclusive rating approach, however, would inflate the overall SAPS score of a patient with dementia and aphasia who has minimal hallucinations.

Raters without experience interviewing patients with schizophrenia may have less familiarity with many of the constructs within each subsection, especially in eliciting the various types of delusions. This could have a significant effect on the validity and reliability of the instrument. The SAPS provides a set of structured interview questions, but experienced raters are aware of the need to probe in greater depth to clarify the presence or absence of a given phenomenon based on information provided by the patient or others, as well as observations of the patient. To that end, the structured interview could yield a scale that is administered reliably but lacks validity.

Final assessment The SAPS fulfills criteria as a **Recommended** scale for rating PD psychosis. While not intended to be used to track changes in treatment, it has been used for this purpose in PD psychosis. It is best used in nondemented populations.

NURSES' OBSERVATION SCALE FOR INPATIENT EVALUATION (NOSIE-30)

Scale description The NOSIE-30 is an inpatient ward behavior rating scale. A first version consisted of 80 items of ward behavior completed by a pair of nursing service members. A revised form, the NOSIE-30, is a selection of 30 items.[76] Each item is rated on a 5-point scale of frequency (0 = *never*; 1 = *sometimes*; 2 = *often*; 3 = *usually*; 4 = *always*). The behavior is rated as observed "in the last three days." Factor analysis has identified six factors, three "positive" (social competence, social interest, and personal neatness) and three "negative" (irritability, manifest psychosis, and retardation).

This scale has been designed to evaluate the behavior of hospitalized schizophrenic patients. The original report on the NOSIE-30 was based upon a sample of 630 schizophrenic *male* patients.

Key evaluation issues The scale has been used in PD psychosis, but only in a few studies, and often with other psychosis rating scales.

Original reports by Honigfeld et al.[76] do not provide adequate psychometric data. There is a weak correlation between the NOSIE psychosis score with Friedberg et al.'s PPRS (0.48). Internal consistency of positive symptom items is fair (KR 0.68), but it is weak for negative symptoms (KR 0.10).[77] Inter-rater reliability is adequate for global score but not for subscores.[78]

Strengths and weaknesses Strengths: The scale is brief (takes under 10 minutes to complete) with simple scoring, focusing on frequency. Raters require little training and simply fill in the responses at the end of the three-day period without having to ask the patient questions. No interpretation of behavior is required (e.g., whether a patient is uncommunicative because of depression, delusional thinking, confusion, etc.), making this a reliable and simple tool for nurses.

It has been used for over 40 years in a large number of published studies on inpatient schizophrenics and shown to be sensitive to changes in therapeutic trials with a high inter-rater reliability.

Weaknesses: The items in the NOSIE-30 were chosen to describe behavior of severe (male) schizophrenic inpatients (and therefore not applicable to the outpatient setting). A number of items do not fit well with PD patients (e.g., "tries to be friendly with others"). It scores frequency, but not severity. Some of the items can be confounded by the motor state or apathy (e.g., "is slow moving or sluggish," "sits, unless directed into activity," etc.).

As mentioned, the NOSIE-30 has been used in only a few studies of PD patients with psychosis[79,80] and often with other psychosis rating scales.

It contains several items focused on social integration and maintaining social norms, assuming normal physical function. It has no items related to delusions, apathy, or anxiety.

Final assessment The NOSIE-30 fulfills criteria as a **Listed** scale for rating PD psychosis.

Other scales used in Parkinson psychosis studies

CLINICAL GLOBAL IMPRESSION SCALE (CGIS)

Scale description The CGIS comprises three subscales: CGI-severity; CGI-improvement; and CGI-therapeutic effect.[81] Each subscale is a single-item rating that is the closest thing to a clinical "gestalt." In CGI-severity, the clinician simply categorizes the severity of the patient's problem using a nominal scoring system with: 0 = *not assessed*; 1 = *normal*; 2 = *borderline ill*; 3 = *mildly ill*; 4 = *moderately ill*; 5 = *markedly ill*; 6 = *severely ill*; 7 = *among the most extremely ill patients*. Similarly, in CGI-improvement, the clinician categorizes the improvement using a similar nominal scoring system from *very much improved* to *very much worse*. The only instruction is to rate this patient within the spectrum of "similar patients." This guideline would be interpreted in the context of PD psychosis as meaning other PD patients with psychosis, excluding, for example, Alzheimer's disease or schizophrenia. The scale does not include a battery of questions, and interpretation of severity encompasses whatever the rater considers important. It may be applied to any illness.

Key evaluation issues The scale has been used extensively in PD psychosis clinical trials, often as a secondary outcome measure, but occasionally as the primary outcome measure.

However, there is limited psychometric information available, despite the scale's being used in several large, randomized PD psychosis clinical trials. Nonetheless, it appears to be sensitive to change.[56,62,82] Guy[83] notes that the limited studies available on psychometrics are quite critical of the scale but that some studies may not have adequately evaluated psychometric properties of the scale by virtue of having included heterogeneous samples, e.g., patients with schizophrenia, depression, and anxiety. Inter-rater reliability for the severity scale is low (0.41 to 0.66). Nonetheless, it has been used in a several PD psychosis studies, either as the primary or secondary outcome measure, and has been found to always correlate with the other more in-depth psychosis scale.[56,62,82] Some guidelines for its use and training are probably needed in order to establish adequate inter-rater reliability, at least in multi-center studies in PD samples.

Strengths and weaknesses Strengths: This scale takes only a few seconds to complete once the history and examination are concluded. The formulation of the score involves no extra effort on the clinician's behalf, as there are no particular questions to ask, and the clinician should have obtained sufficient information in any encounter to be able to complete this question. The scale provides a measure of clinical relevance, which may be a useful addition to the more sophisticated scales with high reliability and sensitivity, but where the clinical relevance of a change may be limited. The scale is in the public domain, making it free to use.

Weaknesses: Whereas the CGIS is a "flexible" and open scale that permits the rater to consider the "whole picture," assessment of single items can easily be confusing. For example, hallucinations of similar degree in different patients may cause markedly different responses in the patients, making it a major problem in one case and a minor problem in another. Raters for the CGI may also confound more than one problem, so that depression, anxiety, or motor dysfunction itself may alter the rater's interpretation of the severity of the illness (i.e., a patient with mild psychosis may have severe anxiety, causing the global impression to have an uncertain interpretation). Importantly, item 3 (*minimally improved*) and 5 (*minimally worse*) do not indicate whether these refer to "minimal" in the sense of the minimal change that is still clinically significant or to "minimal" in the sense of "inconsequential."

Final assessment The CGIS fulfills criteria as a **Suggested** scale for rating PD psychosis. It is best used as an additional outcome measure to complement a more detailed psychosis scale.

UNIFIED PARKINSON DISEASE RATING SCALE (UPDRS) PART I

Scale description Part I of the UPDRS has 4 items ("mentation"; "thought disorders," "depression" and "motivation/initiative"), scored from 0 (*normal*) to 4 (*most severe*), based on the week prior to assessment.[84] It was developed as a subscale of the larger UPDRS with the goal of tapping non-motor phenomena. The ratings for Part I are based on a clinical interview of the patient, although probably best performed with a caregiver present. Some scoring strategies are unclear. Under item 2 (thought disorders), the following are the anchor points: 0 = *none*; 1 = *vivid dreaming*; 2 = *benign hallucinations with insight retained*; 3 = *occasional to frequent hallucinations or delusions, without insight, could interfere with daily activities*; 4 = *persistent hallucinations, delusions, or florid psychosis; not able to care for self.* Thus, item 2 is the most relevant item for psychosis, although cognitive impairment, depression, and reduced motivation frequently co-occur with psychosis. The item combines dreaming phenomena, hallucinations, and delusions in one item. The UPDRS is currently under revision, and this subscale is subject to major changes.

Key evaluation issues The scale is more utilized in the general PD population rather than for specific PD psychosis studies. If used in this population, it is used more as a screening criterion rather than an outcome measure that tracks change.

A major problem is that a "floor effect" may be present in many patients (23%).[85] Inter-rater reliability is questionable. Internal consistency is good (Cronbach's alpha 0.79). Item-to-scale mentation total correlations were moderate (0.57–0.66). Factor structure confirmed; the four items loaded on their own factor (loadings 0.54–0.72). A self-rating version exists, which has demonstrated good reliability with a clinical interview.[86]

Strengths and weaknesses Strengths: The thought-disorder item can be administered and scored very rapidly. Its inclusion in the most widely used PD scale has made it a widely used instrument for assessment of psychiatric symptoms in epidemiological studies, although psychometric studies are wanting. It is brief and easily administered. The anchor points are clear and clinically relevant.

Weaknesses: A single item is obviously not sufficient to explore the variety of psychotic phenomena in PD. The item implicitly assumes that there is a continuum from vivid dreams to formed hallucinations, a point that is controversial, based on current literature. The lumping of dream phenomena, hallucinations, and delusions into one item does not always fit with the clinical presentation. Although less common, it is possible for some patients to experience delusions but not hallucinations. Many symptoms that are not uncommon in PD patients with psychosis, such as auditory or other hallucinations, are not included. Finally, as a screening instrument, it may not be particularly sensitive to change, and to our knowledge, studies addressing this issue do not exist.

Final assessment The UPDRS Part I and item 2 within Part I fulfill criteria as a **Listed** scale for rating PD psychosis.

CONCLUSION AND RECOMMENDATIONS

Several factors are implicit concerns in the assessment of psychosis scales. Validity of any scale is necessarily affected by the rater who conducts the interview. Patients or informants may be more likely to endorse symptoms when asked, for example, by a physician versus a research assistant. Furthermore, knowledge of a patient's history and familiarity with previously reported hallucinations or delusions provides a basis for the physician's inquiry about present symptoms and their impact. Clinical judgement and the experience of the interviewer will influence the consistency of the informant/patient answers and the extent to which the rater probes or notices subtle features of psychosis. As an example, an untrained rater with limited clinical experience may base ratings on the patient's

initial answer to a direct question and miss hallucinatory or delusional phenomena that only become apparent during an open-ended interview or through disclosure that is based on trust in the physician. Some scales attempt to limit this source of variation in symptom ratings by providing scripted screening probes or detailed anchors for scoring the ratings, but these restrictions may in fact underrate behaviors like psychosis that are culturally sensitive.

The source of information also influences ratings, and the various scales use a number of approaches, e.g., self-report, informant-derived information, medical records. Some patients may not reveal their psychotic or affective phenomena to others, diminishing the validity of the instrument when it is administered to an informant only. Conversely, cognitive impairment may limit the information a patient can provide.

Some scales focus only on psychosis, whereas others include a range of psychiatric symptoms in addition to psychosis. Psychosis scales usually provide more detailed description of psychosis, while the latter group provides a broader psychopathological description. A final concern is that most psychosis scales were developed in non-PD samples and have not been psychometrically tested in PD.

Similar to the Quality Standards Subcommittee of the American Academy of Neurology who concluded in their review that there currently are "no validated tools for psychosis screening in PD,"[87] it is evident from this review that none of the current scales used in PD adequately captures the entire phenomenology of PD psychosis. It is important that the current scales do not have the ability to assess the incidence, prevalence, and severity (or impact) of all forms of discrete psychotic phenomena. For treatment studies, it is essential that the scale be useful for assessing individual responses as well as group scores and responses. The BPRS and the SAPS are scales that appear to be sensitive to change. The SAPS is relatively complete, but like most psychosis scales derived from psychiatric research (BPRS, SAPS, PANSS, etc.), several items relevant to schizophrenia are less useful to PD psychosis. The NPI is a good scale in cataloguing the presence or absence of psychotic phenomena. It is a scale with a scripted interview that relies less on the clinician's judgement. Scales with open-ended interviews rely more on the judgement of the rater. As opposed to tremor, which is observable and fairly objective, clinical experience and judgement are needed to classify in a reliable and valid way whether a perception is indeed hallucinatory. Yet, despite the script in the NPI, there are still concerns about how the constructs are interpreted when the scale is used by clinicians who are not psychiatrically trained. Trained raters are better at picking up on cues that the patient does have paranoid ideas or is hallucinating, and notice inconsistencies in responses. The PPRS, PPQ, and the UPDRS Part I were designed specifically for PD but are still inadequate scales for exploring and tracking the entire PD psychosis phenomenology. The Rush Hallucination Inventory, Baylor Hallucination Questionnaire, and UM-PDHQ do not explore delusions. The NOSIE-30 cannot be applied to the majority of PD patients who are community-dwelling. (See Tables 18-2 and 18-3 for the summary of the general properties of each scale reviewed.) While the task force has labeled some scales as "recommended" or "suggested" based on the fulfilling defined criteria, it does not mean that these scales are "ideal."

Based on these limitations, the MDS Task Force actually recommended the development of a new scale of PD psychosis, as none of the current scales contains all the basic content, mechanistic, and psychometric properties desired for the ideal PD psychosis scale. A new task force for the composition and validation of this new PD psychosis scale has been formed. In the meantime, selection of the current scales should be based on the goals of the assessment. Different scales may be better for some settings than others. Any chosen scale should be adapted to use both informant and patient information, and the rater will need to make a judgement as to which information to use when making a final rating. Since one scale may not be able to serve all needs, a scale used to measure clinical response and changes over time (such as the CGIS) may need to be combined with another scale better at cataloguing specific features (such as the NPI or

SAPS). At present, for clinical trials on PD psychosis assessing new treatments, the following are recommended primary outcome scales: NPI (for the cognitively impaired PD population or when a caregiver is required), SAPS, PANSS, or BPRS (for the cognitively intact PD population or when the patient is the sole informant). The CGIS is suggested as a secondary outcome scale to measure change and response to treatment over time.

Acknowledgments

The author would like to thank the following members of the Writing Committee of the MDS Task Force on Scales to Assess Psychosis in Parkinson's Disease, and the Steering Committee of the MDS Task Force for Rating Scales: Dag Aarsland, Giles Fénelon, Joseph H. Friedman, Laura Marsh, Alex I. Tröster, Werner Poewe, Olivier Rascol, Cristina Sampaio, Glenn T. Stebbins, and Christopher G. Goetz.

RECOMMENDED SCALES
NPI (for the cognitively-impaired PD population or when a caregiver is required)
SAPS, Positive and Negative Syndrome Scale (PANSS)
Brief Psychiatric Rating Scale (BPRS) (for the cognitively-intact PD population or when the patient is the sole informant)

References

1. Fernandez HH, Aarsland D, Fenelon G, et al. Scales to assess psychosis in Parkinson's disease: critiques and recommendations. *Mov Disord.* 2008;23(4):484–500.
2. Fenelon G, Mahieux F, Huon R, Ziegler M. Hallucinations in Parkinson's disease: prevalence, phenomenology and risk factors. *Brain.* 2000;123:733–745.
3. Hely MA, Morris JG, Reid WG, Trafficante R. Sydney multicenter study of Parkinson's disease: non-L-dopa-responsive problems dominate at 15 years. *Mov Disord.* 2005;20:190–199.
4. Sanchez-Ramos JR, Ortoll R, Paulson GW. Visual hallucinations associated with Parkinson disease. *Arch Neurol.* 1996;53:1265–1268.

5. Fenelon G, Mahieux F, Huon R, Ziegler M. Hallucinations in Parkinson's disease: prevalence, phenomenology and risk factors. *Brain.* 2000;123:733–745.

6. Papapetropoulos S, Mash DC. Psychotic symptoms in Parkinson's disease. From description to etiology. *J Neurol.* 2005;252: 753–764.

7. Graham JM, Grunewald RA, Sagar HJ. Hallucinosis in idiopathic Parkinson's disease. *J Neurol Neurosurg Psychiatry.* 1997;63:434–440.

8. Inzelberg R, Kipervasser S, Korczyn AD. Auditory hallucinations in Parkinson's disease. *J Neurol Neurosurg Psychiatry.* 1998;64: 533–535.

9. de Maindreville AD, Fenelon G, Mahieux F. Hallucinations in Parkinson's disease: a follow-up study. *Mov Disord.* 2005;20: 212–217.

10. Marsh L. Psychosis in Parkinson's disease. *Curr Treat Options Neurol.* 2004;6:181–189.

11. Fernandez HH, Trieschmann ME, Okun MS. Rebound psychosis: effect of discontinuation of antipsychotics in Parkinson's disease. *Mov Disord.* 2005;20:104–105.

12. Pollak P, Tison F, Rascol O, et al. Clozapine in drug induced psychosis in Parkinson's disease: a randomised, placebo controlled study with open follow up. *J Neurol Neurosurg Psychiatry.* 2004;75:689–695.

13. Factor SA, Feustel PJ, Friedman JH, et al. Longitudinal outcome of Parkinson's disease patients with psychosis. *Neurology.* 2003;60:1756–1761.

14. Aarsland D, Larsen JP, Karlsen K, Lim NG, Tandberg E. Mental symptoms in Parkinson's disease are important contributors to caregiver distress. *Int J Geriatr Psychiatry.* 1999;14:866–874.

15. Aarsland D, Larsen JP, Tandberg E, Laake K. Predictors of nursing home placement in Parkinson's disease: a population-based, prospective study. *J Am Geriatr Soc.* 2000;48:938–942.

16. Goetz CG, Stebbins GT. Mortality and hallucinations in nursing home patients with advanced Parkinson's disease. *Neurology.* 1995;45:669–671.

17. Fernandez HH, Donnelly EM, Friedman JH. Long-term outcome of clozapine use for psychosis in parkinsonian patients. *Mov Disord.* 2004;19:831–833.

18. *Diagnostic and Statistical Manual of Mental Disorders.* 4th ed. Washington, DC: American Psychiatric Association; 1994.

19. First MB, Spitzer RL, Gibbon M, Williams JBW. *Structured Clinical Interview for DSM-IV Axis I Disorders–Patient Edition.* Washington, DC: American Psychiatric Press; 2007.

20. Ravina B, Marder K, Fernandez HH, et al. Diagnostic criteria for psychosis in Parkinson's disease: report of an NINDS/NIMH Work Group. *Mov Disord.* 2007;15;22(8):1061–1068.

21. Nunnally JC. *Psychometric Theory.* 2nd ed. New York: McGraw-Hill; 1978.

22. Sattler JM. *Assessment of Children: Cognitive Applications.* 4th ed. San Diego, CA: Jerome M Sattler Publisher Inc; 2001.

23. Streiner DL, Norman GR. *Health Measurement Scales: A Practical Guide to Their Development and Use.* 2nd ed. Oxford: Oxford University Press; 1995.

24. Friedman JH, Alves G, Hagell P, et al. Fatigue rating scales critique and recommendations by the Movement Disorders Society task force on rating scales for Parkinson's disease. *Mov Disord.* 2010;25(7):805–822.

25. Leentjens AF, Dujardin K, Marsh L, et al. Apathy and anhedonia rating scales in Parkinson's disease: critique and recommendations. *Mov Disord.* 2008;23(14):2004–2014.

26. Papapertropoulos S, Katzen H, Schrag A, et al. A questionnaire-based (UM-PDHQ) study of hallucinations in Parkinson's disease. *BMC Neurol.* 2008;8:21. doi:10.1186/1471-2377-8-21.

27. Friedberg G, Zoldan J, Melamed E. Parkinson Psychosis Rating Scale: a practical instrument for grading psychosis in Parkinson's disease. *Clin Neuropharmacol.* 1998;21:280–284.

28. Brandstaedter D, Spiker S, Ulm G, et al. Development and evaluation of the Parkinson Psychosis Questionnaire: a screening instrument for the early diagnosis of drug-induced psychosis in Parkinson's disease. *J Neurol.* 2005;252:1060–1066.

29. Goetz CG, Leurgans S, Pappert EJ, Raman R, Stemer AB. Prospective longitudinal assessment of hallucinations in Parkinson's disease. *Neurology.* 2001;57:2078–2082.

30. Ondo WG, Tinter R, Voung MA, Lai D, Ringholz G. Double-blind, placebo-controlled, unforced titration, parallel trial of quetiapine for dopaminergic-induced hallucinations in Parkinson's disease. *Mov Disord.* 2005;20(8):958–963.

31. Cummings JL, Mega M, Gray K, Rosenberg-Thompson S, Carusi DA, Gornbein J. The Neuropsychiatric Inventory: comprehensive

assessment of psychopathology in dementia. *Neurology.* 1994;44:2308–2314.

32. Juncos JL, Roberts VJ, Evatt ML, et al. Quetiapine improves psychotic symptoms and cognition in Parkinson's disease. *Mov Disord.* 2004;19:29–35.

33. Breier A, Sutton VK, Feldman PD, et al. Olanzapine in the treatment of dopamimetic-induced psychosis in patients with Parkinson's disease. *Biol Psychiatry.* 2002;52:438–444.

34. Marsh L, Lyketsos C, Reich S. Olanzapine for the treatment of psychosis in patients with Parkinson's disease and dementia. *Psychosomatics.* 2001;42:477–481.

35. Reisberg B, Borenstein J, Salob SP, et al. Behavioral symptoms in Alzheimer's disease: phenomenology and treatment. *J Clin Psychiatry.* 1987;48(suppl 5):9–15.

36. Chacko RC, Hurley RA, Harper RG, Jankovic J, Cardoso F. Clozapine for acute and maintenance treatment of psychosis in Parkinson's disease. *J Neuropsychiatry Clin Neurosci.* 1995;7:471.

37. Auer SR, Monteiro IM, Reisberg B. The empirical behavioral pathology in Alzheimer's disease (BEHAVE-AD) rating scale. *Int Psychogeriatr.* 1996;8:247–266.

38. De Deyn PP, Rabheru K, Rasmussen A, et al. A randomized trial of risperidone, placebo, and haloperidol for behavioral symptoms of dementia. *Neurology.* 1999;53:946–955.

39. Harwood DG, Ownby RL, Barker WW, Duara R. The behavioral pathology in Alzheimer's Disease Scale (BEHAVE-AD): factor structure among community-dwelling Alzheimer's disease patients. *Int J Geriatr Psychiatry.* 1998;13(11):793–800.

40. Overall JE, Gorham DR. The Brief Psychiatric Rating Scale. *Psychol Rep.* 1962;10:799–812.

41. Hedlund JL, Vieweg BW. The Brief Psychiatric Rating Scale (BPRS): a comprehensive review. *J Oper Psychiatry.* 1980;11:48–65.

42. Overall JE, Gorham DR. Brief Psychiatric Rating Scale. In: Handbook of Psychiatric measures Edited by *Task Force for the Handbook of Psychiatric Measures,* . Washington, DC: American Psychiatric Association; 2000: 490–494.

43. Nicholson IR, Chapman JE, Neufeld RW. Variability in BPRS definitions of positive and negative symptoms. *Schizophr Res.* 1995;17(2):177–185.

44. Shafer A. Meta-analysis of the brief psychiatric rating scale factor structure. *Psychol Assess.* 2005;17(3):324–335.

45. Scholtz E, Dichgans J. Treatment of drug-induced exogenous psychosis in parkinsonism with clozapine and fluperlapine. *Eur Arch Psychiatry Clin Neurosci.* 1985;235:60–64.

46. Fernandez HH, Trieschmann ME, Okun MS. Rebound psychosis: effect of discontinuation of antipsychotics in Parkinson's disease. *Mov Disord.* 2005;20(1):104–105.

47. Ostergaard K, Dupont E. Clozapine treatment of drug-induced psychotic symptoms in late stages of Parkinson's disease. *Acta Neurol Scand.* 1988;78:349–350.

48. Friedman J, Lannon M. Clozapine in the treatment of psychosis in Parkinson's disease. *Neurology.* 1990;39:1219–1221.

49. Kahn N, Freeman A, Juncos J, et al. Clozapine is beneficial for psychosis in Parkinson's disease. *Neurology.* 1991;41:1699–1700.

50. Wolk S, Douglas C. Clozapine treatment of psychosis in Parkinson's disease: a report of five consecutive cases. *J Clin Psychiatry.* 1992;53:373–376.

51. Factor S, Brown D. Clozapine prevents recurrence of psychosis in Parkinson's disease. *Mov Disord.* 1992;7(2):125–131.

52. Lew M, Waters C. Clozapine treatment of parkinsonism with psychosis. *J Am Geriatr Soc.* 1993;41:669–671.

53. Factor S, Brown D, Molho ES, Podskalny GD. Clozapine: a 2-year trial open trial in Parkinson's disease patients with psychosis. *Neurology.* 1994;44:544–546.

54. Ford B, Cote L, Fahn S. Risperidone in Parkinson's disease [letter]. *Lancet.* 1994;344:681.

55. Wagner M, Defilippi J, Menza M, et al. Clozapine for the treatment of psychosis in Parkinson's disease: chart review of 49 patients. *J Neuropsychiatry.* 1996;3:276–280.

56. The Parkinson Study Group. Low-dose clozapine for the treatment of drug-induced psychosis in Parkinson's disease. *N Engl J Med.* 1999;340:757–763.

57. Fernandez HH, Friedman JH, Jacques C, Rosenfeld M. Quetiapine for the treatment of drug-induced psychosis in Parkinson's disease. *Mov Disord.* 1999;14(3):484–487.

58. Ellis T, Cudkowicz ME, Sexton PM, Growdon JH. Clozapine and risperidone treatment of psychosis in Parkinson's disease. *J Neuropsychiatry Clin Neurosci.* 2000;12:354–336.

59. Overall JE, Gorham DR. The Brief Psychiatric Rating Scale (BPRS): recent developments in

ascertainment and scaling. *Psychopharmacol Bull.* 1988;24:97–99.

60. Kay SR, Opler LA, Lindermayer JP. The Positive and Negative Syndrome Scale (PANSS): rationale and standardisation. *Br J Psychiatry.* 1989;155(suppl 7):59–65.

61. Chacon JR, Duran E, Duran JA, Alvarez M. Usefulness of olanzapine in the levodopa-induced psychosis in patients with Parkinson's disease. *Neurologia.* 2002;17:7–11.

62. French Clozapine Study Group. Clozapine in drug-induced psychosis in Parkinson's disease. *Lancet.* 1999;353:2041–2042.

63. Kohmoto J, Kihira T, Miwa H, Kondo T. Effect of quetiapine fumarate on drug-induced psychosis in patients with Parkinson's disease. *No To Shinkei.* 2002;54:489–492.

64. Mohr E, Mendis T, Hildebrand K, De Deyn PP. Risperidone in the treatment of dopamine-induced psychosis in Parkinson's disease: an open pilot trial. *Mov Disord.* 2000;15: 1230–1237.

65. Kay SR. Positive-negative symptom assessment in schizophrenia: psychometric issues and scale comparison. *Psychiatr Q.* 1990;61(3):163–178.

66. Bell M, Milstein R, Beam-Goulet J, et al The Positive and Negative Syndrome Scale and the Brief Psychiatric Rating Scale. Reliability, comparability, and predictive validity. *J Nerv Ment Dis.* 1992;180(11):723–728.

67. Norman RM, Malla AK, Cortese L, Diaz F. A study of the interrelationship between and comparative interrater reliability of the SAPS, SANS and PANSS. *Schizophr Res.* 1996;19(1):73–85.

68. Muller MJ, Rossbach W, Davids E, Wetzel H, Benkert O. [Evaluation of standardized training for the Positive and Negative Syndrome Scale (PANSS)]. *Nervenarzt.* 2000;71(3):195–204.

69. Kay SR, Fiszbein A, Opler LA. The positive and negative syndrome scale (PANSS) for schizophrenia. *Schizophr Bull.* 1987;13(2): 261–276.

70. Van den Oord EJ, Rujescu D, Robles JR, et al. Factor structure and external validity of the PANSS revisited. *Schizophr Res.* 2006;82 (2–3):213–223.

71. Andreasen NC. *Scale for the Assessment of Positive Symptoms (SAPS).* Iowa City, Iowa: University of Iowa; 1984.

72. Malla AK, Norman RM, Williamson P. Stability of positive and negative symptoms in schizophrenia. *Can J Psychiatry.* 1993;38(9):617–621.

73. Malla AK, Norman RM, Williamson P, Cortese L, Diaz F. Three syndrome concept of schizophrenia. A factor analytic study. *Schizophr Res.* 1993;10(2):143–150.

74. Andreasen NC, Grove WM. Evaluation of positive and negative symptoms in schizophrenia. *Psychiatry Psychobiol.* 1986;1:108–121.

75. Peralta V, Cuesta MJ. Dimensional structure of psychotic symptoms: an item-level analysis of SAPS and SANS symptoms in psychotic disorders. *Schizophr Res.* 1999;38(1):13–26.

76. Zoldan J, Friedberg G, Livneh M, Melamed E. Psychosis in advanced Parkinson's disease: treatment with ondansetron, a 5-HT3 receptor antagonist. *Neurology.* 1995;45:1305–1308.

77. Dingemans PM. The Brief Psychiatric Rating Scale (BPRS) and the Nurses' Observation Scale for Inpatient Evaluation (NOSIE) in the evaluation of positive and negative symptoms. *J Clin Psychol.* 1990;46(2):168–174.

78. Honigfeld G, Klett CJ, Gillis RD. NOSIE-30: a treatment sensitive ward behaviour scale. *Psychol Rep.* 1966;19:180–182.

79. Wolters EC, Hurwitz TA, Mak E, et al. Clozapine in the treatment of parkinsonian patients with dopaminomimetic psychosis. *Neurology.* 1990;40:832–834.

80. Hafkenscheid A. Psychometric evaluation of the Nurses Observation Scale for Inpatient Evaluation in the Netherlands. *Acta Psychiatr Scand.* 1991;83(1):46–52.

81. Guy W. *1976 ECDEU Assessment Manual for Psychopharmacology.* DHEW Publ ADM-76-338, Rockville, MD: National Institute of Mental Health; 1976: 534–537.

82. Morgante L, Epifanion A, Spina E, et al. Quetiapine and clozapine in parkinsonian patients with dopaminergic psychosis. *Clin Neuropharmacol.* 2004;27:153–156.

83. Guy W. Clinical Global Impressions (CGI) Scale. In: *Task Force for the Handbook of Psychiatric Measures, Handbook of Psychiatric Measures.* Washington, DC: American Psychiatric Association; 2000:100–102.

84. Fahn S, Elton RL; and UPDRS Program Members. Unified Parkinson's Disease Rating Scale. In: Fahn S, Marsden CD, Goldstein M, Calne D, eds. *Recent Developments in Parkinson's Disease.* vol 2. Florham Park, NJ: Macmillan Healthcare Information; 1987: 153–163.

85. Martinez-Martin P, Forjaz MJ. Metric attributes of the Unified Parkinson Disease Rating Scale 3.0 battery: part I, feasibility,

scaling assumptions, reliability and precision. *Mov Disord.* 2006;29:1182–1188.

86. Louis ED, Lynch T, Marder K, Fahn S. Reliability of patient completion of the historical portion of the Unified Parkinson Disease Rating Scale. *Mov Disord.* 1996;11(2):185–192.

87. Miyasaki JM, Shannon K, Voon V, et al. Practice parameter: evaluation and treatment of depression, psychosis and dementia in Parkinson disease (an evidence based review). Report of the Quality Standards Subcommittee of the American Academy of Neurology. *Neurology.* 2006;66:996–1002.

19

DEPRESSION RATING SCALES IN PARKINSON'S DISEASE: CRITIQUE AND RECOMMENDATIONS

Anette Schrag

Summary

Depression is a common comorbid condition in Parkinson's disease and a major contributor to poor quality of life and disability. However, depression can be difficult to assess in patients with PD due to overlapping symptoms and difficulties in the assessment of depression in cognitively impaired patients. The scales to assess depression in PD reviewed here are the Beck Depression Inventory (BDI), Hamilton Depression Scale (Ham-D), Hospital Anxiety and Depression Scale (HADS), Zung Self-Rating Depression Scale (SDS), Geriatric Depression Scale (GDS), Montgomery-Asberg Depression Rating Scale (MADRS), Unified Parkinson's Disease Rating Scale (UPDRS) Part I, Cornell Scale for the Assessment of Depression in Dementia (CSDD), and Center for Epidemiologic Studies Depression Scale (CES-D). In keeping with the previous MDS-commissioned Task Force report, the recommendation is that the most appropriate scale (and cutoff) is dependent on the clinical or research goal. A diagnosis of depressive illness should not be made based on scale scores alone. Overall, observer-rated scales are preferred if the study or clinical situation permits. The Ham-D, MADRS, BDI, HADS, CSDD, and GDS are "Recommended" instruments in dPD for *screening* for dPD. The SDS also fulfilled criteria for "Recommended" but needs further validation studies. The CES-D has not been adequately tested in dPD. The UPDRS and MDS-UPDRS depression item is a single question, and whilst formally fulfilling criteria for a "Recommended" scale, it should be used with caution. For *severity* rating, currently the Ham-D, MADRS, BDI, and SDS are "Recommended." The HADS and the GDS include limited motor symptom assessment and may therefore be most useful in rating depression severity across a range of PD severity; however, these scales appear insensitive in severe depression and have not been sufficiently assessed for rating severity of dPD. To account for overlapping motor and non-motor symptoms of depression, adjusted instrument cutoff scores should be employed in screening for dPD, and scales to assess severity of motor symptoms (e.g., MDS-UPDRS) should be used to adjust for overlapping symptoms in studies assessing depression severity.

INTRODUCTION

Depressive symptoms commonly occur in Parkinson's disease, affecting approximately 40% of patients in cross-sectional studies.[1-3] Depressive symptoms have also been recognized to be a major determinant of health-related quality of life in PD, and also affect functional ability, cognitive functioning, and caregiver quality of life.[4-5] It is therefore important to recognize and assess depressive symptoms in patients with PD adequately. The gold standard for the diagnosis of depressive disorder at present are the criteria of the *Diagnostic and Statistical Manual* (DSM) of the American Psychiatric Association. However, in clinical practice and research studies, particularly in epidemiological studies, surveys and treatment trials measuring severity of depressive symptoms, use of DSM, or similar criteria often are not feasible or useful. A number of rating scales for screening and/or assessment of severity of depression are available and have been used widely to assess depression in patients with and without PD. However, there are many methodological difficulties in assessing depressive symptoms in PD. The Movement Disorder Society (MDS) Task Force on Rating Scales for Parkinson's Disease evaluated commonly used rating scales for depression in PD (dPD), and made recommendations on the utilization of specific scales and their need for modifications or replacement in this population[6]. This assessment made in 2007 has been adapted and updated, and the classification into "Recommended," "Suggested" and "Listed" scales of later similar reviews is adopted here.

METHODS

The methodology of the task force reviews was as described in Chapter 6 In addition, a survey of MDS members explored the members' clinical experience with depression scales in dPD. An extensive appendix on the available literature regarding all concerned scales was published with the manuscript simultaneously on the journal's website.

The assessment was limited to depression-specific scales, as assessment of all multidimensional scales that include assessment of depression was beyond the scope of this project. Scales specifically assessing features that can occur as aspects of depression, such as anxiety, anhedonia, and apathy, were also excluded, but the ability of depression scales to capture these aspects was assessed. Scales that assess short-lived mood states only were also excluded.

Literature search strategy

Medline on PubMed was searched for the relevant papers for all listed publications up to June of 2011. The terms used were "Parkinson's disease" or "Parkinsonism," "depression," and "psychiatric status rating scale," "scale," or "measure." For each scale, a search was also conducted for the terms "Parkinson's disease" (or "Parkinsonism" or "Parkinson disease") and the name of the scale.

RESULTS

Identified problems when using rating scales for dPD

1. Overlap between symptoms of depression and Parkinson's disease.

DSM defines "an episode of major depressive disorder" as the presence of depressed mood or loss of interest or pleasure for at least two weeks, together with at least five other symptoms if they represent a significant change from previous functioning. These other features include change in appetite or weight; insomnia or hypersomnia; psychomotor agitation or retardation (i.e., generalized slowing of thought, speech, and body movements); fatigue or loss of energy; feelings of worthlessness or excessive or inappropriate guilt; diminished ability to think or concentrate, or indecisiveness; recurrent thoughts of death or recurrent suicidal ideation. Importantly, symptoms that are clearly due to a general medical condition are excluded. Rating some of the core symptoms of depression is therefore difficult due to the considerable overlap of symptoms of depression and core symptoms of PD (e.g., cognitive impairment, apathy, psychomotor changes [both retardation and agitation], attentional or concentration changes, loss of appetite, weight change, sleep disturbances, and fatigue; see Table 19-1). It is unclear whether an inclusive approach (i.e., rating all symptoms that are present on a depression scale without judgement of their specific relationship to depression) should be adopted for rating scales as has been suggested when applying diagnostic criteria for depression.[7] The use of scales (and diagnostic criteria) that automatically include all somatic symptoms may lead to inflated depression scores.[8,9] In such cases, patients risk scoring as depressed without the core symptoms of depression. On the other hand, scales that exclude these overlapping symptoms, which may cluster with depression rather than with motor features,[9,10] may have poor criterion validity, particularly at the severe end of the depression spectrum. Current evidence suggests that some somatic symptoms in PD are important and sensitive aspects of dPD and should not be neglected in the assessment of depression in PD.[11]

2. Overlap between symptoms of depression and apathy.

Apathy is one of the core symptoms of depression. However, it may also occur independently of depression as part of a syndrome of apathy. A significant proportion of patients who are not depressed have apathy with loss of interest, motivation, and effortful behavior, but without other cognitive, affective, or somatic symptoms of depression.[12-15]

3. Assessment of cognitively impaired patients.

Cognitive impairment is common in PD and approximately 30% to 40% of patients with PD meet criteria for dementia.[16] The frequent occurrence of dementia complicates accurate diagnosis and monitoring of depression in cognitively impaired PD patients.

4. Differences between depression without PD and dPD.

Depression in PD differs in some aspects from major depression; e.g., with a relative rarity of feelings of guilt, self-blame or worthlessness in PD.[17-19] Furthermore, the majority of patients with PD have depressive symptoms not fulfilling the criteria for a major depressive episode.[20] It is therefore unclear whether the DSM criteria and rating scales for depression are as valid in this population as in non-PD populations.

5. Use for different study purposes.

Depression scales serve different purposes. One purpose is to assess the severity of depression and monitor the patients' response to antidepressant treatment. For this clinical or research task, the validity, reliability, and responsiveness of a scale to mood changes are relevant. Another reason to use rating scales is to screen for the presence of depressive symptoms in patients with PD. For screening purposes, ease of use is important in large epidemiological studies and in clinical settings that employ untrained raters or self-rating scales. Scales with good sensitivity and specificity at appropriate cutoffs may serve as screening tools. Rating scales alone, however, should not be used for the diagnosis of depression, which is reserved for the appropriate "gold standard" diagnostic instrument (i.e., [semi] structured DSM interviews).

6. Timing of assessment.

Rating scales for depression do not usually specify the *timing of assessment*, which is important in PD patients with motor and non-motor fluctuations.

7. Use of collateral information.

Most rating scales are patient-reported or clinician-rated, yet the input of collateral information when assessing PD patients may be important. However, whether or how to incorporate such collateral information from informed others needs to be operationalized.

Identified scales and their utilization in clinical practice and research

Nine scales were identified in multiple publications to assess dPD, including the Hamilton Depression Scale (Ham-D),[21] the Beck Depression Inventory (BDI),[22] the Geriatric Depression Scale (GDS),[23,24], the Zung Self-Rating Depression Scale (SDS),[25] the Hospital Anxiety and Depression Scale (HADS)[26]

Table 19-1. Properties of Depression Scales in Parkinson's Disease

SCALE	SENSITIVITY	SPECIFICITY	CUTOFF SCORE FOR SCREENING IN PATIENTS WITHOUT PD	CUTOFF SCORE FOR SCREENING IN PATIENTS WITH PD	SENSITIVITY TO CHANGE	SOMATIC ITEMS	PSYCHOLOGICAL ITEMS
Ham-D	++	++	7/8 to 11/12. (13/14 for discrimination between cases and non-cases)	9/10 to 11/12. (13/14 to 18/19 for discrimination)	+	***	**
MADRS	++	++	6/7	14/15	+	**	*
BDI	+	+	9/10	13/14	+	**	***
HADS	+	+/-	7/8	10/11	+	*	***
SDS	++	+	50/51	54/55	+	***	***
GDS 30	++	++	9/10	9/10	na	*	***
GDS 15	++	++	2/3	4/5	na	*	***
CSDD	+	+	6/7	7/8	na	**	**
CES-D	na	na	15/16	na	na	*	***
UPDRS Part I	na	na	na	1/2	na	*	*

+/– sensitivity/specificity limited; + some sensitivity/specificity; ++ good sensitivity/specificity; na = not sufficiently assessed in patients with Parkinson's disease; * <25% of items; ** 25–50% of items; *** >50% of items.

the Montgomery- Asberg Depression Rating Scale (MADRS),[27] the Cornell Scale for the Assessment of Depression in Dementia (CSDD)[28] and the Center for Epidemiologic Studies Depression Scale (CES-D).[29] The Unified Parkinson's Disease Rating Scale (UPDRS)[30] and MDS-UPDRS[31] Part I was also included, as it is the most widely used rating scale to assess PD symptoms and includes questions on psychiatric symptoms. Scales that were considered but not included were scales that assess short-lived mood states only, such as the Profile of Mood States (POMS),[32] and multidimensional scales that include a dimension of depression within a wider assessment of psychiatric symptoms, such as the Neuropsychiatric Inventory (NPI)[33]: the assessment was limited to depression-specific scales. Scales that were only used in individual studies (e.g., the Andersen scale[34]) were also not included.

Critique of depression scales

While the limitations of the DSM or other diagnostic criteria, and the recent recommendations to improve these criteria,[7] are recognized, these criteria and structured or semistructured interviews for DSM or ICD 10 diagnoses were used as the available "gold standard" and as a measure of criterion validity in the available literature.

All scales were found to be valid in both genders, although the factor structures may vary and scores may differ.[35-37] No data were available to give recommendations on who should administer the observer-rated scales. However, information on the need for training for each scale is provided. A summary of the properties of the depression scales reviewed is provided in Table 19-2.

Hamilton Depression Rating Scale (Ham-D)

SCALE DESCRIPTION

The interviewer-rated Ham-D is the most widely used and accepted measure for evaluating the severity of depression.[38] Appropriate training in the administration and scoring of the scale

is important for obtaining reliable scores.[39] Several cutoffs have been suggested. The most widely accepted cutoff scores are: <8, normal; 8–13, mild depression; 14–18, moderate depression; 19–22, severe depression, >23, very severe depression. The Ham-D is available in the public domain and has been translated into most European and Asian languages. There are self-rated and over the telephone–administered formats that yield comparable results to the interviewer-administered version.[40] Multiple versions of the scale exist, of which the 17-item version is the most frequently used.

Use in PD: The Ham-D has been used frequently and across the spectrum of severity of PD and of depression.

Use by other investigators: It has been used by multiple authors in patients with and without PD and across different cultures.

CLINIMETRIC PROPERTIES

Depression in non-PD patients It has been shown to have good sensitivity to change in depressed patients.[41-44] Although it covers DSM criteria incompletely, it has acceptable discriminant validity, high sensitivity and high specificity. Furthermore, it has high negative predictive value (NPV), and acceptable positive predictive values (PPV) for a DSM diagnosis of depressive disorder.[45] Its sensitivity and specificity have been shown to be superior to that of the BDI and SDS,[46] and similar to the MADRS.[47] It has good test-retest and inter-rater reliability, although item reliability is poor.[48] Semi-structured versions have been developed, including scoring guidelines that improved item reliability.[49] It has also been shown to be valid in patients with significant cognitive impairment.[50,51] It correlates with biological markers of depression.[52-56]

Depression in Parkinson's disease The Ham-D has been shown to have good sensitivity and specificity[57] Cutoff scores of 9/10[57] ([171]) and 11/12[47] to screen for dPD, and 13/14,[47] 15/16,[57] and 18/19[58] to detect major depressive disorder (although diagnosis using a scale alone is not recommended), have been suggested. Using these cutoffs, sensitivity, specificity, and positive and

Table 19-2. Conclusions Regarding Scale Status to Assess Depression in Parkinson's Disease

SCALE	USE IN PD	USE BY OTHER INVESTIGATORS	ADEQUATE CLINIMETRICS IN PD	CONCLUSION
Ham-D	X	X	X	Recommended for Screening Recommended for Severity Rating
MADRS	X	X	X	Recommended for Screening Recommended for Severity Rating
BDI	X	X	X	Recommended for Screening Recommended for Severity Rating
HADS	X	X	X	Recommended for Screening Suggested for Severity Rating
SDS	X	X	X but limited	Recommended with Limitations for Screening Recommended with Limitations for Severity Rating
GDS	X	X	X	Recommended for Screening Suggested for Severity Rating
CSDD	X	X	X	Recommended for Screening Suggested for Severity Rating
UPDRS and MDS-UPDRS, depression question	X	X	X	Recommended for Screening with Limitations: only one screening question Not Suitable for Severity Rating
CES-D	(X)	X	Not adequately tested	(Suggested for Screening; Suggested for Severity Rating)

negative predictive values for a DSM diagnosis of major depressive disorder in PD have been found to be acceptable. It has been demonstrated to be sensitive to changes in PD patients[59–66] and to correlate with biological markers of dPD.[67–70]

STRENGTHS AND WEAKNESSES

Advantages: The Ham-D is the most widely used and accepted outcome measure for evaluating depression severity and has been validated and used in non-PD and PD patients. It is the most commonly used interviewer-rated outcome

scale in treatment studies (it has been used in about 95% of randomized controlled trials (RCT) of selective serotonin reuptake inhibitors (SSRI)[71] and has been studied extensively. It has good clinimetric properties and assesses frequent comorbid symptoms of depression, such as anxiety and somatic symptoms.[72]

Disadvantages: Somatic symptoms are heavily represented,[72] and its use as a screening measure, particularly in patients with physical illness, has therefore been criticised.[72,73] Thus, almost 60% of the total items could be experienced by a typical patient with PD. There is a lack of consistency at the item level; some items assess multiple symptoms, and some symptoms can be rated on multiple items. In addition, the 17-item version has also been shown to measure more than one dimension.[71] It covers DSM/ICD-10 criteria for depression incompletely, which limits its use as a screening measure.[72]

CONCLUSIONS

The Ham-D fulfils criteria for a "Recommended" scale, well-suited for assessing depression severity in treatment trials of dPD, for correlation studies with biological markers or other Parkinsonism scales, and for the study of the phenomenology of depression.[11,74-76] It also fulfills criteria for a "Recommended" screening measure for dPD, but, like all scales and diagnostic criteria that include somatic items, it overlaps with core PD symptoms. As an observer-rated scale it requires training, and self-report questionnaires may be more appropriate as screening instruments for dPD in routine clinical neurological clinics or in large-scale epidemiological studies.[57]

Montgomery-Asberg Depression Rating Scale (MADRS)

DESCRIPTION OF THE SCALE

The MADRS is an observer-rated scale and requires some clinical experience with depression. It covers all the DSM criteria of a major depressive episode, with the exception of psychomotor retardation/agitation and reverse neurovegetative symptoms (e.g., hypersomnia and increased appetite). When compared to other observer-rated scales, such as the Ham-D, the MADRS has relatively few somatic items. It was designed to measure changes in severity of depressive symptoms during antidepressant clinical trials. It is not usually used for screening. The MADRS is in the public domain (although because of its publication in the *British Journal of Psychiatry* the scale is formally copyrighted by this journal). It has been translated into several European and Asian languages.

Use in PD: The MADRS has been used across the spectrum of PD and severity of depression.

Use by other investigators: It has been used by multiple authors in patients with and without PD and across different cultures.

CLINIMETRIC PROPERTIES

Depression in non-PD patients The MADRS has good face validity, criterion validity, and concurrent validity.[27,77] Inter-rater agreement and internal consistency are high.[27,78] While it has been shown to be valid in older patients with mild cognitive impairment,[79] there are only sparse data on patients with severe cognitive impairment.[80] It is at least as sensitive to change as the Ham-D.[27,81]

Depression in Parkinson's disease Although the MADRS is not usually used for screening purposes, one group[82,83] reported on its use in screening for dPD. Cutoff scores in PD of 14/15 for screening (high sensitivity and high NPV) have been validated in PD against a diagnosis of major depressive disorder.[47] It has been used in medication trials in dPD and been shown to be sensitive to change in the level of severity of depression.[74,84] It has also been used to assess the phenomenology of dPD.[85]

STRENGTHS AND WEAKNESSES

Advantages: The MADRS has been studied in PD and was found to have good concurrent validity with the DSM criteria, and with appropriate cutoff it can be used for screening purposes. Moreover, it was designed to measure change of depression severity and has been proven sensitive to change in PD.

Disadvantages: It is an observer-rated scale and requires some (though not extensive) clinical experience with depression.

CONCLUSIONS

The MADRS fulfils criteria for a "Recommended" scale for screening and severity measurement. It is appropriate for medication trials in PD and for correlation studies with biological markers. It is also suitable for screening when the appropriate cutoff scores are used, and for studying the phenomenology of dPD.

Beck Depression Inventory (BDI)

DESCRIPTION OF THE SCALE

The BDI is one of the most-utilized self-rated instruments for major depression in clinical practice.[86] It has been used both to measure the severity of depression and as a screening instrument in more than 2,000 studies.[87,88] Several modified versions exist for adaptation to DSM criteria. In the revised BDI-II, agitation, concentration difficulties, and loss of energy were added to the original version. However, most validation studies have been performed for the BDI-1A, which is also the most-used version.[89] The scale is generally considered to be in the public domain, but purchase of the scale from the publisher is required for use in large-scale research projects.[90]

Use in PD: The BDI has been used frequently and across the spectrum of severity of PD and of depression.

Use by other investigators: It has been validated and used worldwide. Cross-cultural evaluations suggest that some cultural differences in depression measurements exist, particularly for the psychological aspects,[37,91–93] but the scale has been shown to be valid across cultures.

CLINIMETRIC PROPERTIES

Depression in non-PD patients In a study on ease of comprehension of self-reported depression scales, the BDI had high overall cognitive complexity.[94] Nevertheless, it has high test-retest reliability[95,96] and internal consistency[22,95,96] in a variety of patient groups. Its concurrent and discriminant validity is good.[88,97–99] Although it contains a number of somatic symptoms,[8,9] it is weighted towards psychological symptoms of depression. It has been shown to correlate with biological markers of depression[100] and to be sensitive to change.[101,102] It also appears to be valid in patients with significant cognitive impairment.[103,104]

Depression in Parkinson's disease The BDI has been used widely in PD. It has been used to screen for dPD,[105–108] to measure severity[17,109] and to assess the response to pharmacological or surgical treatment.[110–112] While the most commonly used version of the BDI assesses the state of the patient's mood "during the past week" (or "the past two weeks" for the BDI-II), it has been used to quantify "on-" or "off"-state-dependent mood.[113] However, the use of the BDI as a short-time scale has not been validated. It has good internal consistency and test-retest reliability in dPD.[9,114] Concurrent[62,115,116] and discriminant validity[117,118] and concurrent validity in PD are acceptable. Different cutoff scores have been used, with recommendations from 8/9 for screening for dPD.[117] An optimal cutoff of 13/14 has been suggested with acceptable sensitivity and specificity.[119] Despite concerns about the number of somatic symptoms, it has been shown to have good reliability and validity compared to a DSM diagnosis of major depression in dPD, superior to that of the HADS.[117,120]

STRENGTHS AND WEAKNESSES

Advantages: The BDI is a well-researched scale, for which some validation studies in PD are available.

Disadvantages: The BDI contains numerous somatic items. It has been argued that this may lead to false positives among patients with physical problems.[8] These objections are largely theoretical, however, and not reflected in a reduced reliability or validity. Although there are no directly comparative studies, some validation studies show that the BDI is superior to the HADS.[121] Moreover, it has been demonstrated that some somatic symptoms in PD are sensitive for depression and should not be neglected in the assessment of depression in PD, and that potential overlapping somatic items may cluster with depression rather than with motor features.[122] Most of validation studies used the original version of the BDI, and it is not clear how far these apply to the revised version.

CONCLUSION

The BDI fulfils criteria for a "Recommended" scale for screening and severity measurement. It is suitable for screening if an appropriate cutoff is used. It is also suitable for assessing the severity of depressive symptoms and for monitoring change during treatment, but changes in the severity of PD symptoms should be adjusted for. It can also be used in phenomenological studies of dPD.

Hospital Anxiety and Depression Scale (HADS)

DESCRIPTION OF THE SCALE

The HADS is a short, self-rated scale yielding subscores for depression and anxiety. Anxiety symptoms are rated separately from the depression symptoms, but due to high comorbidity between anxiety and depression, some researchers have used the total HADS as a measure of global mood disorder. The depression subscale is weighted towards the emotional aspects of depression (emphasizing anhedonia rather than sadness)[26] and does not include physical and cognitive symptoms or suicidal ideation. The scale is in the public domain, but for use in large-scale research projects, purchase of the scale from the publisher is required.[123]

Use in PD: The HADS has been used in a number of studies in patients with PD.

Use by other investigators: It has been validated and used in many countries in all parts of the world.[124] However, in a multinational study, it was found that nationality significantly influenced HADS scores.[125] The use of this scale in different countries could be influenced by the different perception and expression of emotions by the patients from different cultural backgrounds.[124]

CLINIMETRIC PROPERTIES

Depression in non-PD patients Face validity is moderate, as some of the core diagnostic criteria for depression are not included in the scale and it excludes items at the severe end of the spectrum of depression, including suicidal ideation, psychotic features, and vegetative symptoms. Nevertheless, sensitivity and specificity for DSM criteria for major depressive disorder and other depression scales were reported as good.[126] The HADS has been reported to have medium overall cognitive complexity or respondent comprehensibility, in between the

BDI (high) and the SDS (low).[94] The internal consistency and test-retest reliability of the scale are good.[126,127] Sensitivity to change has been shown to be good, for studies evaluating both pharmacotherapy and psychotherapy for depression.[124,128–131] It has not been validated in patients with significant cognitive impairment, and has only rarely been used in this population.[132,133]

Depression in Parkinson's disease There is little overlap with non-depression symptoms of PD, as only the item querying about feeling "slowed down" overlaps with core PD symptoms. While this is advantageous in patients with PD with mild depression, it reduces it's the scale's validity in severe depression. It has also been criticized for its use in PD due to its reverse coding of some items, which has been reported to result in frequent cross-outs and inconsistent ratings, perhaps related to problems with concept-shifting.[134] Cutoff scores for the total HADS of 10/11 for screening have been suggested,[120,135] although specificity was low at a cutoff of 10/11.[120] The internal consistency and test-retest reliability of the scale is good in patients with PD.[120,136] The HADS has not been used in PD for treatment trials. However, it has been used to measure the severity of dPD.[137,138]

STRENGTHS AND WEAKNESSES

Advantages: The HADS is quick and easy to administer and a self-rated scale.

Disadvantages: It has questionable face validity and no clear relationship with DSM-IV criteria for depression. Its reverse coding of some items may result in inconsistent ratings in PD, perhaps related to problems with concept-shifting.

CONCLUSIONS

The HADS fulfils criteria for "Recommended" and is moderately suitable for screening purposes for dPD.[120] Its use as a severity measure in PD is controversial, with no clear evidence to support its use in this context, and, as it excludes most somatic symptoms, it may be more suitable for mild to moderate than for more severe depression. Due to its low content validity, it is not suitable for phenomenological studies of depression.

Zung Self-Rating Depression Scale (SDS)

DESCRIPTION OF THE SCALE

The SDS is a short, self-rated scale that assesses psychological and somatic symptoms of depression. It has been widely used to screen for[139–142] and measure severity of depression.[143–145] Several shortened versions are available, but the original version is the most commonly used. There is a large number of somatic items. In order to adjust for an expected higher baseline score in elderly patients seen in medical settings, it has therefore been recommended that the cutoff score be raised from 50 in the general population to 60 or greater in this population.[146] The scale is in the public domain.

Use in PD: The SDS has been used in many studies to screen for and measure severity of depressive symptoms in patients with PD. However, few validation studies in PD are available.

Use by other investigators: It has been used in numerous languages and has been validated in English, Japanese, Chinese, Finnish, and Italian.

CLINIMETRIC PROPERTIES

Depression in non-PD patients It is more easily comprehended than the HADS, CES-D, or BDI.[94] It has good internal consistency[36,147–149] and test-retest reliability.[150] Content and criterion validity are good, as it includes most of the DSM criteria for major depression,[151] and concurrent validity is acceptable.[36,152,153] No data on its use in patients with significant cognitive impairment are available.

Depression in Parkinson's disease Few validation studies in PD are available, and cutoff scores for patients with PD have not been established. It appears to have adequate discriminant validity in patients with PD,[154] and it has been reported to be sensitive to change,[84,155,156] despite the limitation of yes/no answer options. A cutoff

at 54/55 was reported to provide acceptable sensitivity and specificity.[157] Similar to the HADS, the use of reverse coding introduces complexity, particularly for patients with PD who may have difficulty in set-shifting, and there are many somatic items that overlap with PD symptoms.

STRENGTHS AND WEAKNESSES

Advantages: SDS is an internally consistent, highly reliable, valid scale for assessing depression. It correlates well with DSM criteria for depression, and can discriminate both depressed from non-depressed patients and among different kinds of diagnoses.

Disadvantages: Few validation data of the scale in PD patients are available, although it has been applied in a number of studies. It has many somatic items, and the mix of positively keyed and negatively keyed items may confuse some patients and result in higher mean scores and affect factor analytic structure.

CONCLUSIONS

The SDS fulfills criteria for a "Recommended" scale for screening and severity measurement but with the limitation that there are few validation studies in PD and numerous somatic items. It may be suitable to measure change of severity of dPD, but further studies are need to confirm its validity in patients with PD. The large number of somatic items is likely to inflate depression rates, and appropriate cutoffs should be used.

Geriatric Depression Scale (GDS)

DESCRIPTION OF THE SCALE

The GDS is a short, self-report, yes/no screening instrument for depression in the elderly. It focuses on the psychological aspects and social consequences of depression, avoiding symptom overlap with medical disorders or aging in general. Two commonly used versions exist (the 30-item GDS [GDS-30][24] and the 15-item GDS [GDS-15][23]), and they perform equally well.[158] A telephone version has demonstrated good agreement with the self-report questionnaire.[159]

The GDS is in the public domain. It is not usually used as an outcome measure in treatment trials.

Use in PD: The GDS has been used in a number of studies to screen for depressive symptoms in patients with PD. Some validation studies in PD are available.

Use by other investigators: It has been translated in many European and Asian languages and used in numerous languages.

CLINIMETRIC PROPERTIES

Depression in non-PD patients There is limited concordance between GDS items and DSM symptoms of depressive disorder, as it excludes somatic symptoms and suicidal ideation, thus raising questions about the content validity of the instrument. It has nevertheless been reported to have discriminant validity similar to that of the Ham-D and better than the SDS,[24] and correlates highly with other depression scales.[24,160] It also has been shown to have good internal consistency and test-retest reliability.[161] Scores are skewed toward the lower end of the scale, as patients without symptoms of depression commonly score a "0." As each question on the GDS can only be scored "0" or "1," the instrument is not able to capture degrees of severity at the level of individual items. However, there is preliminary evidence that the overall scale may be sensitive to changes in depression severity.[162] While it performs well in patients with mild to moderate cognitive impairment,[163–165] the data on its validity in moderate to severely cognitively impaired patients are conflicting.[164,166–169]

Depression in Parkinson's disease The GDS-30 has been reported to have adequate discriminant validity for a DSM diagnosis of major depressive disorder in PD at a cutoff of 9/10[170] or 10/11.[135] The GDS-15 appears to have adequate discriminant validity for a diagnosis of major and minor depressive disorder at a cutoff of 4/5 (or also reported 7/8[157]), performing comparably to the Ham-D.[171] The GDS avoids many, but not all, symptoms overlapping between depression and PD. It has been reported to perform similarly

to the CSDD in PD patients with dementia,[172] suggesting that it may be a sensitive indicator of depression severity in cognitively impaired patients with PD.

STRENGTHS AND WEAKNESSES

Advantages: The GDS is a reliable and valid self-report screening instrument for depression in the elderly that is short and easily understood, making it appropriate for use in both clinical research and routine clinical care. Research suggests that the GDS-15 performs as well as the GDS-30. GDS items focus on the psychological aspects of depression, thus avoiding symptom overlap with other disorders or aging in general. It performs well as a screening instrument for depression in PD.

Disadvantages: There is limited concordance between GDS items and DSM symptoms of depression, as it excludes somatic symptoms and suicidal ideation.

CONCLUSION

The GDS fulfills criteria for a "Recommended" scale for screening purposes. It is short and easily understood, making it appropriate for use in both clinical research and routine clinical care as a screening instrument for depression in elderly PD patients. It has been insufficiently evaluated for the assessment of severity of dPD, however.

Cornell Scale for Depression in Dementia (CSDD)

DESCRIPTION OF THE SCALE

This interview-based scale was developed specifically for the assessment of depression in patients with dementia and utilizes a caregiver to provide collateral information. The CSDD is therefore appropriate in assessing dPD in patients with comorbid cognitive impairment. The CSDD was developed to measure depression severity, but has also been used to screen for depression in patients with dementia. The CSDD is based on observation and interviews with both an "informed other" and the patient. The instructions do not specify how the information from the informed other is to be weighed in making the final assessment. There is also no formal definition of an informed other, and informants may vary in their relationship to the patient. The CSDD de-emphasizes questions related to motor symptoms of PD, but retains some overlap with PD symptoms (e.g., retardation, physical complaints, sleep, energy). The observer scoring the scale also relies on the informed other to make difficult clinical distinctions about whether symptoms are secondary to PD or dPD (attributional approach). Administration of the scale requires some sophistication in assessing psychiatric symptoms and training in understanding the motor symptoms of PD. The scale may therefore be difficult for neurologists and general physicians to complete accurately without some psychiatric expertise or training. The scale is in the public domain and has been translated into several European and Asian languages.

Use in PD: The CSDD has rarely been used in patients with PD.

Use by other investigators: It has been used in numerous studies.

CLINIMETRIC EVALUATION

Depression in non-PD patients In research studies, internal consistency, inter-rater reliability and concurrent validity were shown to be acceptable,[28,173,174] and the CSDD was shown to have acceptable psychometric properties in severe dementia.[175] Sensitivity to change was demonstrated in a few trials.[176-179] Informed other ratings on the CSDD in patients with dementia were shown to have higher sensitivity for correctly detecting depression than other depression scales, including the BDI, the Ham-D, and the GDS (all modified for caregiver rating).[180] Although there are limited data on the reliability, validity, and sensitivity of the CSDD in non-demented elderly patients,[174] it has also been recommended as a useful scale for screening older adults for a diagnosis of depression.[181]

Depression in Parkinson's disease In one study with patients with PD, a cutoff score greater than or equal to 6 produced a sensitivity of 0.83 and specificity of 0.73; a cutoff score of greater than or equal to 8, a sensitivity of 0.75 and specificity of 0.82. There was no evidence for differential results with respect to cognitive impairment[182]. However, no further validation studies are available.

STRENGTHS AND WEAKNESSES

Advantages: The scale uses reports from both the caregiver and the patient. It de-emphasizes questions related to motor symptoms of PD and potentially decreases the overlap of depression and PD.

Disadvantages: There is a reliance on the caregiver's determining whether symptoms are secondary to PD or depression, and this can be difficult. There is no formal definition of "the caregiver," and it is therefore possible that the rater could rely on multiple caregivers. It was not designed for PD, and there several somatic symptoms that overlap with PD. The interviewer for the CCSD has to have some sophistication in assessing psychiatric symptoms and will need training in this area. The scale was primarily developed for patients with dementia, and has not been properly assessed for its psychometric properties in non-demented patients.

CONCLUSIONS

The CSDD fulfils criteria for a "Recommended" scale for screening in patients with cognitive impairment. It offers an opportunity to assess severity of and screen for depression in patients with dPD and comorbid dementia. The CSDD has shown reasonable psychometric properties in depressed demented patients with and without comorbid PD. However, its administration requires experience and training, and attribution of symptoms to depression or PD is a particular problem in the informed other–rated component of the scale. Further validation studies are needed, particularly with regard to measuring the severity of dPD.

Unified Parkinson's Disease Rating Scale (UPDRS) Part I

DESCRIPTION OF THE SCALE

The first part of the UPDRS[30] comprises four screening questions on "mood, mentation, and behavior," of which only one assesses mood (the other three assess intellectual impairment, thought disorder, and motivation/initiative). The question on mood lumps several symptoms of depression into one question. The revised MDS-UPDRS restricts assessment of mood to low mood, sadness, hopelessness feelings of emptiness or loss of enjoyment, and has separate question on other aspects of mood elsewhere. Both serve as screening tools but have not been used as an outcome measures in clinical trials. The UPDRS and MDS-UPDRS Part I are clinician-rated, requiring training, but a self-rated version of the UPDSR Part I has been validated.[183] It is short and specifically designed for use in patients with PD, but it only includes one aspect of depression (with some additional information in the other three questions). The original UPDRS is in the public domain and has been used in many languages. The MDS-UPDRS is licensed by the Movement Disorders Society.

Use in PD: Numerous studies in multiple languages.

Use by other investigators: Multiple.

CLINIMETRIC EVALUATION

Depression in non-PD patients Not used, as it was designed for patients with PD.

Depression in Parkinson's disease It has limited face and content validity, and construct validity cannot be assessed in a single question. The test-retest and inter-rater reliability and the concordance rates between patient and observer rating of the depression item are fair or moderate in non-depressed PD patients.[184–186] Part I in its entirety has been reported to be sensitive to change in some studies of anti-Parkinsonian drugs with purported antidepressant properties,[187] and a score of 2 or greater on the depression item had 77% sensitivity and 82% specificity to detect major depression as diagnosed with DSM criteria in one study.[188] Another study reported good concurrent validity of the MDS-UPDRS depression item with the HADS and Ham-D[34] but further studies on its screening properties are needed. In addition, depression can only be screened for with either version of the UPDRS, as it is only a single question, but some of the somatic features of depression, as well as apathy, cognitive impairment, anxiety, and sleep disturbances, are also assessed in separate questions of the UPDRS/MDS-UPDRS).

STRENGTHS AND WEAKNESSES

Advantages: The UPDRS and MDS-UPDRS depression item is short, and specifically designed for patients with PD. The UPDRS depression item has been used in numerous studies and is typically assessed as part of the whole UPDRS.

Disadvantages: It has poor face validity and content validity, and it does not screen adequately for DSM-IV criteria of depression. The original version has some ambiguities in the depression item.

CONCLUSIONS

The original UPDRS and the MDS-UPDRS depression items should only be used as screening tools. They are not recommended for measuring severity of depression. In clinical practice, many clinicians complete UPDRS or MDS-UPDRS Part I as they are completing other parts of the scale for the complete examination of patients with PD, using the results to screen for a variety of psychiatric symptoms. The psychometric properties of the MDS-UPDRS Part 1 should be assessed further in clinical studies.

Center for Epidemiologic Studies Depression Scale (CES-D)

DESCRIPTION OF THE SCALE

The CES-D was derived from other depression scales as a screening instrument for depression in older adults with physical illness. It has been used extensively in epidemiological studies.

It does not require training or experience and has been validated in several formats, including face-to-face interviews and self-report. Several versions, including a short version for use in older adults, are available and have similar psychometric properties.[189] It has some face validity but lacks several symptoms of depression included in DSM or ICD 10. It is strongly weighted to the assessment of depressed mood and depressive thinking, somatic symptoms are underrepresented, and no question assesses loss of interest. It is mainly used as a screening tool, but is skewed towards the less severe end of depressive illness. It has rarely been reported as an outcome measure in clinical trials. The CES-D has arguably been subject to wider evaluation than any other depression scale in different populations, age groups, and cultures, particularly in epidemiological studies.

The scale is in the public domain and has been translated and used in multiple European, Middle Eastern, and Asian languages.

Use in PD: It has been used in few studies in patients with PD.

Use by other investigators: It has been used in numerous studies worldwide.

CLINIMETRIC PROPERTIES

Depression in non-PD patients It has medium cognitive complexity, similar to the HADS.[94] It has good internal consistency and acceptable test-retest reliability.[29,190] It has acceptable construct validity[29,190,191] and discriminant validity ("no depression" vs. "major depressive disorder"),[192,193] but it may lack utility in distinguishing between gradations of severity within the clinical range of depression ("minor" vs. "major depression").[194]

Depression in Parkinson's disease The CES-D appears acceptable for use in PD in terms of the language and format. As it contains few somatic items and no item on loss of interest, it is unlikely to be significantly contaminated by non-depressive symptoms of PD and may be useful across the range of PD disease severity. Despite its widespread use in other settings, the CES-D has been used relatively infrequently in PD,[195] and it has not been formally evaluated

for its psychometric properties. However, in one study[196] it has been reported to be sensitive to change. Due to its low number of somatic items, it may not be sensitive at the severe end of the depression severity spectrum, and may be more suitable for patients with mild to moderate depression.

STRENGTHS AND WEAKNESSES

Advantages: The CES-D is short, easy to complete, and has been used widely. Nevertheless, its item content suggests that its primary value would be in as a screening instrument for dysphoric mood. The lack of content relating to loss of interest/anhedonia would have some advantages in studies seeking to assess dysphoria independently of apathy.

Disadvantages: It does not fit well with DSM or other criteria for depression, limiting its use as a screening instrument. The CES-D-Revised may correct these shortcomings, but this version of scale has not yet been adequately evaluated. The primary disadvantage of the CESD for use in PD is the lack of evidence of its psychometric properties in the condition. Therefore, the CES-D should probably be used with caution and alongside other, better characterized scales.

CONCLUSION

The CES-D, or one of its shortened versions, is a suitable screening instrument for depression in older adults with physical illness in community studies or primary care settings. It has limited validity at the more severe end of the spectrum of depression, but it may be particularly useful for the detection of subsyndromal depression. However, further validation studies in PD are needed before it can be recommended for wider use as a primary study tool. Unless further evidence becomes available, it is not recommended for assessing change of depression severity.

CONCLUSIONS AND RECOMMENDATIONS

- The Ham-D, MADRS, BDI, HADS, CSDD, and GDS are "Recommended" instruments in dPD for screening for dPD. The SDS also fulfilled criteria for "Recommended" instruments but with limitations, and it needs further validation studies. The CES-D has not been adequately tested in dPD. The UPDRS and MDS-UPDRS depression question is a single question, therefore, whilst formally fulfilling criteria for a "Recommended" scale, it does so with limitations. For severity rating, the Ham-D, MADRS, BDI, and SDS are "Recommended."

- All the reviewed scales have some utility in the assessment of dPD. Apart from the UPDRS Part I (which is merely a screening instrument in the context of overall assessment of PD symptoms), they are useful in assessing depressive symptoms in PD. The BDI and Ham-D have been validated and widely used in patients with PD, but there are few data available on other scales, particularly the CES-D; therefore, further validation studies are required before their use can be recommended in PD. Overall, observer-rated scales (e.g., Ham-D and MADRS) have better psychometric properties than self-rated scales, and observer-rated scales should therefore be preferred if the study or clinical situation permits.
- Available depression scales serve diverse purposes (e.g., screening instruments vs. instruments used to measure severity and to follow symptoms over time). Different uses require that different scale properties be taken into account, and that adaptations of cutoff scores be made as needed (depending on whether sensitivity, specificity, PPV, or NPV are important to the aims of the study). The diagnosis of depression should not be solely made on the basis of a score on a rating scale. A cutoff score on these instrument cannot comprehensively capture the range of depressive disorders in PD; high scores can occur when somatic symptoms are endorsed even without the two core symptoms of depression (i.e., sad mood and loss of interest or pleasure); low scores can occur despite serious depressive symptoms when somatic or vegetative problems are absent. For this reason, the gold standard for establishing the diagnosis of depression

remains a (semi)structured interview using DSM criteria or its equivalent future diagnostic adaptation.

- Insufficient evidence is available to recommend the best depression rating scales for PD patients with dementia. Current evidence suggests that the MADRS, GDS, and CSDD may be useful, but further studies are required.
- Patients may perceive their own condition differently in an "off" than during an "on" period.[197] "Off" periods may be associated with severe psychiatric symptoms, including depression, anxiety and delusions,[197,198] which usually improve along with motor symptoms and are therefore typically short-lived. As the reviewed scales are designed to assess the preceding one or two weeks and as these off-periods are also not considered the same as untreated PD and may represent rebound worsening after the beneficial effect of L-dopa has worn off[199], it is recommended, in line with common practice, that patients with motor fluctuations be assessed for depression during "on" periods. The scales are therefore also not suitable for specifically assessing fluctuating depressive symptoms during "off" periods versus "on" periods in the same way that motor symptoms or dyskinesia can be monitored.
- All depression scales include items that assess symptoms with overlap between depression, Parkinsonism, cognitive impairment, and apathy; particularly the Ham-D and SDS, and to a lesser degree MADRS and BDI. The scale with one of the highest number of items assessing overlapping symptoms, the Ham-D, has the best psychometric properties compared to DSM criteria at recommended adjusted cutoffs. For most studies, instruments that have been demonstrated to have good psychometric properties are recommended above those with poorer validity or reliability or those not validated in dPD. Appropriately adjusted cutoff scores for patients with PD should be chosen and overlapping symptom areas should be assessed in parallel with a primary PD scale like the UPDRS motor scale. This twofold assessment could allow for adjustment of confounding factors in the assessment of depression. The HADS and GDS have few

overlapping items and may therefore be useful in the comparison of patients with different disease stages and could also be used to monitor change in depression even in the context of changes in underlying Parkinsonism. They have limited content validity and appear insensitive at the severe end of the depression severity spectrum. As such, they may be useful candidates for studies of mild or mild-to-moderate depressive symptoms, the most commonly encountered problem in cross-sectional cases of dPD. They would, however, be less useful in assessing moderate to severe depression.

- In line with the NINDS recommendations,[7] use of "loss of pleasure" (reflecting anhedonia) may be more specific to depression than "loss of interest," which, as a symptom of apathy, may occur in the absence of depression, but this needs to be researched further.

The following unresolved issues require further research:

- Since the publication of the Movement Disorders Society Rating Scale Task Force review, a number of studies have been conducted that improved our knowledge of the validity of these instruments. However, the CES-D and the MDS-UPDRS Part I depression question need further assessment. In addition, for most of the discussed scales, research has focused on their ability to screen for depression, but further studies are needed to assess additional properties of these scales, including their sensitivity to change and more advanced scale properties using Rasch analysis of item response theory. Furthermore, studies that directly compare the performance of these scales would help in choosing the appropriate scale for any given study.
- The assessment of concurrent validity of depression scales is typically made in comparison to DSM-R criteria of major depression. The criteria for assessment of depressive disorder of dPD are undergoing changes,[7] and the validity of depression rating scales using these assessment criteria will need to be established.

- The inclusion of somatic symptoms in depression scales theoretically leads to falsely inflated depression scores in patients with PD and may influence the results of treatment trials of depression in PD (e.g., with anti-Parkinsonian medication). The influence of anti-Parkinsonian treatment on depression scores on these scales needs to investigated further in clinical trials.
- In general, the observer should score answers on the scales using an inclusive approach, and patients should be instructed not to attribute their symptoms to either PD or depression when scoring self-rated scales. An exclusive approach may lead to an underestimation of depression severity. However, some scales require judgement, such as the CSDD and to a lesser degree other observer-rated scales such as the MADRS and Ham-D, and may be conducive to using a more etiological approach. Whilst this should be investigated further, without evidence of advantages of exclusive or etiological approaches, the task force advises investigators to follow an inclusive approach.
- The evaluated instruments were not designed nor are they used to identify minor or subsyndromal depression, and do not reflect the variety of mood disorders seen in PD, including recurrent brief depressive disorder or dysthymia. Thus, further characterization of other types of dPD is required, and cutoffs must be adapted to purpose of the study and time frame specified to include more diverse depressive disorders in PD rather than merely using a cutoff for major depression.
- Further studies are needed on impact of age, cognitive impairment, apathy, and cultural differences on the validity of the depression scales.
- The minimal clinically important change and the minimal clinically important difference has been evaluated for only a few of the evaluated scales.[200]
- In this review, multidimensional scales, which assess depression as part of a wider assessment, were not assessed. However, these scales, such as the POMS or the NPI, may be useful in some circumstances and require validation before their use can be recommended.

Other depression scales, not evaluated here, may in the future be found to be appropriate and valid instruments to assess dPD.

- The role of the caregiver in reporting symptoms of depression should be operationalized, particularly on scales such as the CSDD, which assesses dPD with comorbid dementia.
- The use of scales to measure present state of mood (e.g., for the measurement of short-term mood fluctuations), which requires a change of time scales, needs to be validated before it can be recommended.

RECOMMENDED SCALES for screening
HAM-D
MADRS
BDI
HADS
CSDD
GDS
RECOMMENDED SCALES for severity rating
HAM-D
MADRS
BDI
SDS

References

1. Leentjens AFG. Depression in Parkinson's disease: conceptual issues and clinical challenges. *J Geriatr Psychiatry Neurol.* 2004;17:120–126.
2. McDonald WM, Richard IH, DeLong MR. Prevalence, etiology, and treatment of depression in Parkinson's disease. *Biol Psychiatry.* 2003;54:363–375.
3. Slaughter JR, Slaughter KA, Nichols D, et al. Prevalence, clinical manifestations, etiology, and treatment of depression in Parkinson's disease. *J Neuropsychiatry Clin Neurosci.* 2001;13:187–196.
4. Liu CY, Wang SJ, Fuh JL, et al. The correlation of depression with functional activity in Parkinson's disease. *J Neurol.* 1997;244:493–498.
5. Aarsland D, Larsen JP, Karlsen K, et al. Mental symptoms in Parkinson's disease are important contributors to caregiver distress. *Int J Geriatr Psychiatry.* 1999;14:866–874.
6. Schrag A, Barone P, Brown RG, et al. Depression rating scales in Parkinson's disease: critique and recommendations. Mov Disord. 2007;22:1077-92.
7. Marsh LF, McDonald WM, Cummings J, et al. Provisional diagnostic criteria for depression in Parkinson's disease: report of an NINDS/NIMH Work Group. *Mov Disord.* 2006;21:148–158.
8. Williams AC, Richardson PH. What does the BDI measure in chronic pain? *Pain.* 1993;55:259–266.
9. Levin BE, Llabre MM, Weiner WJ. Parkinson's disease and depression: psychometric properties of the Beck Depression Inventory. *J Neurol Neurosurg Psychiatry.* 1988;51:1401–1404.
10. Starkstein SE, Preziosi TJ, Forrester AW, et al. Specificity of affective and autonomic symptoms of depression in Parkinson's disease. *J Neurol Neurosurg Psychiatry.* 1990;53:869–873.
11. Leentjens AF, Marinus J, Van Hilten JJ, et al. The contribution of somatic symptoms to the diagnosis of depression in Parkinson's disease: a discriminant analytic approach. *J Neuropsychiatry Clin Neurosci.* 2003;15:74–77.
12. Kirsch-Darrow L, Fernandez HF, Marsiske M, et al. Dissociating apathy and depression in Parkinson disease. *Neurology.* 2006;67:33–38.
13. Starkstein SE, Ingram L, Garau LM, et al. On the overlap between apathy and depression in dementia. *J Neurol Neurosurg Psychiatry.* 2005;76(8):1070–4
14. Starkstein SE, Mayberg HS, Preziosi TJ, et al. Reliability, validity, and clinical correlates of apathy in Parkinson's disease. *J Neuropsychiatry Clin Neurosci.* 1992;4:134–139.
15. Richard IH. Apathy does not equal depression in Parkinson disease: why we should care. *Neurology.* 2006;67:10–11.
16. Emre M. Dementia associated with Parkinson's disease. *Lancet Neurol.* 2003;2:229–237.
17. Brown RG, MacCarthy B, Gotham A-M, et al. Depression and disability in Parkinson's disease: a follow-up of 132 cases. *Psychol Med.* 1988;18:49–55.
18. Gotham A-M, Brown RG, Marsden CD. Depression in Parkinson's disease: a quantitative and qualitative analysis. *J Neurol Neurosurg Psychiatry.* 1986;49:381–389.
19. Ehrt U, Bronnick K, Leentjens AF, et al. Depressive symptom profile in Parkinson's disease: a comparison with depression in elderly patients without Parkinson's disease. *Int J Geriatr Psychiatry.* 2006;21:252–258.

20. Tandberg E, Larsen JP, Aarsland D, et al. The occurrence of depression in Parkinson's disease. A community-based study. *Arch Neurol.* 1996;53:175–179.

21. Hamilton M. A rating scale for depression. *J Neurol Neurosurg Psychiatry.* 1960;23:56–62.

22. Beck AT, Ward CH, Mendelson M, et al. An inventory for measuring depression. *Arch Gen Psychiatry.* 1961;4:561–571.

23. Sheikh JI, Yesavage JA. Geriatric Depression Scale (GDS): recent evidence and development of a shorter version. *Clin Gerontol.* 1986;5:165–173.

24. Yesavage JA, Brink TL, Rose TL, et al. Development and validation of a geriatric depression screening scale: a preliminary report. *J Psychiatr Res.* 1982;17:37–49.

25. Zung WWK. A self-rating depression scale. *Arch Gen Psychiatry.* 1965;12:63–70.

26. Snaith RP, Zigmond AS. Hospital Anxiety and Depression Scale (HADS). In: Rush AJ. ed. *Handbook of Psychiatric Measures.* Washington, DC: American Psychiatric Association; 2000:547–548.

27. Montgomery SA, Asberg M. A new depression scale designed to be sensitive to change. *Br J Psychiatry.* 1979;134:382–389.

28. Alexopolous GS, Abrams RC, Young RC, et al. Cornell scale for depression in dementia. *Biol Psychiatry.* 1988;23:271–284.

29. Radloff LS. The CES-D scale: a self-report depression scale for research in the general population. *Appl Psychol Meas.* 1977;1:385–401.

30. Fahn S, Elton RL; and Members of the UPDRS Development Committee. Unified Parkinson's Disease Rating Scale. In: Fahn S, Marsden CD, Goldstein M, et al, eds. *Recent Developments in Parkinson's Disease.* vol. 2. Florham Park, NJ: Macmillan Health Care Information; 1987: 153–163.

31. Gallagher DA, Goetz CG, Stebbins G, Lees AJ, **Schrag** A. Validation of the MDS-UPDRS Part I for nonmotor symptoms in Parkinson's disease. Mov Disord. 2012;27:79-83

32. McNair DM, Lorr M, Droppleman LF. *Profile of Mood States.* San Diego, CA: Educational and Industrial Testing Service; 1971.

33. Cummings JL, Mega M, Gray K, et al. The Neuropsychiatric Inventory: comprehensive assessment of psychopathology in dementia. *Neurology.* 1994;44:2308–2314.

34. Andersen J, Aabro E, Gulmann N, et al. Anti-depressive treatment in Parkinson's disease: a controlled trial of the effect of nortriptyline in patients with Parkinson's disease treated with L-dopa. *Acta Neurol Scand.* 1980;62:210–219.

35. Jolly JB, Wiesner DC, Wherry JN, et al. Gender and the comparison of self and observer ratings of anxiety and depression in adolescents. *J Am Acad Child Adolesc Psychiatry.* 1994;33: 1284–1288.

36. Tanaka-Matsumi J, Kameoka VA. Reliabilities and concurrent validities of popular self-report measures of depression, anxiety, and social desirability. *J Consult Clin Psychol.* 1986;54:328–333.

37. Dion KL, Giordano C. Ethnicity and sex as correlates of depression symptoms in a Canadian university sample. *Int J Soc Psychiatry.* 1990;36:30–41.

38. Guy W. *ECDEU Assessment Manual for Psychopharmacology-Revised.* DHEW publ no. (ADM) 76–338 ed. Rockville, MD: U.S. Department of Health, Education, and Welfare, Public Health Service, Alcohol, Drug Abuse, and Mental Health Administration, NIMH Psychopharmacology Research Branch, Division of Extramural Research Programs; 1976:217–222.

39. Muller MJ, Dragicevic A. Standardized rater training for the Hamilton Depression Rating Scale (HAMD-17) in psychiatric novices. *J Affect Disord.* 2003;77:65–69.

40. Mundt JC, Kobak KA, Taylor LV, et al. Administration of the Hamilton Depression Rating Scale using interactive voice response technology. *MD Comput.* 1998;15:31–39.

41. Cowen PJ, Ogilvie AD, Gama J. Efficacy, safety and tolerability of duloxetine 60 mg once daily in major depression. *Curr Med Res Opin.* 2005;21:345–356.

42. Nunes EV, Levin FR. Treatment of depression in patients with alcohol or other drug dependence: a meta-analysis. *JAMA.* 2004;291:1887–1896.

43. Guaiana G, Barbui C, Hotopf M. Amitriptyline versus other types of pharmacotherapy for depression. *Cochrane Database Syst Rev.* 2003;CD004186.

44. Waugh J, Goa KL. Escitalopram: a review of its use in the management of major depressive and anxiety disorders. *CNS Drugs.* 2003;17: 343–362.

45. Bagby RM, Ryder AG, Schuller DR, et al. The Hamilton Depression Rating Scale: has the gold standard become a lead weight? *Am J Psychiatry.* 2004;161:2163–2177.

46. Bagby RM, Ryder AG, Schuller DR, et al. The Hamilton Depression Rating Scale: has the gold standard become a lead weight? *Am J Psychiatry.* 2004;161:2163–2177.

47. Leentjens AF, Verhey FRJ, Lousberg R, et al. The validity of the Hamilton and Montgomery-Åsberg Depression Rating Scales as screening and diagnostic tools for depression in Parkinson's disease. *Int J Geriatr Psychiatry.* 2000;15:644–649.

48. Bagby RM, Ryder AG, Schuller DR, et al. The Hamilton Depression Rating Scale: has the gold standard become a lead weight? *Am J Psychiatry.* 2004;161:2163–2177.

49. Williams JB. A structured interview guide for the Hamilton Depression Rating Scale. *Arch Gen Psychiatry.* 1988;45:742–747.

50. Migliorelli R, Teson A, Sabe L, et al. Prevalence and correlates of dysthymia and major depression among patients with Alzheimer's disease. *Am J Psychiatry.* 1995;152:37–44.

51. Chemerinski E, Petracca G, Sabe L, et al. The specificity of depressive symptoms in patients with Alzheimer's disease. *Am J Psychiatry.* 2001;158:68–72.

52. Rafter D. Biochemical markers of anxiety and depression. *Psychiatry Res.* 2001;103:93–96.

53. Neumeister A, Nugent AC, Waldeck T, et al. Neural and behavioral responses to tryptophan depletion in unmedicated patients with remitted major depressive disorder and controls. *Arch Gen Psychiatry.* 2004;61: 765–773.

54. Muck-Seler D, Pivac N, Sagud M, et al. The effects of paroxetine and tianeptine on peripheral biochemical markers in major depression. *Prog Neuropsychopharmacol Biol Psychiatry.* 2002;26:1235–1243.

55. Isogawa K, Nagayama H, Tsutsumi T, et al. Simultaneous use of thyrotropin-releasing hormone test and combined dexamethasone/corticotropine-releasing hormone test for severity evaluation and outcome prediction in patients with major depressive disorder. *J Psychiatr Res.* 2005;39:467–473.

56. Brouwer JP, Appelhof BC, Hoogendijk WJ, et al. Thyroid and adrenal axis in major depression: a controlled study in outpatients. *Eur J Endocrinol.* 2005;152:185–191.

57. Naarding P, Leentjens AFG, van Kooten F, et al. Disease-specific properties of the Hamilton Rating Scale for depression in patients with stroke, Alzheimer's dementia, and Parkinson's disease. *J Neuropsychiatry Clin Neurosci.* 2002;14:329–334.

58. Serrano-Duenas M, Soledad SM. Concurrent validation of the 21-item and 6-item Hamilton Depression Rating Scale versus the DSM-IV diagnostic criteria to assess depression in patients with Parkinson's disease: an exploratory analysis. *Parkinsonism Relat Disord.* 2008;14:233–238.

59. Dell'Agnello G, Ceravolo R, Nuti A, et al. SSRIs do not worsen Parkinson's disease: evidence from an open-label, prospective study. *Clin Neuropharmacol.* 2001;24:221–227.

60. Ceravolo R, Nuti A, Piccinni A, et al. Paroxetine in Parkinson's disease: effects on motor and depressive symptoms. *Neurology.* 2000;55:1216–1218.

61. Dragasevic N, Potrebi A, Damjanovi A, et al. Therapeutic efficacy of bilateral prefrontal slow repetitive transcranial magnetic stimulation in depressed patients with Parkinson's disease: an open study. *Mov Disord.* 2004;17:528–532.

62. Fregni F, Santos CM, Myczkowski ML, et al. Repetitive transcranial magnetic stimulation is as effective as fluoxetine in the treatment of depression in patients with Parkinson's disease. *J Neurol Neurosurg Psychiatry.* 2004;75: 1171–1174.

63. Lemke MR. Effect of reboxetine on depression in Parkinson's disease patients. *J Clin Psychiatry.* 2002;63:300–304.

64. Rampello L, Chiechio S, Raffaele R, et al. The SSRI, citalopram, improves bradykinesia in patients with Parkinson's disease treated with L-dopa. *Clin Neuropharmacol.* 2002;25:21–24.

65. Steur EN, Ballering LA. Combined and selective monoamine oxidase inhibition in the treatment of depression in Parkinson's disease. In: Stern GM, ed. *Parkinson's Disease: Advances in Neurology.* vol. 80. Philadelphia, PA: Lippincott Williams & Wilkins; 1999:505–508.

66. Tesei S, Antonini A, Canesi M, et al. Tolerability of paroxetine in Parkinson's disease: a prospective study. *Mov Disord.* 2000;15:986–989.

67. Mellers JD, Quinn NP, Ron MA. Psychotic and depressive symptoms in Parkinson's disease. A study of the growth hormone response to apomorphine. *Br J Psychiatry.* 1995;167:522–526.

68. Frochtengarten ML, Villares JC, Maluf E, et al. Depressive symptoms and the dexamethasone suppression test in parkinsonian patients. *Biol Psychiatry.* 1987;22:386–389.

69. Kostic VS, Covickovic-Sternic N, Beslac-Bumbasirevic L, et al. Dexamethasone suppression test in patients with Parkinson's disease. *Mov Disord.* 1990;5:23–26.

70. Kostic VS, Lecic D, Doder M, et al. Prolactin and cortisol responses to fenfluramine in Parkinson's disease. *Biol Psychiatry.* 1996;40:769–775.

71. Licht RW, Qvitzau S, Allerup P, et al. Validation of the Bech-Rafaelsen Melancholia Scale and the Hamilton Depression Scale in patients with major depression; is the total score a valid measure of illness severity? *Acta Psychiatr Scand.* 2005;111:144–149.

72. Zimmerman M, Posternak MA, Chelminski I. Is it time to replace the Hamilton Depression Rating Scale as the primary outcome measure in treatment studies of depression? *J Clin Psychopharmacol.* 2005;25:105–110.

73. Bech P. The Hamilton disorders. *Psychother Psychosom.* 1993;60:113–115.

74. Leentjens AF, Vreeling FW, Luijckx GJ, et al. SSRIs in the treatment of depression in Parkinson's disease. *Int J Geriatr Psychiatry.* 2003;18:552–554.

75. Leentjens AF, Van den AM, Metsemakers JF, et al. Higher incidence of depression preceding the onset of Parkinson's disease: a register study. *Mov Disord.* 2003;18:414–418.

76. Khan A, Brodhead AE, Kolts RL. Relative sensitivity of the Montgomery-Asberg depression rating scale, the Hamilton depression rating scale and the Clinical Global Impressions rating scale in antidepressant clinical trials: a replication analysis. *Int Clin Psychopharmacol.* 2004;19:157–160.

77. Davidson J, Turnbull CD, Strickland R, et al. The Montgomery-Asberg Depression Scale: reliability and validity. *Acta Psychiatr Scand.* 1986;73:544–548.

78. Davidson J, Turnbull CD, Strickland R, et al. The Montgomery-Asberg Depression Scale: reliability and validity. *Acta Psychiatr Scand.* 1986;73:544–548.

79. Gabryelewicz T, Styczynska M, Pfeffer A, et al. Prevalence of major and minor depression in elderly persons with mild cognitive impairment—MADRS factor analysis. *Int J Geriatr Psychiatry.* 2004;19:1168–1172.

80. Muller-Thomsen T, Arlt S, Mann U, et al. Detecting depression in Alzheimer's disease: evaluation of four different scales. *Arch Clin Neuropsychol.* 2005;20:271–276.

81. Khan A, Brodhead AE, Kolts RL. Relative sensitivity of the Montgomery-Asberg depression rating scale, the Hamilton depression rating scale and the Clinical Global Impressions rating scale in antidepressant clinical trials: a replication analysis. *Int Clin Psychopharmacol.* 2004;19:157–160.

82. Slawek J, Derejko M, Lass P. [Depression in patients with Parkinson's disease]. *Neurol Neurochir Pol.* 2003;37:351–364.

83. Slawek J, Derejko M. Depression and dementia: the most frequent non-motor symptoms of Parkinson's disease. *Neurol Neurochir Pol.* 2003;37:103–115.

84. Rektorova I, Rektor I, Bares M, et al. Pramipexole and pergolide in the treatment of depression in Parkinson's disease: a national multicentre prospective randomized study. *Eur J Neurol.* 2003;10:399–406.

85. Leentjens AF, Marinus J, Van Hilten JJ, et al. The contribution of somatic symptoms to the diagnosis of depressive disorder in Parkinson's disease: a discriminant analytic approach. *J Neuropsychiatry Clin Neurosci.* 2003;15:74–77.

86. Watkins CE, Campbell VL, Nieberding R, et al. Contemporary practice of psychological assessment by clinical psychologists. *Prof Psychol Res Pract.* 1995;26:54–60.

87. Steer RA, Beck AT, Garrison B. Applications of Beck Depression Inventory. In: Sartorius N, Ban T, eds. *Assessment of Depression.* New York: Springer; 1986:123–142.

88. Richter P, Werner J, Heerlein A, et al. On the validity of the Beck Depression Inventory; a review. *Psychopathology.* 1998;31:160–168.

89. McDowell I, Newell C. *Measuring Health—A Guide to Rating Scales and Questionnaires.* 2nd ed. New York: Oxford University Press; 1996.

90. Harcourt Assessment—The Psychological Corporation, 555 Academic Court, San Antonio, TX 78204-2498. (Phone: 800-211-8378), 2005.

91. Rader KK, Adler L, Schwibbe MH, et al. [Validity of the Beck Depression Inventory for cross-cultural comparisons. A study of German and Egyptian patients]. *Nervenarzt.* 1991;62:697–703.

92. Azocar F, Arean P, Miranda J, et al. Differential item functioning in a Spanish translation of the Beck Depression Inventory. *J Clin Psychol.* 2001;57:355–365.

93. Rader KK, Krampen G, Sultan AS. [Locus of control of depressive patients in a cross-cultural comparison]. *Fortschr Neurol Psychiatr.* 1990;58:207–214.

94. Shumway M, Sentell T, Unick G, et al. Cognitive complexity of self-administered depression measures. *J Affect Disord.* 2004;83:191–198.

95. Beck AT, Epstein N, Brown G, et al. An inventory for measuring clinical anxiety: psychometric properties. *J Consult Clin Psychol.* 1988;56:893–897.

96. Beck AT, Steer RA. Beck Depression Inventory. In: Rush AJ, ed. *Handbook of Psychiatric*

Measures. Washington, DC: American Psychiatric Association; 2000:519–523.

97. Groth-Marnat G. *The Handbook of Psychological Assessment.* 2nd ed. New York: John Wiley & Sons; 1990.

98. Steer RA, Beck AT, Brown G, et al. Self-reported depressive symptoms that differentiate recurrent-episode major depression from dysthymic disorders. *J Clin Psychol.* 1987;43:246–250.

99. Andrade L, Gorenstein C, Vieira Filho AH, et al. Psychometric properties of the Portuguese version of the State-Trait Anxiety Inventory applied to college students: factor analysis and relation to the Beck Depression Inventory. *Braz J Med Biol Res.* 2001;34:367–374.

100. Gold SM, Zakowski SG, Valdimarsdottir HB, et al. Higher Beck depression scores predict delayed epinephrine recovery after acute psychological stress independent of baseline levels of stress and mood. *Biol Psychol.* 2004;67:261–273.

101. O'Reardon JP, Chopra MP, Bergan A, et al. Response to tryptophan depletion in major depression treated with either cognitive therapy or selective serotonin reuptake inhibitor antidepressants. *Biol Psychiatry.* 2004;55:957–959.

102. Richter P, Werner J, Bastine R, et al. Measuring treatment outcome by the Beck Depression Inventory. *Psychopathology.* 1997;30:234–240.

103. Powell R. Psychometric properties of the Beck Depression Inventory and the Zung Self Rating Depression Scale in adults with mental retardation. *Ment Retard.* 2003;41:88–95.

104. Logsdon RG, Teri L. Depression in Alzheimer's disease patients: caregivers as surrogate reporters. *J Am Geriatr Soc.* 1995;43:150–155.

105. Tandberg E, Larsen JP, Aarsland D, et al. The occurrence of depression in Parkinson's disease. A community-based study. *Arch Neurol.* 1996;53:175–179.

106. Schrag A, Jahanshahi M, Quinn NP. What contributes to depression in Parkinson's disease? *Psychol Med.* 2001;31:65–73.

107. Shulman LM, Taback RL, Bean J, et al. Comorbidity of the nonmotor symptoms of Parkinson's disease. *Mov Disord.* 2001;16: 507–510.

108. Shulman LM, Taback RL, Rabinstein AA, et al. Non-recognition of depression and other non-motor symptoms in Parkinson's disease. *Parkinsonism Relat Disord.* 2002;8:193–197.

109. Huber SJ, Freidenberg DL, Paulson GW, et al. The pattern of depressive symptoms varies with progression of Parkinson's disease. *J Neurol Neurosurg Psychiatry.* 1990;53:257–258.

110. Funkiewiez A, Ardouin C, Caputo E, et al. Long term effects of bilateral subthalamic nucleus stimulation on cognitive function, mood, and behaviour in Parkinson's disease. *J Neurol Neurosurg Psychiatry.* 2004;75:834–839.

111. Hauser RA, Zesiewicz TA. Sertraline for the treatment of depression in Parkinson's disease. *Mov Disord.* 1997;12:756–759.

112. Avila A, Cardona X, Martin-Baranera M, et al. Does nefazodone improve both depression and Parkinson disease? A pilot randomized trial. *J Clin Psychopharmacol.* 2003;23:509–513.

113. Troster AI, Fields JA, Wilkinson S, et al. Effect of motor improvement on quality of life following subthalamic stimulation is mediated by changes in depressive symptomatology. *Stereotact Funct Neurosurg.* 2003;80:43–47.

114. Visser M, Leentjens AF, Marinus J, et al. Reliability and validity of the Beck depression inventory in patients with Parkinson's disease. *Mov Disord.* 2006;21:668–672.

115. Fernandez HH, Tabamo RE, David RR, et al. Predictors of depressive symptoms among spouse caregivers in Parkinson's disease. *Mov Disord.* 2001;16:1123–1125.

116. Mauduit N, Schuck S, Allain H, et al. [Rating scales and questionnaires in Parkinson's disease]. *Rev Neurol (Paris).* 2000;156 (suppl 2, pt 2):63–69.

117. Leentjens AF, Verhey FRJ, Luijckz G-J, et al. The validity of the Beck Depression Inventory as a screening and diagnostic instrument for depression in patients with Parkinson's disease. *Mov Disord.* 2000;15:1221–1224.

118. Visser M, Leentjens AF, Marinus J, et al. Reliability and validity of the Beck depression inventory in patients with Parkinson's disease. *Mov Disord.* 2006;21:668–672.

119. Visser M, Leentjens AF, Marinus J, et al. Reliability and validity of the Beck depression inventory in patients with Parkinson's disease. *Mov Disord.* 2006;21:668–672.

120. Leentjens AFG, Lousberg R, Verhey FRJ. The psychometric properties of the Hospital Anxiety and Depression Scale in patients with Parkinson's disease. *Acta Neuropsychiatrica.* 2001;13:83–85.

121. Leentjens AF, Verhey FRJ, Luijckz G-J, et al. The validity of the Beck Depression Inventory as a screening and diagnostic instrument for depression in patients with Parkinson's disease. *Mov Disord.* 2000;15:1221–1224.

122. Levin BE, Llabre MM, Weiner WJ. Parkinson's disease and depression: psychometric properties of the Beck Depression Inventory. *J Neurol Neurosurg Psychiatry.* 1988;51: 1401–1404.

123. Nfer-Nelson, Darville House, 2 Oxford Road East, Windsor, Berkshire SL4 IDF, England (email: information@nfer-nelson.co.uk); 2005.

124. Herrmann C. International experiences with the hospital anxiety and depression scale; a review of validation data and clinical results. *J Psychosom Res.* 1997;42:17–41.

125. Jones PW. Quality of life, symptoms and pulmonary function in asthma: long-term treatment with nedocromil sodium examined in a controlled multicentre trial. Nedocromil Sodium Quality of Life Study Group. *Eur Respir J.* 1994;7:55–62.

126. Bjellard I, Dahl AA, Tangen Haug T, et al. The validity of the Hospital Anxiety and Depression Scale. An updated literature review. *J Psychosom Res.* 2002;52:69–77.

127. Mykletun A, Stordal E, Dahl AA. Hospital Anxiety and Depression (HAD) scale: factor structure, item analyses and internal consistency in a large population. *Br J Psychiatry.* 2001;179:540–544.

128. Friedman S, Samuelian JC, Lancrenon S, et al. Three-dimensional structure of the Hospital Anxiety and Depression Scale in a large French primary care population suffering from major depression. *Psychiatry Res.* 2001;104:247–257.

129. Kenn C, Wood H, Kucyj M, et al. Validation of the Hospital Anxiety and Depression Rating Scale (HADS) in an elderly psychiatric population. *Int J Geriat Psychiatry.* 1987;2: 189–193.

130. Wu KK. Use of eye movement desensitisation and reprocessing for treating post-traumatic stress disorder after a motor vehicle accident. *Hong Kong J Psychiatry.* 2002;12:20–24.

131. Tignol JA. A double-blind, randomized, fluoxetine-controlled, multicenter study of paroxetine in the treatment of depression. *J Clin Psychopharmacol.* 1993;13:18S–22S.

132. Shah A, Hoxey K, Mayadunne V. Suicidal ideation in acutely medically ill elderly inpatients: prevalence, correlates and longitudinal stability. *Int J Geriatr Psychiatry.* 2000;15:162–169.

133. Wands K, Merskey H, Hachinski VC, et al. A questionnaire investigation of anxiety and depression in early dementia. *J Am Geriatr Soc.* 1990;38:535–538.

134. Leentjens AFG. *Parkinson's Disease, Depression, and Serotonin.* Maastricht, Netherlands: Datwyse/Universitaire Pers Maastricht; 2002.

135. Mondolo F, Jahanshahi M, Grana A, et al. The validity of the hospital anxiety and depression scale and the geriatric depression scale in Parkinson's disease. *Behav Neurol.* 2006;17:109–115.

136. Marinus J, Leentjens AFG, Visser M, et al. Evaluation of the Hospital Anxiety and Depression Scale in patients with Parkinson's disease. *Clin Neuropharmacol.* 2002;6: 318–324.

137. Serrano-Duenas M, Martinez-Martin P, Vaca-Baquero V. Validation and cross-cultural adjustment of PDQL-questionnaire, Spanish version (Ecuador) (PDQL-EV). *Parkinsonism Relat Disord.* 2004;10:433–437.

138. Martinez-Martin P, Valldeoriola F, Tolosa E, et al. Bilateral subthalamic nucleus stimulation and quality of life in advanced Parkinson's disease. *Mov Disord.* 2002;17:372–377.

139. Passik SD, Kirsh KL, Donaghy KB, et al. An attempt to employ the Zung Self-Rating Depression Scale as a "lab test" to trigger follow-up in ambulatory oncology clinics: criterion validity and detection. *J Pain Symptom Manage.* 2001;21:273–281.

140. Zung WW, Richards CB, Short MJ. Self-rating depression scale in an outpatient clinic. Further validation of the SDS. *Arch Gen Psychiatry.* 1965;13:508–515.

141. Turner JA, Romano JM. Self-report screening measures for depression in chronic pain patients. *J Clin Psychol.* 1984;40:909–913.

142. Raft D, Spencer RF, Toomey T, et al. Depression in medical outpatients: use of the Zung scale. *Dis Nerv Syst.* 1977;38: 999–1004.

143. Brodaty H, Luscombe G, Peisah C, et al. A 24-year longitudinal, comparison study of the outcome of depression. *Psychol Med.* 2001;31:1347–1359.

144. Bremner JD, Narayan M, Anderson ER, et al. Hippocampal volume reduction in major depression. *Am J Psychiatry.* 2000;157:115–118.

145. Raison CL, Borisov AS, Broadwell SD, et al. Depression during pegylated interferon-alpha plus ribavirin therapy: prevalence and prediction. *J Clin Psychiatry.* 2005;66:41–48.

146. Okimoto JT, Barnes RF, Veith RC, et al. Screening for depression in geriatric medical patients. *Am J Psychiatry.* 1982;139:799–802.

147. Jegede RO. Psychometric properties of the Self-Rating Depression Scale (SDS). *J Psychol*. 1976;93:27–30.

148. Toner J, Gurland B, Teresi J. Comparison of self-administered and rater-administered methods of assessing levels of severity of depression in elderly patients. *J Gerontol*. 1988;43:136–140.

149. Kaneda Y. Usefulness of the Zung self-rating depression scale for schizophrenics. *J Med Invest*. 1999;46:75–78.

150. Kaneda Y. Usefulness of the Zung self-rating depression scale for schizophrenics. *J Med Invest*. 1999;46:75–78.

151. Chida F, Okayama A, Nishi N, et al. Factor analysis of Zung Scale scores in a Japanese general population. *J Psychiatry Clin Neurosci*. 2004;58:420–426.

152. Faravelli C, Albanesi G, Poli E. Assessment of depression: a comparison of rating scales. *J Affect Disord*. 1986;11:245–253.

153. Biggs JT, Wylie LT, Ziegler VE. Validity of the Zung Self-Rating Depression Scale. *Br J Psychiatry*. 1978;132:381–385.

154. Happe S, Schrodl B, Faltl M, et al. Sleep disorders and depression in patients with Parkinson's disease. *Acta Neurol Scand*. 2001;104:275–280.

155. Indaco A, Carrieri PB. Amitriptyline in the treatment of headache in patients with Parkinson's disease. *Neurology*. 1988;38: 1720–1722.

156. Pellecchia MT, Grasso A, Biancardi LG, et al. Physical therapy in Parkinson's disease: an open long-term rehabilitation trial. *J Neurol*. 2004;251:595–598.

157. Chagas MH, Tumas V, Loureiro SR, et al. Validity of a Brazilian version of the Zung self-rating depression scale for screening of depression in patients with Parkinson's disease. *Parkinsonism Relat Disord*. 2010;16:42–45.

158. Burke WJ, Roccaforte WH, Wengel SP. The short form of the Geriatric Depression Scale: a comparison with the 30-item form. *J Geriatr Psychiatry Neurol*. 1991;4:173–178.

159. Burke WJ, Roccaforte WH, Wengel SP, et al. The reliability and validity of the Geriatric Depression Rating Scale administered by telephone. *J Am Geriatr Soc*. 1995;43:674–679.

160. Scogin F. The concurrent validity of the Geriatric Depression Scale with depressive older adults. *Clin Gerontol*. 1987;7:23–31.

161. Yonkers KA, Samson J. Mood disorders measures. In: Rush AJ, Pincus HA, First MB, et al, eds. *Handbook of Psychiatric Measures*. Washington, DC: American Psychiatric Association; 2000:544–546.

162. Raskin J, Goldstein DJ, Mallinckrodt CH, et al. Duloxetine in the long-term treatment of major depressive disorder. *J Clin Psychiatry*. 2003;64:1237–1244.

163. Burke WJ, Houston MJ, Boust SJ, et al. Use of the Geriatric Depression Scale in dementia of the Alzheimer type. *J Am Geriatr Soc*. 1989;37:856–860.

164. Feher EP, Larrabee GJ, Crook TH. Factors attenuating the validity of the Geriatric Depression Scale in a dementia population. *J Am Geriatr Soc*. 1992;40:906–909.

165. Harper RG, Kotik-Harper D, Kirby H. Psychometric assessment of depression in an elderly general medical population: over- or underassessment. *J Nerv Ment Dis*. 1990;178:113–119.

166. Montorio I, Izal M. The Geriatric Depression Scale: a review of its development and utility. *Int Psychogeriatr*. 1996;8:103–112.

167. McGivney SA, Mulvihill M, Taylor B. Validating the GDS depression screen in the nursing home. *J Am Geriatr Soc*. 1994;42:490–492.

168. Kafonek S, Ettinger WH, Roca P, et al. Instruments for screening for depression and dementia in a long-term care facility. *J Am Geriatr Soc*. 1989;37:29–34.

169. Brink TL. Limitation of the G.D.S. *Clin Gerontol*. 1984;2:60–61.

170. McDonald WM, Holtzheimer PE, Haber M, et al. Validity of the 30-item geriatric depression scale in patients with Parkinson's disease. Mov Disord. 2006;21:1618–22

171. Weintraub D, Oehlberg KA, Katz IR, et al. Test characteristics of the 15-item geriatric depression scale and Hamilton depression rating scale in Parkinson disease. *Am J Geriatr Psychiatry*. 2006;14:169–175.

172. Burn DJ, Rowan EN, Minett T, et al. Extrapyramidal features in Parkinson's disease with and without dementia and dementia with Lewy bodies: a cross-sectional comparative study. *Mov Disord*. 2003;18:884–889.

173. Muller-Thomsen T, Arlt S, Mann U, et al. Detecting depression in Alzheimer's disease: evaluation of four different scales. *Arch Clin Neuropsychol*. 2005;20:271–276.

174. Alexopoulos GS, Abrams RC, Young RC, et al. Use of the Cornell scale in nondemented patients. *J Am Geriatr Soc*. 1988;36:230–236.

175. Muller-Thomsen T, Arlt S, Mann U, et al. Detecting depression in Alzheimer's disease:

evaluation of four different scales. *Arch Clin Neuropsychol.* 2005;20:271–276.

176. Teri L, Gibbons LE, McCurry SM, et al. Exercise plus behavioral management in patients with Alzheimer disease: a randomized controlled trial. *JAMA.* 2003;290:2015–2022.

177. van Weert JC, van Dulmen AM, Spreeuwenberg PM, et al. Behavioral and mood effects of snoezelen integrated into 24-hour dementia care. *J Am Geriatr Soc.* 2005;53:24–33.

178. Steinberg M, Tschanz JT, Corcoran C, et al. The persistence of neuropsychiatric symptoms in dementia: the Cache County Study. *Int J Geriatr Psychiatry.* 2004;19:19–26.

179. Ballard CG, O'Brien JT, Swann AG, et al. The natural history of psychosis and depression in dementia with Lewy bodies and Alzheimer's disease: persistence and new cases over 1 year of follow-up. *J Clin Psychiatry.* 2001;62:46–49.

180. Logsdon RG, Teri L. Depression in Alzheimer's disease patients: caregivers as surrogate reporters. *J Am Geriatr Soc.* 1995;43:150–155.

181. Sharp LK, Lipsky MS. Screening for depression across the lifespan: a review of measures for use in primary care settings. *Am Fam Physician.* 2002;66:1001–1008.

182. Williams JR, Marsh L. Validity of the Cornell scale for depression in dementia in Parkinson's disease with and without cognitive impairment. Mov Disord. 2009 Feb 15;24(3):433-7.

183. Louis ED, Lynch T, Marder K, et al. Reliability of patient completion of the historical section of the Unified Parkinson's Disease Rating Scale. *Mov Disord.* 1996;11:185–192.

184. Martinez-Martin P, Gil-Nagel A, Gracia LM, et al. Unified Parkinson's Disease Rating Scale characteristics and structure. The Cooperative Multicentric Group. *Mov Disord.* 1994;9:76–83.

185. Siderowf A, Newberg AB, Chou KL, et al. [99mTc] TRODAT-1 SPECT imaging correlates with odor identification performance in early Parkinson's disease. Neurology. 2005;64:1716–20; .

186. Louis ED, Lynch T, Marder K, et al. Reliability of patient completion of the historical section of the Unified Parkinson's Disease Rating Scale. *Mov Disord.* 1996;11:185–192.

187. Allain H, Cougnard J, Neukirch H-C, et al. Selegiline in de novo parkinsonian patients: the French selegiline multicenter trial (FSMT). *Acta Neurol Scand.* 1991;84 (suppl 136):73–78.

188. Starkstein SE, Merello M. The Unified Parkinson's Disease Rating Scale: validation study of the mentation, behavior, and mood section. *Mov Disord.* 2007;22:2156–2161.

189. Andresen EM, Malmgren JA, Carter WB, et al. Screening for depression in well older adults: evaluation of a short form of the CES-D (Center for Epidemiologic Studies Depression Scale). *Am J Prev Med.* 1994;10:77–84.

190. Devins GM, Orme CM, Costello CG, et al. Measuring depressive symptoms in illness populations: psychometric properties of the Center for Epidemiologic Studies Depression (CES-D). *Psychology and Health.* 1988;2: 139–156.

191. Sheehan TJ, Fifield J, Reisine S, et al. The measurement structure of the Center for Epidemiologic Studies Depression Scale. *J Pers Assess.* 1995;64:507–521.

192. Beekman AT, Deeg DJ, van Limbeek J, et al. Criterion validity of the Center for Epidemiologic Studies Depression scale (CES-D): results from a community-based sample of older subjects in the Netherlands. *Psychol Med.* 1997;27:231–235.

193. Parikh RM, Eden DT, Price TR, et al. The sensitivity and specificity of the Center for Epidemiologic Studies Depression Scale in screening for post-stroke depression. *Int J Psychiatry Med.* 1988;18:169–181.

194. Schein RL, Koenig HG. The Center for Epidemiological Studies-Depression (CES-D) Scale: assessment of depression in the medically ill elderly. *Int J Geriatr Psychiatry.* 1997;12:436–446.

195. Fenelon G, Mahieux F, Huon R, et al. Hallucinations in Parkinson's disease: prevalence, phenomenology and risk factors. *Brain.* 2000;123(pt 4):733–745.

196. Happe S, Berger K. The association of dopamine agonists with daytime sleepiness, sleep problems and quality of life in patients with Parkinson's disease—a prospective study. *J Neurol.* 2001;248:1062–1067.

197. Nissenbaum H, Quinn NP, Brown RG, et al. Mood swings associated with the "on-off" phenomenon in Parkinson's disease. *Psychol Med.* 1987;17:899–904.

198. Raudino F. Non motor off in Parkinson's disease. *Acta Neurol Scand.* 2001;104:312–315.

199. Quinn NP. Classification of fluctuations in patients with Parkinson's disease. *Neurology.* 1998;51(suppl 2):S25–S29.

200. Visser M, Leentjens AF, Marinus J, et al. Reliability and validity of the Beck depression inventory in patients with Parkinson's disease. *Mov Disord.* 2006;21:668–672.

20

NOCTURNAL SLEEP

Birgit Högl

Summary

There is a broad spectrum of sleep disturbances observed in Parkinson's disease and a variety of scales have been applied to the evaluation of PD sleep, but only three have been assessed specifically for clinimetric properties in the PD population. These are the Parkinson's Disease Sleep Scale (PDSS), the Pittsburgh Sleep Quality Index (PSQI) and the SCOPA-SLEEP scale (SCOPA). All are recommended for rating overall sleep problems and for screening and measure severity.

INTRODUCTION

Sleep disturbances are common in patients with Parkinson's disease, affecting more than 75% of patients.[1] The sleep disturbances that may occur more frequently in PD than in healthy, age-matched controls include insomnia, sleep fragmentation, rapid eye movement (REM) behavior disorder (RBD), sleep apnea syndromes, neuropsychiatric disturbance, motor disabilities, restless legs syndrome (RLS)/periodic limb movements (PLM), and nocturia.[2] As PD advances, nighttime sleep disturbances increase.[3] It is therefore important that sleep disturbances in PD patients be recognized and assessed.

Nocturnal sleep can be evaluated by history and scales (often considered to be subjective tools), or by neurophysiological methods such as polysomnography (PSG), which evaluates nocturnal sleep structure and allows quantification of sleep disturbance. However, PSG is both costly and time-consuming and requires specialized hospital-based settings. There has been intense discussion of whether this dichotomization into *subjective* and *objective* is justified— first of all, because scales reflect real life and in a certain way also try to evaluate objectively. Nevertheless, a sometimes-high discrepancy between subjective and objective assessment results is often present in insomnia (e.g., sleep state misperception, paradoxical insomnia).[4,5] While the diagnosis of insomnia is based exclusively on subjective criteria (patient's impairment due to symptoms),[6,7] the use of subjective criteria alone has sometimes been considered insufficient in daytime sleepiness, when lacking awareness may contribute to accidents.[4] In addition, objective tests may not adequately capture the fluctuating nature of some of the sleep disturbances in PD. Hence, more practical and specific tools are needed to screen for sleep disturbances.

The multifactorial and multidimensional nature of sleep disturbances in PD precludes using a single instrument to assess sleep. Furthermore, medications as well as the occurrence of motor symptoms, fatigue, cognitive impairment, depression, and medication side effects in PD may confound the outcome of sleep scales that were developed for a non-Parkinsonian population. It is therefore necessary to identify whether the scale focuses on insomnia, daytime sleepiness, or other specific sleep disturbances reported in PD. For PD patients, not only specific sleep disorders but also various nocturnal motor and psychiatric problems contribute to nighttime disturbance.

In insomnia, the phenomenon of sleep state misperception[8] refers to a subject's thinking he or she has been awake all night, but the bed partner (or objective PSG) attests the contrary. Several other sleep items cannot be assessed by the patient alone (e.g., snoring and apneas are not perceived, and patients are often unaware of RBD unless it causes them injury), so assessment with the bed partner or caregiver is useful. It should always be specified if someone other than the patient contributed to answering scale questions.

Depression is also a common feature of PD, and both hypersomnia and insomnia are associated with depression.

Between 30% and 40% of PD patients suffer from cognitive decline associated with the disease.[9] This limits the use of self-assessment scales in these patients, and a caregiver or bed partner is required to help answer questions about the patient's sleep habits and sleep disturbances.

This chapter is an adaptation of a peer-reviewed manuscript published previously (Högl et al.) and uses the same methodology as described in Chapter 6.

PDSS AND PDSS-2

Scale description

STRUCTURE

The original PDSS is a self-rated scale designed to measure nocturnal problems, sleep disturbance, and excessive daytime sleepiness in PD over the previous week.[10] It was used to screen for daytime sleepiness and to ascertain the prevalence of general "sleep disturbance" in PD. A revised version of the PDSS, the PDSS-2, was recently validated and extends the original scale from a visual

analogue scale to a frequency measure scale with five categories, and encompasses unmet needs such as evaluating certain sleep disturbances in PD, like those caused by restless legs syndrome, akinesia, pain, and sleep apnea.[11] The PDSS-2 also measures treatment effects better by integrating nocturnal disturbances and disabling symptoms. Questions on daytime sleepiness and "sleep attacks" were removed from the PDSS-2. The PDSS-2 consists of 15 questions, addressing 15 commonly reported symptoms associated with various sleep and nocturnal disturbances occurring in PD patients.

Several of the items are not related to sleep per se, but to nocturnal disability impacting sleep. These are rated by the patients using one of five categories, from 0 (never) to 4 (very frequent). PDSS-2 total score ranges from 0 (no disturbance) to 60 (maximum nocturnal disturbance).

In the PDSS-2 validation study, the mean (SD) total score was 16.5 (±8.9). The distribution of this score indicated that most patients from the sample had mild or moderate sleep problems.[11] Only 6.3 % of the sample had a PDSS-2 total score greater than 30.

HANDLING COMORBIDIITES

As the PDSS was specifically designed to address sleep problems, any impact of non–sleep-related comorbidities should be minimal. There are, however, many sleep-related comorbidities in Parkinson's disease such as depression and dementia, how much these comorbidities affect sleep cannot be differentiated or separated by the scale alone.

Key evaluation issues

USE IN PD AND APPLICATIONS ACROSS THE DISEASE SPECTRUM

The PDSS-2 has been specifically designed for use in PD patients and has been validated in patients with Hoehn and Yahr stages I–V.

USE BY MULTIPLE AUTHORS

Although the original PDSS was not designed to be used to monitor treatment effects, it has been applied for this purpose in several trials,[12-14] and has been validated in several languages, including Spanish, Japanese, and Chinese.[15-17] The PDSS-2 has been validated in English and German.[11]

CLINIMETRIC ISSUES

Reliability The alpha coefficient for the total score as a measure of internal consistency was 0.73, and for the subscores was as follows: 0.66 for the motor symptoms at night (subscale 1), 0.65 for PD symptoms at night (subscale 2), and 0.47 for patients' disturbed sleep (subscale 3).

The test-retest reliability (ICC) for the total score was sufficiently high at 0.80. The three subscores indicated a high test-retest reliability between 0.69 and 0.77.

Validity The validity of the PDSS-2 was assessed by convergent validity and discriminative validity.

The highest correlations (≥ 0.50) with the PDSS-2 total score were found for the Medical Outcomes Study MOS "sleep disturbance" scale and the Sleep Problems Index I and II, the PDQ-39 "mobility," "activities of daily living," and "cognition," and the summary Index. There were no significant correlations for the MOS "snoring" and "optimal sleep" scales, for the PDQ-39 subscale "social support," or for UPDRS IV.B "clinical fluctuations."

The motor symptoms at night (subscale 1) correlated significantly with the MOS "sleep disturbance" and "short of breath" scales and Sleep Problems Index II. There were marked correlations with most of the PDQ-39 subscales (except "stigma," "social support," and "communication"). For PD symptoms at night (subscale 2), there were high correlations with all PDQ-39 subscales, but not with the MOS subscales. Subscale 3, (disturbed sleep), however, was highly significantly correlated to the MOS subscales (except for the "snoring" scale). There were moderate but significant correlations between the disturbed sleep symptoms and the PDQ-39 subscales, as well as for the UPDRS III–V (except the PDQ-39 subscale "social support" and the UPDRS IV.B "clinical fluctuations"). Subscale 3's score was also highly correlated with CGI severity.

As far as discriminative validity is concerned, there were significant differences in the PDSS-2 total scores, depending on CGI and Hoehn and Yahr severity levels. The SEM value was 3.98 (< 0.5 SD = 4.45).

The comparison between patients and their bed partners or caregivers shows a high correlation in almost all items except for the extent of "sleep disruptions with waking periods during the night" and "difficulties turning in bed at night" due to nocturnal akinesia.

Responsiveness The original PDSS has been extensively used in the PD population and differentiates between PD subgroups in early and advanced stages of the disease.[13]

MCRD and MCRID The minimal clinically relevant difference (MCRD) and minimal clinically relevant incremental difference (MCRID) have not been assessed.

Strengths and weaknesses: additional considerations

The PDSS-2 is simple to use and easy to complete. The original PDSS has been widely used. The PDSS-2 has been validated in the PD population and was specifically designed for PD patients and for their disabilities.

The PDSS in its original version[11] was intended as a self-assessment tool and did not include a caregiver questionnaire, nor did it assess sleep apnea, snoring, or sleep problems derived from respiratory disturbances.[14] This has now been remedied by the PDSS-2. The PDSS-2 addresses the multidimensional nature of sleep problems in PD, which makes it a very specific instrument.

Final assessment

The PDSS-2 is in the public domain and has been translated and validated in English and German. It has been shown to have satisfactory internal consistency, stability, construct validity, and precision. The PDSS-2 is particularly valuable for sleep screening, and due to the application of a sum score, is potentially a treatment-responsive tool for measuring nocturnal disabilities and sleep disorders in PD.

PITTSBURGH SLEEP QUALITY INDEX (PSQI)

Scale description

STRUCTURE

The PSQI was developed by psychiatrists with the objective of covering psychiatric clinical practice and research activities. It is a self-rating questionnaire designed to evaluate sleep quality and examine sleep habits and disturbances "during the previous month." It consists of 19 questions that are combined to form seven component scores (subjective sleep quality, sleep latency, sleep duration, habitual sleep efficiency, sleep disturbances, use of sleeping medication, and daytime dysfunction), each of which can be scored from 0 to 3 (from *no difficulty* to *severe difficulty*), yielding a possible maximum score of 21. A higher score indicates more severe difficulties in the specific areas. A further five questions are available to be answered by the bed partner or roommate and provide clinical information, but they do not contribute to the final score.

HANDLING COMORBIDITIES

The SCOPA scale questions are unspecific, therefore, confounding with comorbidities is possible.

ADDITIONAL POINTS

Key evaluation issues Use in PD and applications across the disease spectrum
As the PSQI is self-administered, it has been difficult to use to assess sleep quality in patients with PD and dementia.[12] It would be useful to evaluate whether the bed partner or caregiver's completion of the scale is reliable.

Some items in the PSQI are ambiguous and may be confusing. In particular, the respiratory question may not be specific, and could include a variety of different problems, including dyspnea,

choking, coughing, snoring, or apneas. Similarly, frequent awakenings during the night and early morning awakenings are included in one question, although they are indicative of different features of sleep disturbance.

USE BY MULTIPLE AUTHORS

The PSQI has been widely used in the PD population to examine sleep quality. It has been also used to assess the sleep quality in PD patients with RLS,[18] with sleep disturbances in general,[19] in consecutive PD patients where 43% to 65% showed a PSQI score greater than 5,[20,21] in PD subjects with associated dementia,[12] with excessive daytime sleepiness,[22,23] *de novo* versus treated patients,[23,24] with depression and anxiety,[25] and with hallucinations.[26]

CLINIMETRIC ISSUES

Reliability A Cronbach's alpha of between 0.80 and 0.83 has been reported for the PSQI in different studies and different populations,[19,20] indicating a high degree of internal consistency and internal homogeneity. Individual items are strongly correlated with each other.[27] The PSQI has also been shown to be internally consistent and stable across time.[20,21] PSQI has been shown to have adequate internal consistency and test-retest reliability in patients with primary insomnia. The PSQI global score Pearson's correlation coefficient for test-retest reliability was 0.87.[28] This is a measure of association and not agreement, and may overestimate the intra-class correlation used to measure test-retest reliability.

Validity One study showed the validation of a three-factor scoring model in 417 depressed and non-depressed adults (age > 60 yrs). Results yielded a three-factor scoring model that obtained a measure of perfect fit and was significantly better fitted than either the original single-factor model or a two-factor model. Components of the three factors were characterized by the descriptors *sleep efficiency, perceived sleep quality,* and *daily disturbances.* These findings provide a measure of validation for the factor structure of the PSQI and suggest that a three-factor score should be used to assess disturbances in three separate domains of subjective sleep reports.[29] The clinimetric and clinical properties of the PSQI suggest its utility in both psychiatric clinical practice and research activities.

Scores on the PSQI have been compared to polysomnography (PSG). A *t*-test showed no differences, but the PSQI estimates of sleep duration and efficiency were greater than those obtained by PSG. Pearson correlation demonstrated no significant positive correlations between PSQI estimates and polysomnographic results, except in sleep latency for the total subject pool. Based on these analyses, it does not appear that the PSQI is a surrogate for polysomnographic measures.[27]

The PSQI correlates with ratings of sleepiness using the scale's "beliefs and attitudes about sleep" (BAS) and the "sleep impairment rating scales" (SIRS).[24,25] A high correlation was noted between PSQI score and sleep log data, but less with PSG data.[28] The PSQI has been compared to the SCOPA-SLEEP scale, which evaluates nighttime sleep and daytime sleepiness in PD. The correlation between the scales was 0.83; the coefficient of variation was higher in the SCOPA-SLEEP than in the PSQI, suggesting a better ability to detect differences between individuals when using the SCOPA-SLEEP scale.[30] A correlation has been reported between the PSQI and the visual analogue measures of sleep duration, global sleep quality, and daytime sleepiness, but not with sleep latency. The PSQI score does not correlate with the Epworth Sleepiness Scale ESS.[9]

Responsiveness A global cut-off score greater than 5 for the PSQI distinguishes between "good" and "poor" sleepers with a diagnostic sensitivity of 89.6% and a specificity of 86.5%.[27] In patients with traumatic brain injury, with and without insomnia, a PSQI global score greater than 8 was found to have sensitivity and specificity of 93% and 100%, respectively, and a diagnosis of insomnia based exclusively on a PSQI-derived sleep variable had 83% sensitivity and 100% specificity.[27] Control subjects tended to overestimate their ability to sleep, while insomniacs tended to underestimate it.[27] A PSQI

global score greater than 5 resulted in a sensitivity of 98.7 and specificity of 84.4 as a marker for poor sleep quality in insomnia patients versus controls.[28]

A study of non-demented PD patients with self-reported sleep disturbances ($n = 40$) reported an increased PSQI (>5) in 83% of the patients. Each patient had at least one component score that was abnormal (>0). The mean value was 9.8, leading the authors to conclude that the PSQI was a sensitive indicator of sleep dysfunction in patients with PD.[19]

The PSQI component and global scores have been reported to improve after pharmacological treatment[31] and after subthalamic deep brain surgery,[32] and to increase following one year of treatment with dopaminergic drugs, although the number of "bad sleepers" did not.[33]

MCRD and MCRID The minimal clinically relevant difference and minimal clinically relevant incremental difference have not been assessed.

Strengths and weaknesses: additional considerations

In addition to the points mentioned above concerning the limits of the PSQI in patients with dementia, and the confounding of certain items with other PD symptoms, the PSQI is also limited in its use in PD because it is heavily weighted towards sleep habits with inadequate coverage of sleep disturbances. RLS, PLMS, and RBD are not covered at all. The PSQI does not provide information about the frequency, duration, or nature of specific problems. However, it can be useful in screening patients for the presence of an important sleep alteration. It has been shown to be a reliable, accurate, reproducible instrument for evaluating complex clinical phenomena such as sleep quality, but it remains a subjective test and has not been found to correlate strongly with objective measures such as PSG.

Final assessment

The PSQI is in the public domain. It can be used to screen for the presence of an important sleep alteration and to rate its severity. Based on its widespread used inside and outside the PD population, and available clinimetric data, the PSQI has been recommended by the MDS for use in PD to assess overall sleep abnormalities.

SCOPA-SLEEP (SCOPA)

Scale description

STRUCTURE

The SCOPA (Scales for Outcomes in PD) is a short, practical, self-rating scale designed to evaluate sleep quality and daytime sleepiness in patients with PD,[30] but it has not been widely used. The SCOPA includes three subscales: a nighttime scale, a single-item quality-of-sleep scale, and a daytime sleepiness scale, and also incorporates the concept of "sleep attacks" (or sudden onset of sleep). The daytime sleepiness scale is covered in another chapter and therefore not discussed further here.

The nighttime scale is a five-item scale with four response options that address nighttime disturbances that "occurred in the previous month." Subjects indicate the extent to which they were disturbed on a scale of 0 (*not at all*) to 3 (*very much*). The five items include sleep initiation, sleep fragmentation, sleep efficiency, sleep duration, and early wakening. The maximum score of this scale is 15, with higher scores reflecting more severe sleep problems.

In addition, quality of sleep is assessed using an additional question that evaluates overall sleep quality on a seven-point scale (ranging from *slept very well* to *slept very badly*). The score on this item is not included in the score of the nighttime scale but is used separately as a global measure of sleep quality.

HANDLING COMORBIDITIES

The SCOPA scale questions are unspecific; therefore, confounding with comorbidities is possible.

ADDITIONAL POINTS

None.

Key evaluation issues

USE IN PD AND APPLICATIONS ACROSS THE DISEASE SPECTRUM

The SCOPA does not include specific sleep problems of PD patients such as pain or nocturia. Given that it is a self-administered rating scale, it cannot be used in demented patients with PD.

USE BY MULTIPLE AUTHORS

The SCOPA has been assessed and used by two studies in PD patients, which concluded that it is reliable and valid instrument for assessing nighttime sleep.[30,34]

CLINIMETRIC ISSUES

Reliability The SCOPA was assessed in the original study describing the scale ($n = 142$ patients; 100 controls)[30] and in a Spanish study ($n = 68$).[34] The score distribution covers the full score range, and there are no anticipated floor or ceiling effects. However, in the Spanish study, a mild ceiling effect was seen (22.1%).[34]

The reliability of the nighttime scale has been judged as "good" in evaluations: The internal consistency was demonstrated in the original study[30] where the Cronbach's alpha was 0.88 (corrected item scale correlations, 0.48–0.85), and 0.84 in the Spanish study.[34] The test-retest reliability of the total score was good (intra-class correlation coefficient [ICC] 0.94 [0.82–0.9]).[30]

Factor analysis revealed one factor that accounted for 68.1% of the variance. This indicates that the scale measures one construct, allowing the calculation of a sumscore.[30]

Validity The score on the SCOPA nighttime scale correlated with the PSQI ($r = 0.83$, $P < 0.001$). The correlation between the scale and the PSQI total score in a patient group was 0.83 ($P < 0.001$), and the correlation with the separate subscales of the PSQI ranged from 0.38 to 0.73 (all $P < 0.001$). The correlation between the scale and the global sleep quality score was 0.85 ($P < 0.001$), whereas this was 0.78 ($P < 0.001$)

for the PSQI with the global score. There was a high correlation between the scale and the PDSS (r = −0.70), and between the scale and the PDSS questionnaire by caregiver (rs = −0.53). However, a weak association was found between the scale and health-related quality of life measures (HRQoL).[34]

Responsiveness The score that differentiates good sleepers (score 0–3 PSQI) from poor sleepers (scores 4–6 PSQI) was 6/7 (sensitivity of 0.97 and specificity of 0.80).[30]

MCRD and MCRID The minimal clinically relevant difference and minimal clinically relevant incremental difference have not been assessed.

Strengths and weaknesses: additional considerations

The strengths of the SCOPA are that it is short, it can be completed in five minutes, and it has been validated in the PD population. The sensitivity of the SCOPA to change over time or to treatment has not been examined, and therefore its suitability for use in clinical trials is not known. It does not include any questions about specific sleep problems of PD patients such as RLS or RBD.

Final assessment

The SCOPA is a short, easy-to-use scale that has been used in two studies of PD patients. The scale is in the public domain. The original validation study was conducted using a Dutch version, which was then officially translated into English for publication. A Spanish version is available in the above-mentioned Spanish study.[34]

It is suitable for screening for sleepiness and sleep quality. It is also useful for rating severity of nighttime sleep disturbance. The MDS has recommended the SCOPA in PD for rating overall sleep impairment and daytime sleepiness. Table 20-1 provides an overview of descriptive characteristics for each of the 3 scales reviewed

in this chapter, and Table 20-2 summarizes the key evaluation points of each table.

CONCLUSION

The above three scales are useful in assessing aspects of sleep in PD, and have been used to varying degrees in the PD population. All scales have been studied clinimetrically, validated for use in PD, and used by multiple investigators besides those who originally developed the scale. These scales have in common that they are weighted towards severity more than the mere presence of a sleep disturbance.

None of the scales can replace a clinical interview on sleep disorders and nocturnal problems in PD, but they can assist in rating severity and enabling comparisons within different patient groups. The PDSS-2 can be used as a screening instrument for several sleep disturbances in PD.

It is important to remember that when assessing sleep in PD, the input of a bed partner or caregiver should be sought because of the well-known discrepancies between perception of sleep and sleep insomnia, and the impossibility for an individual to be aware of his or her snoring and nocturnal behavior (unless informed by another). This is particularly the case in patients with PD and dementia, where it is difficult for them to evaluate their sleep quality. It would therefore be useful for the PSQI and the SCOPA to undergo further studies to validate their use by caregivers or bed partners based on their perception of the patients' sleep. It has been shown in the non-PD population that patients usually self-rate their sleepiness lower than do their partners.[35]

The length of time for which sleep is evaluated varies among the scales. The PSQI and the SCOPA refer to "the last month," and the PDSS refers to "the last week."

A scale cannot replace a full sleep history with the patient and/or caregiver, and in selected cases an overnight sleep-study PSG: further educational efforts are required to ensure that physicians are competent in taking a full sleep history.

Table 20-1. Descriptive Characteristics of Nocturnal Sleep Scales

SCALE	# ITEMS/ SELF-COMPLETED	SLEEP DISORDER ASSESSED	INFORMATION FROM PARTNER/ CAREGIVER	PRESENCE OR SEVERITY, PROPOSED CUTOFF	TIMING OF ASSESSMENT	STATE
PDSS-2	15 items, self-completed	Nocturnal disabilities and sleep disorders in PD	No, although they are allowed to help	Weighted towards severity No cutoff published	Over previous week	Recommended for overall sleep impairment as a screening tool, a measure of severity, and as a treatment-responsive tool.
PSQI	19 items, self-completed	Sleep quality	Five extra items (not added in score)	Presence and severity Cutoff 5	Over previous month	Recommended for overall sleep impairment as a screening tool and as a measure of severity.
SCOPA-SLEEP Nighttime scale	5 items, self-completed	Sleep quality, nighttime sleep disturbances	No, but could be helpful for daytime sleepiness	Presence/Severity Cutoff 5/6 suggested to distinguish good from bad sleepers	Over previous month	Recommended for overall sleep impairment as a screening tool and as a measure of severity.

Table 20-2. Key Evaluation Points

SCALE	APPLICABILITY IN PD	USE BY MULTIPLE GROUPS	CLINIMETRICS
PDSS-2	Specifically designed for use in PD	Original PDSS used in many clinical trials. PDSS-2 validated in English and German.	Good acceptability, reliability, internal consistency, and reproducibility.
PSQI	Only applicable to assess global sleep quality. Not applicable to assess and to detect sleep disturbances	Validated in many studies in both PD and non-PD populations.	Good acceptability, reliability, internal consistency, and reproducibility.
SCOPA-SLEEP Nighttime scale	Specifically designed for use in PD	Validated in two groups.	Good acceptability, reliability, internal consistency, and reproducibility.

RECOMMENDED SCALES
Parkinson's disease sleep scale (PDSS)
Pittsburgh sleep quality index (PSQI)
SCOPA-sleep scale (SCOPA)

References

1. Factor SA, McAlarney T, Sanchez-Ramos JR, Weiner WJ. Sleep disorders and sleep effect in Parkinson's disease. *Mov Disord.* 1990;5:280–285.
2. Lowe AD. Sleep in Parkinson's disease. *J Psychosom Res.* 1998;44:613–617.
3. Diederich NJ, Vaillant M, Mancuso G, Lyen P, Tiete J. Progressive sleep "destructuring" in Parkinson's disease. A polysomnographic study in 46 patients. *Sleep Med.* 2005;6:313–318.
4. Merino-Andreu M, Arnulf I, Konofal E, Derenne JP, Agid Y. Unawareness of naps in Parkinson's disease and in disorders with excessive daytime sleepiness. *Neurology.* 2003;60:1553–1554.
5. Engleman HM, Hirst WS, Douglas NJ. Under reporting of sleepiness and driving impairment in patients with sleep apnoea/hypopnoea syndrome. *J Sleep Res.* 1997;6:272–275.
6. American Sleep Disorders Association. *The International Classification of Sleep Disorders, Revised: Diagnostic and Coding Manual.* Rochester, MN: American Sleep Disorders Association; 1997.
7. American Psychiatric Association. *Task Force on DSM-IV. Diagnostic and Statistical Manual of Mental Disorders: DSM-IV.* 4th ed. Washington, DC: American Psychiatric Association; 1994.
8. Edinger JD, Fins AI. The distribution and clinical significance of sleep time misperceptions among insomniacs. *Sleep.* 1995;18:232–239.
9. Emre M. What causes mental dysfunction in Parkinson's disease? *Mov Disord.* 2003;18 (suppl 6):S63–S71.
10. Chaudhuri KR, Pal S, DiMarco A, et al. The Parkinson's disease sleep scale: a new instrument for assessing sleep and nocturnal disability in Parkinson's disease. *J Neurol Neurosurg Psychiatry.* 2002;73:629–635.
11. Trenkwalder C, Kohnen R, Högl B, et al. Parkinson's Disease Sleep Scale—validation of the revised version PDSS-2. *Mov Disord.* 2010;26(4):644–652.
12. Boddy F, Rowan EN, Lett D, O'Brien JT, McKeith IG, Burn DJ. Subjectively reported sleep quality and excessive daytime somnolence in Parkinson's disease with and without dementia, dementia with Lewy bodies and Alzheimer's disease. *Int J Geriatr Psychiatry.* 2007;22:529–535.
13. Dhawan V, Dhoat S, Williams AJ, et al. The range and nature of sleep dysfunction in untreated Parkinson's disease (PD). A comparative controlled clinical study using the Parkinson's disease sleep scale and selective polysomnography. *J Neurol Sci.* 2006;248:158–162.
14. Tse W, Liu Y, Barthlen GM, et al. Clinical usefulness of the Parkinson's disease sleep scale. *Parkinsonism Relat Disord.* 2005;11:317–321.

15. Martinez-Martin P, Salvador C, Menendez-Guisasola L, et al. Parkinson's Disease Sleep Scale: validation study of a Spanish version. *Mov Disord.* 2004;19:1226–1232.

16. Uemura Y, Nomura T, Inoue Y, Yamawaki M, Yasui K, Nakashima K. Validation of the Parkinson's disease sleep scale in Japanese patients: a comparison study using the Pittsburgh Sleep Quality Index, the Epworth Sleepiness Scale and Polysomnography. *J Neurol Sci.* 2009;287:36–40.

17. Wang G, Cheng Q, Zeng J, et al. Sleep disorders in Chinese patients with Parkinson's disease: validation study of a Chinese version of Parkinson's disease sleep scale. *J Neurol Sci.* 2008;271:153–157.

18. Nomura T, Inoue Y, Nakashima K. Clinical characteristics of restless legs syndrome in patients with Parkinson's disease. *J Neurol Sci.* 2006;250:39–44.

19. Pal PK, Thennarasu K, Fleming J, Schulzer M, Brown T, Calne SM. Nocturnal sleep disturbances and daytime dysfunction in patients with Parkinson's disease and in their caregivers. *Parkinsonism Relat Disord.* 2004;10:157–168.

20. Shulman LM, Taback RL, Rabinstein AA, Weiner WJ. Non-recognition of depression and other non-motor symptoms in Parkinson's disease. *Parkinsonism Relat Disord.* 2002;8: 193–197.

21. Ferreira JJ, Desboeuf K, Galitzky M, et al. Sleep disruption, daytime somnolence and "sleep attacks" in Parkinson's disease: a clinical survey in PD patients and age-matched healthy volunteers. *Eur J Neurol.* 2006;13:209–214.

22. Stevens S, Cormella CL, Stepanski EJ. Daytime sleepiness and alertness in patients with Parkinson disease. *Sleep.* 2004;27:967–972.

23. Fabbrini G, Barbanti P, Aurilia C, Vanacore N, Pauletti C, Meco G. Excessive daytime sleepiness in de novo and treated Parkinson's disease. *Mov Disord.* 2002;17:1026–1030.

24. Kaynak D, Kiziltan G, Kaynak H, Benbir G, Uysal O. Sleep and sleepiness in patients with Parkinson's disease before and after dopaminergic treatment. *Eur J Neurol.* 2005;12:199–207.

25. Borek LL, Kohn R, Friedman JH. Mood and sleep in Parkinson's disease. *J Clin Psychiatry.* 2006;67:958–963.

26. Goetz CG, Wuu J, Curgian LM, Leurgans S. Hallucinations and sleep disorders in PD: six-year prospective longitudinal study. *Neurology.* 2005;64:81–86.

27. Buysse DJ, Reynolds CF III, Monk TH, Berman SR, Kupfer DJ. The Pittsburgh Sleep Quality Index: a new instrument for psychiatric practice and research. *Psychiatry Res.* 1989;28:193–213.

28. Backhaus J, Junghanns K, Broocks A, Riemann D, Hohagen F. Test-retest reliability and validity of the Pittsburgh Sleep Quality Index in primary insomnia. *J Psychosom Res.* 2002;53:737–740.

29. Cole JC, Motivala SJ, Buysse DJ, Oxman MN, Levin MJ, Irwin MR. Validation of a 3-factor scoring model for the Pittsburgh sleep quality index in older adults. *Sleep.* 2006;29:112–116.

30. Marinus J, Visser M, van Hilten JJ, Lammers GJ, Stiggelbout AM. Assessment of sleep and sleepiness in Parkinson disease. *Sleep.* 2003;26:1049–1054.

31. Juri C, Chana P, Tapia J, Kunstmann C, Parrao T. Quetiapine for insomnia in Parkinson disease: results from an open-label trial. *Clin Neuropharmacol.* 2005;28:185–187.

32. Iranzo A, Valldeoriola F, Santamaria J, Tolosa E, Rumia J. Sleep symptoms and polysomnographic architecture in advanced Parkinson's disease after chronic bilateral subthalamic stimulation. *J Neurol Neurosurg Psychiatry.* 2002;72:661–664.

33. Fabbrini G, Barbanti P, Aurilia C, Pauletti C, Vanacore N, Meco G. Excessive daytime somnolence in Parkinson's disease. Follow-up after 1 year of treatment. *Neurol Sci.* 2003;24:178–179.

34. Martinez-Martin P, Cubo-Delgado E, Aguilar-Barbera M, et al. [A pilot study on a specific measure for sleep disorders in Parkinson's disease: SCOPA-Sleep]. *Rev Neurol.* 2006;43:577–583.

35. Kumru H, Santamaria J, Belcher R. Variability in the Epworth sleepiness scale score between the patient and the partner. *Sleep Med.* 2004;5:369–371.

INDEX